DRUGGING
FRANCE

INTOXICATING HISTORIES
Series Editors: Virginia Berridge and Erika Dyck

Whether on the street, off the shelf, or over the pharmacy counter, interactions with drugs and alcohol are shaped by contested ideas about addiction, healing, pleasure, and vice and their social dimensions. Books in this series explore how people around the world have consumed, created, traded, and regulated psychoactive substances throughout history. The series connects research on legal and illegal drugs and alcohol with diverse areas of historical inquiry, including the histories of medicine, pharmacy, consumption, trade, law, social policy, and popular culture. Its reach is global and includes scholarship on all periods. Intoxicating Histories aims to link these different pasts as well as to inform the present by providing a firmer grasp on contemporary debates and policy issues. We welcome books, whether scholarly monographs or shorter texts for a broad audience focusing on a particular phenomenon or substance, that alter the state of knowledge.

DRUGGING FRANCE

SARA E. BLACK

Mind-Altering Medicine in
the Long Nineteenth Century

McGill-Queen's University Press
Montreal & Kingston ◆ London ◆ Chicago

ISBN 978-0-2280-1143-9 (cloth)
ISBN 978-0-2280-1164-4 (paper)
ISBN 978-0-2280-1251-1 (ePDF)
ISBN 978-0-2280-1252-8 (ePUB)

Legal deposit third quarter 2022
Bibliothèque nationale du Québec

This book has been published with the help of a grant from the Canadian Federation for the Humanities and Social Sciences, through the Awards to Scholarly Publications Program, using funds provided by the Social Sciences and Humanities Research Council of Canada.

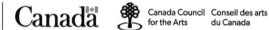

Funded by the Government of Canada   Financé par le gouvernement du Canada   Canada Council for the Arts   Conseil des arts du Canada

We acknowledge the support of the Canada Council for the Arts.
Nous remercions le Conseil des arts du Canada de son soutien.

LIBRARY AND ARCHIVES CANADA CATALOGUING IN PUBLICATION

Title: Drugging France : mind-altering medicine in the long nineteenth century / Sara E. Black.
Names: Black, Sara E., author.
Series: Intoxicating histories ; 5.
Description: Series statement: Intoxicating histories ; 5 | Includes bibliographical references and index.
Identifiers: Canadiana (print) 20220227047 | Canadiana (ebook) 2022022711X | ISBN 9780228011644 (paper) | ISBN 9780228011439 (cloth) | ISBN 9780228012511 (ePDF) | ISBN 9780228012528 (ePUB)
Subjects: LCSH: Psychotropic drugs—France—History—19th century. | LCSH: Psychopharmacology—France—History—19th century. | LCSH: Drugs of abuse—France—History—19th century. | LCSH: Narcotics—France—History—19th century.
Classification: LCC RM315 .B536 2022 | DDC 615.7/88094409034—dc23

CONTENTS

FIGURES

ACKNOWLEDGMENTS

This book would not have been possible without the support of countless individuals over the years. At McGill-Queen's University Press, I would like to thank Kyla Madden for her steadfast support through the publication process, Alison Jacques for her meticulous copyediting, and Virginia Berridge and Erika Dyck for including this book as part of the Intoxicating Histories series. I would also like to thank the anonymous reviewers for their helpful feedback on the manuscript.

The Andrew W. Mellon Foundation, the Social Sciences and Humanities Research Council of Canada, the Federation for the Humanities and Social Sciences, Christopher Newport University, the Rutgers Graduate School of Arts and Sciences, the Rutgers Center for Historical Analysis, and the Christopher Newport University History Department provided generous financial support that made this project possible. I would also like to thank the archivists and librarians at the Archives Nationales; the Archives de la Ville de Paris; the Bibliothèque Nationale de France; the Bibliothèque Interuniversitaire de Santé; the Bibliothèque Charcot at Salpêtrière Hospital; the Bibliothèque Henri Ey at Sainte-Anne Hospital; the Archives de la Préfecture de Police de Paris; the Archives de l'Assistance Publique, Hôpitaux de Paris; the Bibliothèque Centrale du Service de Santé at Val-de-Grâce; and the Archives Nationales d'Outre Mer in Aix-en-Provence. I would particularly like to thank Jérôme van Wijland at the Bibliothèque de l'Académie Nationale de Médecine for going beyond the call of duty.

I am incredibly grateful for the numerous conversations with colleagues that have influenced this project and shaped my own intellectual growth as a historian. In particular, I would like to thank Kate Imy, Allison Finkelstein, Danielle Bradley, Belinda Davis, Carla Yanni, James Delbourgo, Toby Jones, Charlotte Cartwright, Laura Puaca, John Hyland, David Stenner, Jaime Allison, Andrew Falk, Bill Connell, Brian

Puaca, Phil Hamilton, Deirdre Harshman, Matt Harshman, Sheri Shuck-Hall, Xiaoqun Xu, Nigel Sellers, Kathryn Cole, Bill McNamara, Yücel Yanikdağ, Margaret McColley, Gail Bossenga, Katherine Preston, Patrick De Oliveira, and Elizabeth Della Zazzera. I am especially indebted to Seth Koven, Judith Surkis, and Philip Nord for their intellectual rigour and insightful feedback on the manuscript. Bonnie Smith realized this project's potential far before I did. I offer her my sincerest thanks for her intellectual generosity and for many years of invaluable expertise, support, and guidance.

While I conducted research in Paris, the Degons welcomed me into their home and treated me as part of the family. We shared many evenings of laughter and stimulating conversation that made my archival experience enjoyable as well as productive. During the research and writing process, my friends and family have been a source of constant support and encouragement. Thank you to Lauren, Mary, Kate, Allison, Diana, Bethany, Amaya, Julia, Cindy, Roland, Alex, Jared, Eléna, Molson, and Oscar. My grandmother, Marilyn Black, has cheered me on from afar every step of the way and I am so grateful for her encouragement and enthusiasm. Finally, none of this would have been possible without my mum and dad. I would like to thank them for their unshakable confidence in me.

Last, but not least, I would like to thank my husband, Chris. Over the years, he has endured, with patience and good humour, countless conversational digressions as my mind wandered to the nineteenth century. He has celebrated each milestone along the way, and I am deeply grateful for his love and support.

DRUGGING FRANCE

To Carole Black, for 18 minutes,
and to Evan Black, for 110 percent.

INTRODUCTION

In the nineteenth century, France was a nation on drugs. Opium pills relieved insomnia. Morphine calmed agitated nerves. Chloroform obliterated the agony of amputation. Psychotropic drugs offered French citizens a new way to transcend the day-to-day aches, pains, and miseries of modern life. The isolation of new plant alkaloids, the discovery of anesthetic gases, and the industrialization of pharmaceutical production ushered in a dynamic new pharmaceutical economy that supplied a wider variety of products than ever before.[1] Within this emerging psychotropic society, it was no longer necessary to suffer the caprices of a body in pain.[2]

This world of drugs did not emerge out of thin air. Before these substances could become integrated into the everyday lives of French citizens, they had to be transformed into consumable pharmaceuticals. The production of France's psychotropic society depended upon a vast community of knowledge producers – scientists, agriculturalists, entrepreneurs, doctors, and pharmacists, among others – who transformed exotic plant substances and mysterious laboratory gases into the familiar consumer commodities that formed the basis of modern therapeutic medicine. Extensive research created a medical marketplace in which doctors prescribed and patients requested an ever-expanding array of drugs. From the laboratory tests of solitary chemists to fiery debates in the Academy of Sciences about the safety of anesthetic gases, the normalization of psychotropic drugs within French society was contingent upon an immense scientific apparatus.

The chemical enhancement of modern life became a new norm in nineteenth-century France. Opium, morphine, ether, chloroform, cocaine, and hashish all have the capacity to control pain, to produce pleasure, and to modify consciousness.[3] At various points, these multivalent substances served as key technologies of therapeutic innovation, as tools for igniting sexual passion, and as conduits for self-exploration. They enabled individuals to transcend physical pain. However, the enigmatic nature of their psychotropic power made them remarkably versatile commodities. From the pharmacy counter to the boudoir, from the courtroom to the operating theatre, from the battlefield to the birthing chamber, psychotropic drugs reconfigured how individuals perceived and experienced their own minds and bodies.

Swallowing a pill to treat pain, anxiety, or depression has become a normal part of everyday life in the twenty-first century. For most people, it does not involve philosophical reflection. We have come to accept pharmaceutical solutions to these problems. Historically, however, the efficient management of pain was not something that French citizens could take for granted. During the nineteenth century, new therapeutic practices and rituals of consumption fundamentally transformed the ways in which individuals experienced their own bodies. An aching tooth could be soothed with opium extract or extracted painlessly with a few inhalations of chloroform. Pain, rather than being an inevitable burden, became an element over which one had a measure of control.

Psychotropic drugs served as tools of bodily regulation even as they liberated people from pain. A diverse range of individuals, from doctors to journalists to legislators, attempted to harness this regulatory power and appropriate psychotropic drugs for their own ends. Enterprising pharmacists distributed these effective and lucrative medicines to improve profits and defend their legal monopoly over pharmaceutical commerce. Through the practice of medical prescriptions, doctors strove to position themselves as the logical gatekeepers of substances that had such a powerful impact over the minds and bodies of patients. However, patients' own knowledge of and experiences with this psychotropic power also encouraged practices of self-medication and self-experimentation that did not fit into doctors' medicalized vision of pain relief. Individuals sought out drugs on their own to treat ailments, to experience pleasure, and to produce altered states of consciousness. The individual consuming psychotropic substances engaged in an act of bodily regulation by shaping his or her own sensations. At the same time, doctors, pharmacists, and the state sought to mobilize these substances to relieve pain in the hospital wards, restore sanity in the asylum, and shore up their own authority over the bodies of citizens. Nevertheless, psychotropic substances frequently eluded attempts to harness their power toward a specific regulatory end.

The cultural baggage of the twentieth-century "War on Drugs" has shaped how historians have approached the history of drugs. Most drug histories are written through the lenses of regulation and criminalization, focusing on the processes by which certain drugs came to be demonized as dangerous and illicit commodities.[4] Such accounts treat the history of drugs in the nineteenth century as a precursor to the history of drug regulation in the twentieth.[5] Rather than asking why certain drugs and certain kinds of recreational drug use became stigmatized at a particular moment in time, I find the more compelling question to be this: How did drugs become so pervasive in the first place? *Drugging France* is first and foremost a story of normalization. It traces the processes by which psychotropic drugs became commonplace consumer commodities. To be sure, doctors, patients, courts, and society at large still had to confront the problems that drugs generated. However, issues like addiction can only be fully understood within their larger historical context – in this case, a context in which the psychotropic management of pain, sensation, and consciousness had become an accepted social norm. Therefore, *Drugging France* treats the history of drugs in the nineteenth century not as an initial chapter in the history of drug regulation but rather as the foundational period in the history of our current psychotropic society, where pharmaceutical consumption is woven seamlessly into the fabric of everyday life. The story of the normalization of drugs is bound up with the emergence of modern ideas about scientific protocols and ways of knowing, conceptions of the self, and international networks of medical production, trade, and consumption.

Paris was the capital of scientific medicine in the first half of the nineteenth century.[6] During the Enlightenment, Paris's scientific culture and institutions of medical research, which enjoyed royal and church patronage, laid the foundations for this later dominance. However, the early nineteenth century witnessed the dramatic reformation of this Enlightenment inheritance.[7] During the French Revolution, the government confiscated church property and expelled the religious orders from the hospitals. In the name of freedom and individual rights, it opposed professional elitism by eliminating corporations and thereby abolishing institutions like the Faculty of Medicine and the Academy of Sciences.[8] Although France later reorganized these institutions and allowed the nuns to return to the hospitals, the Revolution's radical transformations unfettered the French medical community from traditional authorities.[9] Paris rapidly became the centre of a new form of clinical medicine. Foreign medical students flocked to Paris to profit from the anatomy lessons, modern diagnostic techniques, and bedside clinical observations in the capital's numerous modernized hospitals.[10] This dynamic clinical environment was an ideal location for research on psychotropic drugs.

The medical community had limited knowledge of the effects of psychotropic drugs at the beginning of the nineteenth century. Nevertheless, they recognized their enormous therapeutic potential. For centuries, opium had been one of the only reliable remedies for pain. With the isolation of its alkaloids, particularly morphine, and the introduction of new production techniques in the pharmaceutical industry, opium could be transformed and moulded into a plethora of new remedies for combatting the aches and pains of everyday life. Ether and chloroform had the potential to revolutionize surgical practice by ushering the patient into a state of painless unconsciousness. Hashish produced bizarre hallucinations and sensory distortions that gave asylum doctors reason to hope it might be useful as a treatment for mental illness. Paradoxically, the incredible psychotropic power that made these substances so appealing for medical therapeutics was the very quality that made them dangerous. The ancient Greeks used the term *pharmakon* to describe a substance that was both remedy and poison. The psychotropic pharmacopoeia depended upon a delicate balance of dosage. Too low a dose and the drug would be ineffective. Too high a dose risked acute crisis and even death. Doctors counteracted this intrinsic danger through extensive research. In the process, they constructed a massive body of knowledge about psychotropic drugs.

The enigmatic power of psychotropic drugs over the human body and mind incited a wide range of experiments. While scientists could isolate plant alkaloids and purify anesthetic gases with calculated precision in a laboratory, investigations into the psychosomatic effects of these substances required a far more intimate encounter with psychotropic power. When news of ether's anesthetic potential crossed the Atlantic in 1847, members of the French Academy of Sciences launched into an experimental frenzy to explore its physiological effects, employing the most readily available experimental tool at their disposal: their own bodies. By experimenting with ether and chloroform, doctors documented the feeling of slipping out of consciousness. They witnessed a bizarre disconnect between sight and sensation, watching without pain as their colleagues burned them with hot wax and jabbed them with pins. Self-experimentation provided a foundation of crucial, albeit sometimes befuddling and contradictory, information about the power of these substances over the human organism.

The pursuit of scientific knowledge fuelled most of these accounts of psychotropic self-experimentation. Doctors, pharmacists, chemists, and others portrayed their own self-experimentation with psychotropic drugs as a means of developing a base of practical and generalizable knowledge about their psychosomatic effects. Nevertheless, experimenters could not escape the fact that they were experimenting on a particular subject. Psychotropic self-experimentation transformed the mind of the scientist, the instrument responsible for recording observations, into the site of experimentation. In so doing, psychotropic self-experimentation blurred the boundaries between subject and object, mind and body, self and other.

Extensive research and personal experience gave doctors confidence in the effects of the drugs they prescribed. Doctors increasingly turned to pharmaceutical intervention in therapeutic practice even as medical theories of disease shifted significantly over the course of the nineteenth century. In the early nineteenth century, doctors had understood illness as an imbalance of a "natural" state specific to a particular individual and environment.[11] They treated this imbalance using heroic remedies such as purging and bloodletting, which acted upon the whole system. By mid-century, however, ideas about illness had begun to shift. Instead of a systemic imbalance, doctors began to understand illness as a deviation from a standard, "normal" state of health common to all patients. Therapeutics became more focused, targeting specific symptoms and physiological processes.[12] As opium and other psychotropic drugs had a manifest impact on pain and other symptoms, they became staples of therapeutic medicine.

Psychotropic drugs maintained their prominent position in therapeutics even after widespread acceptance of the germ theory of disease in the 1880s. Popularized by Louis Pasteur's bacteriological research, germ theory held that disease was caused by tiny living organisms known as "microbes" rather than by putrid emanations or miasmas.[13] However, despite this dramatic shift in disease etiology, the medical community still had few remedies that could combat the microbes directly before the introduction of sulfa drugs and antibiotics in the first half of the twentieth century.[14] Therefore, they turned to remedies that demonstratively relieved pain. Psychotropic drugs enabled doctors to treat patients' symptoms effectively, even in cases where the underlying cause of the illness remained unknown or untreatable.

This power over pain had larger social implications for the medical profession. Doctors deployed psychotropic drugs as practical tools of professional legitimacy. From the beginning of the nineteenth century, the practice of medicine and pharmacy in France reflected a complex revolutionary legacy that combined elements of liberalism and regulation. Two laws from 1803 established the legal parameters of medical practice. The Law of 19 Ventôse An XI (10 March 1803) and the Law of 21 Germinal (11 April 1803) granted doctors and pharmacists a legal monopoly over the practice of medicine and the distribution of medicinal substances.[15] In practice, however, these laws were not strictly enforced and the realities of the nineteenth-century medical marketplace often exceeded the boundaries of "official medicine."[16] Doctors faced competition from illegal practitioners, midwives, members of religious orders, quacks, and other empirics. They also experienced skepticism and hostility from their patients, particularly those in rural areas.[17] Through the prescription of psychotropic drugs, doctors presented themselves as masters of pain, bolstering their authority over the bodies of patients. However, this claim to power depended upon patients' acceptance of psychotropic pain relief as both normal and desirable. Patients were key agents in the production of new ideas, practices, and norms of drug consumption. In response to their everyday demands, the pharmaceutical management of the miseries and discomforts of modern life became desirable and, eventually, indispensable.

France's psychotropic society emerged at a time when the French state was becoming increasingly invested in the bodies of its citizens. While population size had served as an important measure of France's wealth under the Old Regime, it took on increasing significance in post-Revolutionary France as a marker of the nation's economic and military strength in an era punctuated by regime change and political turbulence.[18] Yet, the health of France's population gave officials cause for concern. In the 1820s and 1830s, industrialization and urbanization exacerbated overcrowding and deplorable sanitary conditions for the poor and working classes.[19] In response, France developed the first nationalized public health movement rooted in scientific expertise.[20] The French state had deployed scientific experts in the name of rational governance since the last decades of the Old Regime, reflecting a broader turn toward empiricism.[21] However, ideas about the centralized state's responsibility to act in the interest of its citizens' health clashed with the liberalism of the July Monarchy (1830–48), which abhorred unnecessary state intervention. This ensured that the early public health movement focused less on policies and solutions and more on diagnosing public health problems through statistical analysis.[22] Despite these shortcomings, the public health movement reflected the French state's close ties to the medical community during the nineteenth century.[23]

Slow population growth also gave the state cause for concern. French mortality and fertility rates had declined since the end of the eighteenth century. While Malthusians had celebrated these lower birth rates in the early nineteenth century as a sign of progress, France's humiliating defeat in 1870 during the Franco-Prussian War illustrated the military costs of sluggish population growth.[24] During the Third Republic (1870–1940), amid heightened alarm over the diminishing quality and quantity of France's population, the individual body took on increasing significance as a site of social and political contestation. France's demographic crisis and emerging fears of physical and moral degeneration inspired public health initiatives and natalist measures designed to combat depopulation and degeneration.[25] This bound the fate of the national social body to the individual sexual body. Therefore, according to social reformers, the inherently unruly body of the liberal subject had to be regulated, controlled, and guided toward productive and reproductive ends.[26] Although the revolutionaries of 1789 had envisioned health as a fundamental individual right, liberal opposition to state intervention thwarted efforts to introduce programs of medical assistance for the poor at a national level until 1893.[27] Fearing that degeneration tolled

France's geopolitical decline, the Third Republic finally invested in the health of its citizens.[28]

Psychotropic drugs occupied a paradoxical position in relation to the degeneration crisis. On the one hand, emerging medical research on morphine addiction and an increasingly visible population of addicts suggested that drugs were yet another catalyst of national decline, contributing to decadence, criminality, and unhealthy and literally unproductive sexual libertinism. Yet, amid the Third Republic's belief in the power of science to improve society, doctors explored ways in which drugs could be used to treat mental illness and sexual dysfunction.[29] They also deployed drugs on the battlefield and in the birthing chamber to relieve pain, mediating the experiences of men and women who were suffering in service to the French nation.[30] Furthermore, drugs encouraged broader social, ethical, and philosophical debate. Medical investigations into and public discussions about psychotropic drugs served as platforms for grappling with pressing concerns about sexual mores and depopulation, free will and criminal responsibility, and selfhood and the role of the individual within modern society.

France's turbulent political history informed these debates about drugs and the free-willing liberal subject. Between 1840 and 1920, France experienced four different political regimes, punctuated by revolutionary insurrection, dramatic social transformations as a result of industrialization, and persistent religious tensions as the Catholic Church fought to maintain its position in the face of secularization.[31] The French Revolution had eliminated the privileges of birth that characterized the Old Regime's corporate order. Instead, the revolutionaries created a new nation of legally equal (male) citizens who enjoyed freedom and individual rights. Sexual difference, rather than birth, became the key organizing principle of this new social order.[32] According to the ideology of separate spheres, while men exercised their political rights in the public sphere, women's proper role was to take care of the family in the private "domestic" sphere. There, they played a crucial role as mother-educators, moulding their children into virtuous and autonomous citizens.[33]

Individual free will was a central tenet of political citizenship. Throughout the nineteenth century, French women were denied the vote on the grounds that their individual free will was constrained by their subordination to their husbands within the family. As such, they lacked the individual liberty necessary for "active" political citizenship and were instead relegated to the status of "passive" citizens.[34] In post-Revolutionary France, the desire to combat instability and maintain the social order frequently clashed with the Revolution's legacy of individual rights and freedoms.[35] During the July Monarchy, the state hoped to foster social stability by reforming the *lycée* philosophy curriculum to promote Victor Cousin's new vision of the self.[36] Cousin believed that the flimsy, fragmented self of eighteenth-century sensationalist philosophy had made the individual vulnerable to excesses of imagination, which could lead to revolutionary uprisings.[37] Instead, to check the unruly imagination and encourage social stability, he promoted a unified, active, morally accountable vision of the self governed by free will.[38] By cultivating free will and restraint through introspection, the individual could demonstrate his worthiness as a citizen.

Individual free will remained at the heart of conceptions of republican citizenship, judicial responsibility, public education, and the quest for universal suffrage throughout the nineteenth century.[39] However, psychotropic drugs exposed the fragility and contingency of the individual will. In theory, the consumption of psychotropic substances enabled French citizens to master bodily pain and alter consciousness at will. For example, intentionally consuming a psychotropic substance, such as opium syrup, to mitigate the pains of a stomach ulcer could be considered a conscious act of a willful, thinking subject utilizing the tools at his disposal to take control over his sensations and perceptions of pain. However, the opium's psychotropic action over his mind and body disrupted this notion of control. As it modified his physiology, consciousness, and sensation, the locus of power in this act of consumption shifted from the will of the individual subject onto the action of the material object. Medical research on psychotropic drugs exposed the crucial role that the body played in determining individual behaviour. Free will did not exist in the abstract. Self-experimenters, patients, and a wide variety of other psychotropic consumers demonstrated how individual free will was mediated through and contingent upon an embodied self. Therefore, psychotropic consumption revealed the free will of the liberal subject to be inherently unstable.

For all the philosophical questions they posed, psychotropic drugs were material commodities that were grown, transported, processed, sold, and consumed. The normalization of psychotropic consumption entangled individuals in increasingly interdependent relationships with things.[40] Historians of material and consumer culture have emphasized the significance of material commodities and their consumption to the construction of individual, gender, national, and class identities.[41] As integral elements in the experience of everyday life in modern society, these consumer commodities assisted in the production and expression of modern selfhood. *Drugging France* examines the relationship between individuals and a specific type of material commodity involved in a highly intimate act of consumption. It focuses on six material substances used to control pain, produce pleasure, and modify consciousness: opium, hashish, morphine, cocaine, ether, and chloroform. A mixture of ancient plant medicines, modern alkaloids refined from medicinal plants, and gases produced through chemical synthesis, these substances all had a similar psychotropic action upon the human organism when consumed.

The term "psychotrope" refers to a medicine or substance "that chemically acts on the psyche."[42] Although it originated in the mid-twentieth century, "psychotropic" is a useful term for categorizing the particular nature of the power that these substances have over the mind because it emphasizes the material roots of this chemical action within the body. Ingested, injected, and inhaled, psychotropic substances are incorporated into the body to act upon the mind, modifying sensation and consciousness in a fusion of subject and object.

The six drugs explored in this book were certainly not the only psychotropic substances widely consumed during the nineteenth century. For example, although wine is arguably the most quintessentially French psychotrope, this book does not focus on alcohol, which has its own patterns of consumption and unique socio-cultural history.[43] *Drugging France* centres medicine in the history of psychotropic consumption. While I draw parallels with the history of alcohol and other drugs when relevant, I have chosen to focus on opium, morphine, cocaine, hashish, ether, and chloroform because of their significance in nineteenth-century medical research and therapeutic practice.[44] Therefore, I have resisted modern legal classifications of these substances.

Before 1916, morphine, cocaine, and hashish had no special legal distinction from many other pharmaceutical commodities and the state did not regulate their consumption. The rise of international drug regulations in the early twentieth century created a new group of substances classified in France as "stupéfiants."[45] Unlike other drug descriptors, such as "depressants" or "stimulants," the term "stupéfiants" was not a classification based on a drug's specific chemical properties or physiological effects. Instead, the designation was a matter of legal status. It distinguished these particular drugs as illegal substances of abuse.

By isolating the drugs that have become illegal substances of abuse as subjects of historical study, historians risk producing a teleological history of the nineteenth century filtered through the mentality of modern drug regulation. For this reason, it is necessary to explore opium, cocaine, morphine, and hashish alongside ether and chloroform. These last two substances emerged as medicinals rather than illicit recreational substances in the popular imagination of the twentieth century. However, such distinctions did not apply before the advent of international drug regulations. In the nineteenth century, all six of these substances functioned both as therapeutic medicines and as tools for enhancing pleasure and producing oblivion, albeit to different degrees. Medical professionals classified ether and chloroform alongside opium, morphine, cocaine, and hashish because of their similar psychotropic action. Eschewing the licit/illicit and medical/recreational binaries that have informed popular imaginings of what a "drug" is in the twentieth and twenty-first centuries permits a nuanced and more representative exploration of the entangled medical and cultural history of psychotropic commodities in the nineteenth century.

Although nineteenth-century medical practitioners did not view psychotropic substances through contemporary legal/illegal and medicinal/recreational binaries, this is not to suggest that they were naïve about the potential dangers. Between 1845 and 1916, opium, morphine, chloroform, cocaine, and hashish were, in fact, subject to government regulation. Under the 1845 Poisonous Substances Law, only licensed pharmacists could sell these substances – and only with a specific written prescription from a physician.[46] While such a system seems to anticipate twentieth-century drug regulations, nineteenth-century drug legislation functioned quite differently in terms of both logic and practice.[47] First, it operated on a different rationale. The 1845 legislation controlled the *distribution* of psychotropic substances like opium by classifying them as poisons alongside arsenic and other potentially lethal pharmaceuticals. The goal of the legislation was not to protect society against the dangers of addiction, which were not fully recognized at the time; rather, it sought to protect the individual consumer from the dangers of acute poisoning and accidental death. Although social concerns about the dangers of addiction began to emerge in the 1880s and 1890s, it was not until the law of 1916 that the logic of French drug regulation shifted to incorporate these concerns by regulating *consumption*.[48] Second, while the government inspected pharmacies on an annual basis, it lacked both the infrastructure and the desire to strictly enforce the poisonous substances legislation. Nevertheless, however unevenly enforced, the 1845 poisonous substances legislation codified medical authority over the consumption of psychotropic commodities.

Psychotropic consumption was not synonymous with addiction. Most people who consumed psychotropic drugs did not become "addicted" to them. In fact, "addiction" was not a stable or even recognizable concept for much of the nineteenth century. Although doctors had long observed that individuals who regularly consumed opiates could become accustomed to them, the understanding of drug addiction as a social pathology emerged only during the early years of the Third Republic.[49] In the nineteenth century, French citizens engaged in myriad acts of psychotropic consumption: grand and ephemeral, desperate and mundane. In recognition of this remarkable diversity, this book decentres addiction as *the* defining experience. Instead, it situates the history of addiction on a broader spectrum of psychotropic consumption. It explores the quotidian nature of psychotropic consumption as an integral part of medical and pharmaceutical practice. It highlights the complexities and paradoxes of individuals' everyday experiences with drugs in modern French society in connection with medical knowledge production, social regulation, industrialization, and professionalization.

This is in many ways a global story. Imperial and global networks of scientific exchange intersected in France to produce a psychotropic society. Opium grown in Turkey became the gold standard for French pharmaceutical preparations. American anesthetic experiments and South American coca contributed to the development of anesthetic procedures that revolutionized French surgical practice. In exploring the history of drugs in the nineteenth century, I attend to the particular and distinct histories of each drug, charting the various moments when it became an object of fascination, therapeutic medicine, popular consumption, imperial power, social outrage, and legislation. By differentiating among the specific histories of each of these substances even as I explore the points at which they converge, I demonstrate the ways in which some were deeply rooted in the empire while others remained commodities of domestic production.

Doctors, scientists, pharmacists, and other knowledge producers left an incredibly rich archive for mapping out the complex layers of France's industrializing pharmaceutical economy. By examining import statistics, therapeutic manuals, pharmaceutical codices, laboratory observations, medical theses, and scientific debates, I trace the processes by which psychotropic substances were studied, cultivated, refined, produced, distributed, and consumed. The normalization of psychotropic consumption was contingent upon this extensive medical and scientific research that transformed enigmatic psychotropic substances into consumable commodities. However, while medical and pharmaceutical texts form the basis of this book's archive, France's psychotropic society did not emerge solely from the pages of medical journals and debates on the floor of the Academy of Sciences. It came into being with the proliferation of new practices of psychotropic consumption among French citizens, many of whom lacked a platform for conveying their experiences first-hand.[50] Mapping out the entangled medical and cultural history of psychotropic drugs in nineteenth-century France requires reading medical journals, police reports, and pharmacy catalogues against the grain in order to access the experiences of the asylum inmate and the society woman, to peer over the pharmacy counter and into the family medicine cabinet.[51]

Drugging France reframes the history of drugs and the making of modern society. It does not treat the history of drugs primarily as the rise of a social crisis. Instead, it documents the production of a new biomedical norm. It explores the history of drugs in nineteenth-century France as a crucial step in the development of France's modern pharmaceutical economy. Rather than fixating on regulation, criminalization, and deviance, *Drugging France* demonstrates the ways in which psychotropic consumption became an integral practice of everyday life.

Drugging France explores the ways in which psychotropic power operated both within French society and within the individual bodies of French citizens. Psychotropic drugs' widespread availability and popularity in medical therapeutics enabled patients to transcend the quotidian discomforts of modern life and exercise a newly conceived right to freedom from pain. Yet this freedom came at a high potential cost for a nation that saw itself as a collection of liberal subjects. Psychotropic consumption exposed inherent contradictions in constructions of the liberal self as autonomous, rational, and driven by free will. Instead, these substances revealed that self to be malleable, sometimes passive, and mediated through the body's chemical needs and desires.

With prolonged consumption, morphine's addictive power alters the chemical equilibrium of the human organism, creating a new normal state contingent upon its presence in the body. In a similar manner, France's industrializing pharmaceutical economy altered the equilibrium of French society. It offered French citizens the previously elusive promise of freedom from pain. Pharmaceutical control became the new normal in France's psychotropic society. This norm has persisted into the twenty-first century. France continues to be one of the largest consumers of psychotropic pharmaceuticals in the world.[52] A 2006 parliamentary report found that about one in four French citizens had consumed at least one psychotropic medication during the previous year. This consumption was about twice as high as in other European countries including the United Kingdom, Germany, and even that paragon of drug culture, the Netherlands.[53] A 2013 study found that 32 per cent of French people used some form of psychotropic medication on a regular basis.[54] France is still a nation on drugs. Like morphine for the addict, psychotropic consumption has proved impossible to quit.

{ 1 }

PSYCHOTROPIC PHARMACEUTICALS

When it comes to the primary cause that gives this product
the power to soothe pain and bring on irresistible sleep,
we must undoubtedly resign ourselves never to know.
It's one of those thousand mysterious forces ... man uses
its effects without knowing its essence.
– J. Constantin Decharme, on opium (1855)

Drugs became increasingly ubiquitous commodities in nineteenth-century France. However, their incredible power to modify consciousness and relieve pain was contingent upon a delicate balance of dosage. The wrong dose could lead to dire, or even fatal, consequences. Frustratingly, dosing was not an exact science in the 1840s, as the quality and potency of drugs like opium could vary widely on the international market. As a result, psychotropic drugs both fascinated and frightened the medical practitioners who wielded them.

Psychotropic drugs were important legitimizing instruments of the medical and pharmaceutical professions. While doctors and pharmacists officially had a legal monopoly over medical practice in France, in the daily exercise of their professions they faced competition from a litany of unofficial healers and purveyors of drugs. Doctors and pharmacists distinguished themselves through university education and state monopoly, while patients often measured their worth based on their ability to cure the patients' ills and alleviate their symptoms. So, medical professionals sought to control these powerful pain-relieving drugs. They regulated the composition of psychotropic remedies, transforming exotic botanicals and pharmaceutical mixtures of inconsistent potency into reliable, standardized pharmaceutical commodities. However, they also tried to supervise patients' access to these substances within the pharmaceutical marketplace, positioning themselves as gatekeepers of pain relief.

Doctors' and pharmacists' growing control over drugs in French society was bound up with transformations in drug production. During the nineteenth century, the preparation of pharmaceutical remedies became more science than art. In 1818, the Paris Faculty of Medicine published the first official Codex, which established a standardized set of rules, procedures, and formulas for preparing pharmaceutical remedies for all of France.[1] New editions of the national Codex appeared in 1837, 1866, 1884, and 1908 as pharmacists developed new medicines and refined procedures for their preparation.[2] Furthermore, the introduction of industrial manufacturing techniques for mass production made psychotropic drugs even more reliable.

This chapter documents the production of a psychotropic economy. Using opium as the primary case study, it traces the production, circulation, and consumption of psychotropic substances as a quotidian part of everyday life in nineteenth-century France. Through domestic cultivation schemes and industrial production techniques, pharmacists, agriculturalists, and entrepreneurs transformed opium from an unpredictable foreign import into a reliable staple of French industry. Opiate remedies transformed pain. Doctors and pharmacists attempted to control the production and exchange of these substances in French society. However, both within and beyond the boundaries of "official" medicine, patients harnessed the psychotropic power of these drugs to surmount the quotidian discomfort, acute agony, and psychological toll of living with illness.

CULTIVATING RELIABILITY

Opium is one of the world's oldest remedies. Human civilizations have cultivated it as a medicine and a stimulant for over six thousand years.[3]

It is produced by extracting and refining the juice from opium poppies (*Papaver somniferum*). For centuries, it was used in Europe as a base ingredient for theriac and other analgesic concoctions.[4] However, with the introduction of new chemical processes scientists began to isolate alkaloids, the nitrogen-based substances that constitute the active principles of plant medicines. In 1804, German chemist Friedrich Wilhelm Sertürner first isolated morphine, opium's primary alkaloid.[5] Doctors used opium and its alkaloid morphine in a wide range of pharmaceuticals including extracts, pills, salves, enemas, and laudanum, a mixture of opium and alcohol. The remarkable flexibility and efficacy of opium for relieving pain made it the nineteenth century's pharmaceutical analgesic par excellence.

Opium was ubiquitous, but it was also unreliable. The morphine content of opium varied widely based on the type of opium poppy, the climate in which it was grown, and the method of cultivation. For example, Egyptian opium could contain almost twice as much morphine as Persian opium. Turkish opium sold at the market in Smyrna, the modern-day city of Izmir, was famous for having the highest morphine content of any opium sold on the international market, usually at least 10 per cent.[6] Therefore, the vast majority of the opium that France imported was this Turkish variety (Figure 1.1).[7] However, as opium fetched such a high price, cultivators found creative ways to increase their opium's weight and volume using additives like wax, rubber, raisins, flour, egg yolks, and dates.[8] French pharmacists who sought to create reliable standardized pharmaceutical remedies were frustrated by the widespread adulteration of this "exotic opium."[9]

The often unpredictable quality of this imported botanical substance posed challenges to the French pharmaceutical profession's quest for scientific precision. In the early 1850s, pharmacist Hector Aubergier collected twenty-four samples of opium from various druggists and pharmacists in Paris and in the countryside. Chemical analysis revealed that their morphine content varied significantly, from 2.84 per cent to 12.66 per cent.[10] This wide variation was dangerous. An overly strong sample might cause a patient to overdose. A weaker sample might not work effectively to relieve pain. For this reason, the Pharmacie Centrale des Hôpitaux de Paris, the central pharmacy that supplied Paris hospitals, rejected any opium that was not at least 9 per cent morphine.[11]

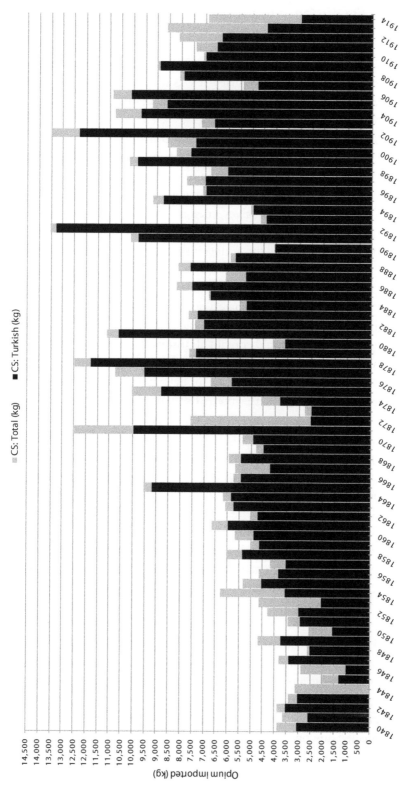

1.1 Opium imported for domestic consumption in France, 1840–1914. Turkish opium comprised the vast majority of France's opium imports during this period. *Source:* Statistics collected from the Direction Générale des Douanes, *Tableau général du commerce* (Paris: Imprimerie Nationale, 1840–1914).

Therefore, finding a reliable source of high-quality raw opium was vital to French pharmacy.

While opium's unpredictable quality posed a scientific challenge, its status as a foreign import posed an economic one. In the ten years between 1827 and 1836, France imported a total of 114,259 kilograms of opium, valued at 3,680,288 francs.[12] This heavy reliance on a foreign import undermined France's long-standing aspirations for economic self-sufficiency. During the Napoleonic Wars when Britain blockaded French ports to try to weaken the French military machine, Napoleon responded by instituting the Continental System, which banned British-manufactured goods and products of British trade.[13] Then, the emperor appealed to the patriotism of men of science to turn their craft to the service of France's economic interests, calling on them to find substitutes for exotic products that could be produced on French soil.[14] Many scientists and entrepreneurs went to work to develop substitutes for colonial commodities like coffee and sugar, which depended on British-dominated sea commerce.[15] For his part, M. Loiseleur-Deslongchamps performed numerous experiments on indigenous poppies to develop medicines that would reduce France's reliance on foreign opium.[16]

In the early nineteenth century, a group of enterprising French pharmacists and agriculturalists saw a golden opportunity to reduce France's reliance on foreign imports and stimulate agricultural revenues by cultivating opium domestically.[17] Many French pharmacists lauded indigenous opium cultivation as a way to standardize opium's morphine content for medical use. Using French science and agricultural techniques, they believed they could avoid the adulteration they perceived to be characteristic of "exotic opium" from the "Orient."[18] Their research focused on two interrelated questions. The first was whether opium cultivated in France contained sufficient quantities of morphine to be competitive with Turkish opium from Smyrna for use in medical therapeutics. The second was whether the profits of this new industry would outweigh the costs of cultivation and enable France to become a self-sufficient producer. If France hoped to develop a domestic source of high-quality opium, it had to ensure that the venture would be both effective and profitable.

Pharmacists and chemists could only measure the quantity of morphine in a given sample of opium through chemical analysis.[19] In 1818,

Louis Nicolas Vauquelin conducted the first chemical analysis of two samples of indigenous opium cultivated by French naturalist Palissot de Beauvois and surgeon Jean-Baptiste-Jacques Thillaye of the Paris Faculty of Medicine. He determined that the French opium contained exactly the same substances as exotic opium.[20] In 1827, Lieutenant General Jean Maximilien Lamarque, who had fought for Napoleon at Austerlitz, decided to cultivate opium poppies in various parts of his lands in the Landes with the hope that France could "escape a foreign tribute." The samples of opium he produced contained between 10 and 14 per cent morphine.[21] While these high levels of morphine provoked skepticism from some pharmacists, they also stimulated further experimentation.

Although most considered "opium poppies" to be the white poppies grown in Anatolia (*Papaver somniferum album*), French researchers discovered that other types of poppies also contained usable quantities of morphine. In 1842, Hector Aubergier began cultivating three different types of poppies in Clermont-Ferrand: *pavot blanc*, or "white poppies"; *pavot pourpre*, or "purple poppies"; and *pavot à oeillette*, black poppies grown for the production of poppyseed oil.[22] He wanted to determine which variety might be most profitably exploited for French agriculture and, as a pharmacist, he had a vested interest in making sure that this locally produced opium had a morphine content that was sufficient for medical use. He concluded that *pavot pourpre* consistently yielded opium with 10 per cent morphine over five years of harvests – twice the morphine content of white poppies – while also producing more seeds.[23] Aubergier saw small-scale cultivation as the key to opening up this new agriculture venture, explaining that "each farmer will add a couple kilos of opium to his poppy seed harvest" as a means of producing unadulterated, morphine-rich domestic opium for the medical marketplace.[24]

While indigenous opium had to pass the muster of laboratory analysis for quality and consistency, it also had to prove its worth by effectively treating patients in pain. In 1853, Professor Bouchardat, chief pharmacist at the Hôtel-Dieu Hospital in Paris, published a report confirming the efficacy of Aubergier's indigenous opium. He cited two Paris physicians, Augustin Grisolle at Pitié Hospital and Pierre Rayer at Charité Hospital, who had extensively studied the effects of indigenous opium on patients to determine its effectiveness at producing pain relief and inducing sleep. Together, they tested indigenous opium on over one hundred patients suffering from conditions ranging from cancer to rheumatism. Based on their patients' reactions, the doctors determined that Aubergier's French opium was at least as effective as "exotic opium" from Anatolia, if not more so. One woman at Pitié who suffered from uterine cancer habitually took opium to manage pain and help her sleep. She found that a 4-centigram dose of indigenous opium calmed her pain just as well as a 5-centigram dose of exotic opium, suggesting that the French opium might have been even more potent than the exotic variety.[25]

At Charité, Rayer set up an experiment to rule out the placebo effect. He administered patients suffering from painful chronic illnesses first with indigenous opium, then with exotic opium, and finally with granules of the same volume as the first two substances but that "contained no medical substance."[26] The patients never experienced lower sedative effects while taking indigenous opium instead of exotic opium. However, when they took the inert placebo substance, their pain and sleeplessness returned.[27] This suffering proved that the patients' responses were not just a product of their own expectations of relief. By testing French opium against an inert placebo, Rayer determined that it actually produced the same sedative effects as Turkish opium.

As French pharmacists and doctors began to experiment with opium cultivation domestically, colonial agriculturalists and pharmacists explored the possibility of transforming opium into a cash crop for colonial Algeria. In 1830, Charles X of France had invaded Algeria as a last-ditch attempt to shore up support for his monarchy amid a widespread crisis of political legitimacy.[28] Although the plan failed and his regime was overthrown, his successor, Louis-Philippe d'Orléans, continued the imperial project in Algeria under the July Monarchy, reframing colonization as a matter of national pride. However, the huge expense of the conquest and occupation remained a source of political tension among its opponents.

The goal of "restoring" Algeria's fertile agricultural lands to their mythical former glory under ancient Rome shaped France's vision of a settler colony in Algeria.[29] The warm climate made men of science enthusiastic about the prospect of growing opium poppies. In Algeria, "our compatriots will be able to engage in experiments with the cultivation of *Papaver somniferum*, under a latitude little different from that of Anatolia, where we have long obtained the best varieties of medicinal opium."[30]

This would give France greater control over its opium supply and enable colonial cultivators to produce a high-quality opium that could meet France's medicinal demand. Paris pharmacist J.-B. Caventou, then the vice-president of the National Academy of Medicine, even suggested that Algerian opium cultivation might offer further advantages. Not only would opium cultivation provide an economic benefit to France by increasing colonial resources, Caventou explained, but it would also "create another powerful argument against those who claim that this glorious conquest of Algiers, consolidated since 1830 with so much gold and blood, thus far has only given France ... some highly questionable political benefits in return."[31] Profitable opium cultivation, he implied, could serve to justify the entire colonial project.

During the 1840s and 1850s, the French government sponsored scientific investigations into how to transform Algeria's existing subsistence farming into capitalist agricultural production.[32] Maréchal Soult, the French minister of war, was enthusiastic about the possibility of cultivating high-quality opium in Algeria, so the French government began supporting agricultural research in 1841. Researchers sent their reports to the French Academy of Sciences. M. Hardy, director of the Central Nursery in Algeria, conducted a small-scale experiment in 1843. From the ninety poppy heads he cultivated, he obtained a 50-gram sample of opium, which contained 5.02 per cent crystalized morphine – unfortunately, only about half the potency of Turkish opium.[33]

Undeterred, the minister of war sent another researcher to Algeria the next year to plant and harvest opium, to determine whether it could be exploited profitably for medicinal purposes.[34] The new researcher, M. Simon, claimed that his opium contained 12 per cent morphine and concluded that Algerian opium was much more potent than exotic commercial varieties.[35] However, when the chief pharmacist of the Central Pharmacy of Algiers tested the sample of Simon's opium he found that it contained only 10.075 per cent morphine, making it roughly equivalent to the Turkish opium used as the medicinal standard.[36] While these initial attempts were somewhat ambiguous in their results, the intriguing possibility of Algerian opium cultivation sparked considerable interest among government officials.[37] The minister of war sent these initial reports to the minister of the interior and invited him to publish their content in the *Moniteur Algérien*, the official journal of the colony. Soult hoped that disseminating this information would provoke further experimentation in the other government plant nurseries, in Bône, Philippeville, Constantine, and Oran.[38] Several cultivators rose to the challenge. At the 1855 Exposition Universelle in Paris, Algeria supplied samples of opium grown by farmers in Montpensier, Bou-Ismaïl, and Béjaïa in addition to samples from the government nurseries in Algiers and Constantine.[39]

French officials were eager to capitalize on Algeria's potential as a space for cultivating "tropical" commodities such as indigo, cotton, tobacco, and opium to reduce France's dependence on foreign markets.[40] However, although the government had offered incentives to colonial opium cultivators in Algeria since 1841, by the mid-1850s large-scale Algerian opium cultivation had still made little progress. The protective tariffs that the French government established on Algerian agricultural products in the 1830s might have contributed to undermine these efforts in the early years.[41] French opium cultivators attributed the lack of progress to the meticulous care needed to extract opium, which increased labour costs.[42] However, opium was not alone. Although Algerian cotton production became profitable temporarily in the 1860s as a result of the embargo during the American Civil War, none of the tropical crops did particularly well in the long term. French officials struggled to make agricultural schemes profitable in Algeria.[43] Even the dramatic rise of the Algerian wine industry in the 1880s owed its commercial success in large part to phylloxera's decimation of France's own vineyards.[44] While individuals continued to experiment with opium production in Algeria throughout the nineteenth century, large-scale opium production never seemed to make headway.[45]

The setbacks in Algeria did not discourage French pharmacists from their quest for economic self-sufficiency. Not only did opium offer new avenues for entrepreneurs, but scientists believed it also offered a way to make France's existing domestic agricultural production even more profitable. In the mid-1850s, a group of French pharmacists in Amiens sought to encourage opium production on small farms in the Nord that were already devoted to the cultivation of poppyseed oil from *pavot à oeillette*.[46] Rather than attempting to stimulate a brand-new agricultural industry, J.-P. Bénard, a professor at the Amiens Preparatory School of Medicine and Pharmacy, and C. Collas, a Paris pharmacist, hoped to persuade small-scale poppy farmers that they could increase the revenues gleaned from their production of poppyseed oil simply by investing a little in extra labour, for an additional harvest of opium taken from the same plants. According to statistics from 1857, the *département* of the Somme contained 12,702 hectares of land devoted to poppyseed oil cultivation, which produced a harvest of about 140,000 hectolitres of seed valued at 4,480,000 francs.[47] While opium cultivation was labour intensive, it would only require farmers to make minor adjustments to their existing process. Rather than scattering seeds at random, farmers would need to plant seeds in lines to facilitate opium collection. They would also need to hire a few extra workers for the ten to fifteen days of the opium harvest to incise the capsules and collect the poppy juice.[48]

Bénard and Collas provided a detailed analysis of the costs and profits of adding opium production to an existing poppyseed farm in order to convince farmers that the additional expense was in their best interests. They found that opium produced from *pavot à oeillette* in Amiens contained extremely high levels of morphine: between 15 and 20 per cent depending on the year.[49] They hoped to encourage poppy farmers to produce opium as a means of "doubling the value of their field[s]."[50] At that time, the cost of the labour for preparing, manuring, sowing, hoeing, and harvesting *pavot à oeillette* was 278.50 francs for each hectare of land. The eleven hectolitres of seeds thereby produced could be sold for 346.50 francs, leaving the farmer a profit of 68 francs per hectare from seed production.[51] However, if a farmer decided to invest an additional fortnight of labour into his land before collecting the seeds, to produce opium, he could sell it to nearby pharmacists or send it to Bénard in Amiens or Collas in Paris and be compensated for the opium "according to its richness in morphine," valued at a minimum of 60 francs per kilo and sold for as much as 80 or even 100 francs per kilo.[52] A local cutler had developed a special incising instrument that would prevent workers from cutting too deeply and spoiling the poppy seeds during opium collection. Therefore, Bénard and Collas argued, farmers could employ the unskilled labour of women, schoolchildren, and orphans for between 75 centimes and 1 franc per day to reduce costs further. Assuming that workers would collect approximately 1.5 francs worth of opium per day, this would yield a minimum profit of 50 to 75 centimes per worker per day.[53] These incredibly detailed financial estimations demonstrate Bénard and Collas's serious commitment to producing high-quality French opium to supply France's pharmacies while simultaneously bolstering local agriculture.

Another staunch proponent of domestic cultivation, Constantin Decharme, estimated that it could contribute millions of francs of additional revenue to France as well as providing an additional five to six hundred days of work per hectare of poppy fields for French workers in the Nord during the period of unemployment that preceded the normal seed harvest.[54] Following the example of Bénard and Collas, in 1862 Alphonse Odeph, an enterprising pharmacist from Champlitte in Haute-Saône, published a simple, straightforward guide to cultivating and harvesting opium poppies in *Union Pharmaceutique*.[55] The same year, his article was republished as a pamphlet titled *Practical Summary on the Farming of Indigenous Opium, to Serve as a Guide for Inhabitants of the Countryside*.[56] Proponents of indigenous cultivation deployed French ideals of economic efficiency and profitability in an attempt to normalize opium, transforming an adulterated foreign import into a reliable product of domestic agriculture.

Chemical analyses of French opium found it to be quite rich in morphine. In 1862, Professor Guibourt of the Paris Pharmacy School published an exhaustive study. He found that samples of French opium contained between 11.3 per cent and 22.88 per cent morphine, levels comparable to or higher than the typical content of Smyrna opium.[57] While French doctors celebrated the efficiency and quality of French scientific agriculture, these high yields of morphine did not solve the problem of standardization. Medicines made with French opium could still vary dramatically in potency, which could be dangerous for patients. Pharmacist P. Berthé claimed that out of two different samples of opium gathered from the same field of poppies, one might yield 16 per cent morphine and the other only 6 per cent.[58] If pharmacists used this opium as a base ingredient in compounded medicines, they could never be sure how much morphine it contained. Therefore, he argued that pharmacists should prepare medicines only with the pure alkaloid, morphine, so they could be confident in their remedies.[59]

Guibourt compared the samples of French opium with foreign opium sold on the international market. He found opium from Egypt, Persia, and India to be of low or inconsistent quality.[60] However, despite widespread assumptions that opium from the "Orient" was rife with adulterants, Guibourt founded that samples of Anatolian opium collected from various pharmacies and wholesale druggists in Paris contained a minimum of 9.6 per cent morphine and that most samples contained between 12.4 per cent and 14.7 per cent morphine. This potency was entirely consistent with the levels of morphine found in samples of opium that M. Della-Sudda, one of the major Turkish opium suppliers, had sent to display at the 1855 Universal Exposition in Paris, suggesting that the Anatolian opium sold in Paris had not been adulterated.[61] Berthé noted that opium merchants in Smyrna employed experts who were responsible for testing the quality of each chest of opium. These experts collected samples of each loaf of opium in the chest and set aside any that looked suspicious. Typically, they discarded about 75 per cent of the suspicious samples as unfit for sale.[62] Later in the century, quality control became even more accurate through chemical analysis in laboratories installed in the major opium houses in Anatolia.[63]

The French Pharmaceutical Codex of 1866 reflected the pharmaceutical profession's concerns about producing reliable and standardized remedies. It listed Smyrna opium as the standard opium to use as a base ingredient in pharmaceutical preparations and individually compounded medicines because it had the most consistent quality, at about 10 per cent morphine.[64] The Codex also advised pharmacists to reject, as very inferior in quality, opiums from Egypt, Persia, and India." While it mentioned French opium cultivation from *pavot à oeillette*, it noted that "this opium, which often contains more than 20 per cent morphine, should be reserved for the extraction of the alkaloid" rather than used to prepare opium-based remedies.[65]

During the second half of the nineteenth century, then, Smyrna opium became the gold standard for French pharmaceutical production for its quality and consistency. According to the records of the French Directorate-General of Customs, from 1840 to 1920 France imported between 2,000 and 12,000 kilograms of opium annually, the vast majority of which was supplied by the Ottoman Empire.[66] Until 1914, Turkish opium typically represented over 90 per cent of France's total opium imports (Figure 1.1).[67] French pharmacists also continued to cultivate opium domestically, presumably for use in the production of alkaloids. In 1872, a doctor hoping to cultivate opium in Germany claimed that France had been a pioneer in European opium production that produced indigenous opium "on a large scale." He noted that France cultivated 50,000 acres of poppy fields that yielded 2 million francs of opium per year.[68]

Colonial opium cultivation also remained an attractive possibility for expanding the profitability of France's empire. Later in the century, French pharmacists and naturalists periodically returned to this concept. In 1885, naval pharmacist Édouard Raoul proposed a mission to travel to Madagascar, Réunion, New Caledonia, Indochina, French Oceania, and several other Pacific islands in order to introduce new plants, including rubber and opium, for cultivation in France's colonies.[69] Raoul designed this mission to boost the flagging profitability of France's sugar islands, which faced a loss of profits from agricultural diseases and increased competition from beetroot sugar. He believed that opium production would flourish in colonies like Réunion.[70] Although the Minister of the Navy and Colonies granted funding for Raoul's mission, undertaken between 1886 and 1888, it is unclear from the archival records whether opium production made serious inroads in France's colonies in the Pacific and Indian Oceans.[71] However, opium certainly played a large role in financing France's colonial regime in Indochina. There, France instituted a monopoly over the import and sale of opium designed for recreational smoking, which paid for France's colonial administration through indirect taxes.[72] While colonial opium cultivation may not have lived up to France's expectations, in Indochina at least, the opium monopoly demonstrates that colonial officials continued to view its exchange as a useful strategy for financing imperial rule.

French opium cultivators reimagined opium as a profitable product of domestic and colonial agriculture, lauding its high quality as a source of national pride and economic self-sufficiency. In so doing, they helped to transform opium from an exotic botanical commodity into a reliable base material of the French pharmaceutical industry. France continued to buy high-quality Turkish opium. However, domestic cultivation supplemented these imports and contributed to the normalization of opium as a pharmaceutical commodity. As French pharmacists increased their control over the properties and composition of their opium-based products by standardizing their potency, they reduced the mystery of these commodities while increasing their own reputations as exacting men of science.

STANDARDIZING PRODUCTION

Quality control was a major concern in the practice of pharmacy. Pharmacists in France had a legal monopoly over the production and distribution of medicines, set out in the Law of 21 Germinal, An XI (11 April 1803).[73] While pharmacy students completed coursework in medicine, botany, pharmacy, and chemistry, practical skills were paramount. They had to intern in established pharmacies and pass a practical examination in front of a jury of doctors, surgeons, and pharmacists to demonstrate their ability to produce the medicines necessary to run a pharmacy. The Germinal Law also ensured that the pursuit of scientific ideals was not the only factor motivating pharmacists to produce high-quality products. Once a pharmacist had established his dispensary, he was required to submit it for an annual inspection by a committee of doctors and pharmacists, accompanied by a police commissioner, to verify the quality of the drugs and remedies that he sold. The police commissioner would seize any drugs that were poorly prepared or deteriorated so that they could not be sold to unwitting customers.[74] Therefore, pharmacists distinguished themselves as professionals largely through the precision and reliability of their products.

During the nineteenth century, the pharmaceutical profession adopted increasingly precise and standardized production techniques. The French Codex began to eliminate inert ingredients from pharmaceutical formulas. Instead, it moved toward simpler preparations that isolated the active therapeutic properties of the ingredients. With each successive edition of the Codex, the methods listed for preparing a given remedy became more precise and scientific in accordance with the emerging epistemological ideals of objectivity.[75]

The recipe for "cynoglosse pills," which doctors prescribed as a sleep aid and pain reliever, serves to illustrate this shift. Cynoglosse pills contained opium, houndstooth, henbane, saffron, myrrh, frankincense, and castoreum. The 1818 Codex lists the quantities of ingredients needed in "gros," an old unit of mass equal to ⅛ ounce. Opium appeared in two forms: 4 "gros" of opium wine or laudanum, which was itself a preparation from the Codex, as well as "a sufficient quantity" of opium syrup, left to the judgment of the individual pharmacist.[76] By 1837, the ingredients and proportions for the pills were the same except for the laudanum, which had been replaced by opium extract, a more concentrated form of opium that did not contain extraneous ingredients.[77] In the 1866 Codex, the ingredients were listed for the first time in grams, instead of gros. The formula called for precisely 10 grams of opium extract, no longer relying on a particular pharmacist's judgment as to what constituted a "sufficient" quantity of this powerful psychotropic ingredient. Once the pharmacist had followed the specific instructions for preparation, he had to divide the substance "into 20-centigram pills, each of which contains 0.02gr (2 centigrams) of opium extract."[78] Over time, the formula and procedure for preparing "cynoglosse pills" became more precise. It established increasingly objective standards of measurement, eliminating the pharmacists' subjective judgment from the process.[79]

Pharmacists had to follow official guidelines and specific formulas to prepare medicines. However, it was quite challenging for a pharmacist to produce the wide variety of standardized, reliable products in a small pharmacy laboratory.[80] Pharmacy students were scarce, laboratory equipment was expensive and bulky, and fresh plants were often difficult to acquire when they were needed. It would have been both costly and impractical for the typical pharmacist to produce all of the remedies required for running a profitable dispensary from base ingredients by following the recipes from the Codex.[81] Yet, cutting corners was risky. Medicines prepared with old or rancid ingredients might be less effective or even dangerous for consumers. Therefore, pharmacists had to determine how to keep their pharmacies stocked with all of the necessary medications without compromising on quality.

Although pharmacists in the second half of the nineteenth century lamented a supposed "golden age" of artisanal pharmaceutical production that followed the Germinal Law of 1803, this ideal of the independent dispensary pharmacist was more myth than reality.[82] Industrialized production techniques were already beginning to transform the business of pharmacy at the beginning of the nineteenth century. Independent pharmacists continued to prepare medicines in their dispensary laboratories to a doctor's exact specifications when presented with a unique (magisterial) prescription. However, they increasingly turned to wholesalers to supply standard simple remedies and composite medicines from the Codex. For reasons of practicality

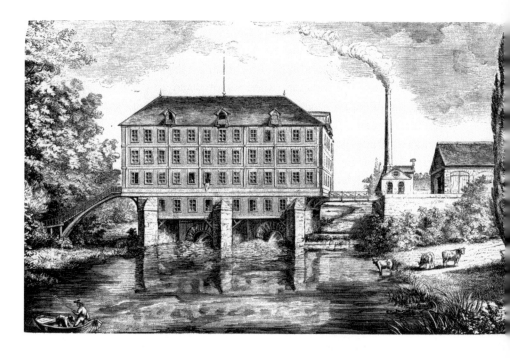

1.2 The hydraulic factory of the Maison Centrale de Droguerie
at Noisiel-sur-Marne. This old mill was purchased by
J.-A.-B. Ménier in 1824.

and profitability as much as pharmaceutical purity, pharmacists relied
more and more upon commercial chemical laboratories to produce their
pharmaceutical products.[83]

One of the largest pharmaceutical manufacturers in the early nineteenth century was the Ménier Company's Maison Centrale de Droguerie.[84]
In 1816, Jean-Antoine-Brutus Ménier (1795–1853), founder of the famous
French chocolate firm, established a small enterprise devoted to pulver-
izing vegetable and mineral medicines, which he expanded in 1824 after
purchasing an old mill in Noisiel on the Marne River (Figure 1.2). In this
new "hydraulic factory," Ménier installed steam-powered machinery
and began to produce high-quality pharmaceutical products in mass
quantities.[85] Unlike pharmacists, who dealt directly with clientele, the
Maison Ménier was a wholesale *droguerie* that manufactured products
in bulk to supply to pharmacies and dispensaries in the Ile-de-France

region. The business expanded through new investors, partnerships, and medals from national and international expositions, and in the 1840s it became known as the Maison Centrale de Droguerie of Ménier et Cie.[86]

The main promotional tool of the Maison Centrale de Droguerie was its price catalogue, first published in 1832, which listed all of its products, ranging from powders, balms, and poultices to surgical equipment and bandages.[87] As the price catalogue demonstrates, the Maison Centrale de Droguerie was far more than a wholesale warehouse of basic pharmaceutical ingredients. Its declared goal was to provide pharmacists with a "central and universal provisioning establishment."[88] The Ménier Company offered pharmacists fair prices for standardized products, which it manufactured on a large scale using hydraulic pulverization and evaporation machines. In addition to the raw opium one would expect a wholesale druggist to supply, Ménier's price catalogue from 1845 includes a wide array of opium-based remedies, including powdered opium, opium extract, opium syrup, and laudanum.[89] The Ménier Company assured pharmacists that "we follow the formulas of the Codex religiously; because, if the fidelity of pharmaceutical preparations is a duty, it is also the only way to maintain the confidence of the pharmacist who wants to have the same absolute faith in the medication that he buys as if he had prepared it himself."[90] Its reputation for quality gave the Maison Centrale de Droguerie considerable commercial reach. The Ménier Company had at least 7,500 customer accounts in 1844, one-fifth of which were international, representing a revenue of over 2 million francs.[91]

Although the Germinal Law granted pharmacists a monopoly over the preparation and sale of medicines, by the mid-nineteenth century they felt that both elements of this monopoly were under threat. Their monopoly over the preparation of medicines diminished as they began to purchase more and more manufactured pharmaceutical products from wholesalers. Furthermore, their commercial monopoly was being threatened by herbalists, doctors, nuns, grocers, and other unsanctioned distributors of medicines.[92] Professional journals began to complain of a "crisis of pharmacy" as unlawful competition and industry whittled away at pharmacists' monopoly over the material exchange of medicines.[93] In 1852, pharmacist François Dorvault (1815–1879) founded the Pharmacie Centrale des Pharmaciens, which he envisioned to be an industrial cooperative of pharmacists that would act as both laboratory and wholesale drug supplier, in order to supply France's dispensaries with standardized, high-quality pharmaceutical preparations produced under the supervision of pharmacists.[94] Supported by subscription, the Pharmacie Centrale had 354 members, representing approximately 9 per cent of the pharmacists in France, in 1852.[95] As a sign of confidence, in August 1855 the members renamed the cooperative the Pharmacie Centrale de France (PCF) and increased its funds to 4 million francs.[96] It rapidly became the most important manufacturer of pharmaceutical products in France. In 1867, it purchased Ménier's Maison Centrale de Droguerie along with its factory in Saint-Denis.[97] Historian Nicolas Sueur has argued that the PCF made its goal "the defence of the pharmacist's monopoly by means of industrialization."[98] With a regular supply of effective, high-quality remedies purchased wholesale from the PCF, the pharmacist could devote more of his attention to the commercial success of his dispensary.

From the mid-nineteenth century onward, French pharmacists increasingly turned to the PCF to supply them with high-quality pharmaceutical products at a fair price.[99] As Ménier et Cie had done before it, the PCF published a pharmaceutical catalogue that united all of the products it offered in a single volume. The PCF offered pharmacists an enormous selection of products. The 1877 price catalogue lists well over one hundred psychotropic remedies for sale, varying from raw botanical products, such as Cannabis indica (8 francs per kilo) and coca (14 francs per kilo), to chemical anesthetics such as ether (9 francs per kilo) and chloroform (16 francs per kilo). In addition to high-quality base ingredients, pharmacists could purchase a plethora of manufactured opium remedies, including "black drops," opium-infused cold cream, sugar-coated pills, extracts, narcotic oil, opium ointment, laudanum, powders, syrups, tinctures, and any number of pharmaceutical specialties.[100] The PCF offered the pharmacist quality and variety so that he could maintain his professional reputation among his clients.

Certain pharmaceutical products, particularly those emerging from chemical processes, were particularly well suited to industrial production. Ether and chloroform, both gases produced through chemical synthesis, have a powerful anesthetic effect when inhaled. In the sixteenth century, Leipzig chemist Valerius Cordus (1515–1544) first synthesized the substance known in the nineteenth century as ether by distilling alcohol with oil of vitriol (sulfuric acid) and called it "sweet oil of vitriol."[101] Chloroform ($CHCl_3$) was discovered in 1831 simultaneously by three chemists: Eugène Souberian, Justus von Liebig, and Samuel Guthrie.[102] In January 1847, in a flurry of clinical research and self-experimentation, French doctors began to use ether as a general anesthetic for surgical procedures.[103] Two months later, French chemist Marie-Jean-Pierre Flourens (1794–1867) discovered that chloroform inhalations produced a similar effect. By 1848, chloroform anesthesia had become a standard procedure in surgical practice.[104] In addition to their surgical uses, ether and chloroform were used in pharmaceutical practice as analgesics and antispasmodics.

Chloroform and ether quickly became part of the purview of industrial rather than artisanal production, because of their extreme volatility. Although industrial production was rapidly expanding by mid-century, the 1866 Codex still included specific preparation instructions for the pharmacist who wished to produce chloroform in his own laboratory by boiling, distilling, and decanting water, quicklime, dry lime chloride, and alcohol.[105] By 1884, however, the Codex specified that it would only include the method of preparation for products that pharmacists should make themselves, and not for products they should purchase wholesale.[106] Therefore, the 1884 Codex does not list the complex instructions for preparing chloroform in a small pharmacy laboratory. Instead, it includes a detailed description of this "colourless, highly mobile liquid," with its "smooth, ethereal odour" and sickly sweet taste, as well as instructions for "modifying" commercial chloroform for dispensary use.[107] While the instructions for making ether remained in 1884, by 1908 the Codex included only a detailed description of anesthetic ether, a list of preparations that called for it, instructions for testing its quality, and warnings about its extreme flammability.[108] Presumably, by 1908 pharmacists were purchasing anesthetic ether from wholesalers like the PCF rather than attempting to produce the volatile liquid in their own laboratories.

By the turn of the twentieth century, plant alkaloids like morphine and cocaine were also frequently purchased wholesale. Pharmacists had isolated morphine in the first decade of the nineteenth century, but doctors did not widely prescribe morphine as a medical therapeutic in France until much later.[109] Professor Behier of the Hôtel-Dieu Hospital is credited with introducing the technique of subcutaneous morphine injection in 1859, which precipitated morphine's popularity in French medical practice.[110] Injecting a solution of morphine dissolved in water under the skin introduced the alkaloid gradually into the bloodstream, which provided swift and effective pain relief that extended beyond the injection site. Although the manner of chemically extracting morphine from opium changed somewhat with each successive edition of the French Codex, the basic procedure involved macerating opium in water to produce a liquid opium extract and then treating the solution several times with alcohol and chemicals, through boiling, filtration, and evaporation.[111] The solution yielded crystals that the chemist or pharmacist would crush into a powder and treat further using the same processes. Initially grey in colour, the crystals became clearer and more refined with each successive chemical treatment and filtration. The 1884 Codex still included instructions for the preparation of morphine and morphine hydrochloride (the primary form used for hypodermic injections), but the 1908 Codex included only descriptive information for these commodities, indicating that by that point they were manufactured in factories and sold wholesale.[112]

Cocaine was another plant alkaloid that pharmacists purchased wholesale. Cocaine is extracted from the leaves of the coca plant (*Erythroxylum coca*), a Peruvian shrub also cultivated in the warm climates of Bolivia, Columbia, and Brazil in the nineteenth century.[113] German chemist Albert Niemann first isolated cocaine in 1860.[114] While the coca leaf had been a staple of traditional South American medicine for millennia, cocaine became popular in European medical practice in the 1880s after two Austrian doctors, Sigmund Freud and his colleague Carl Koller, discovered it was effective as a local anesthetic.[115] The 1884 French Codex listed "coca" as a botanical medicinal substance and included instructions for simple coca preparations – coca extract, powdered coca, coca tincture, a coca tisane, and coca wine – but no instructions for preparing the alkaloid.[116] The first time "cocaine" appeared in the French Codex in its alkaloid form was in 1908, by which point the Codex merely listed a description of its properties, indicating that pharmacists would have purchased it wholesale rather than producing it themselves.

The desire for increasingly standardized and mechanized pharmaceutical products led to the extension of pharmaceutical laboratories into factories designed for such mass production. By 1880 the production of pills and capsules was mechanized, further standardizing their dose and appearance. By the turn of the twentieth century, the PCF's factory in Saint-Denis (Figure 1.3) employed over six hundred people and several other French pharmaceutical laboratories had factories, including Poulenc in Ivry, Adrien and Company in Courbevoie, Darasse and Company in Fontenay sous Bois, and Léon Midy's laboratory and factory in Paris.[117]

While pharmacists made fewer products in their own laboratories, some managed to combine their role as producers of medicines with the resources of the pharmaceutical industry by engaging in the entrepreneurial production of pharmaceutical "specialties." These were pre-prepared medicines whose specific recipes were the property of their inventors instead of formulas from the Codex. Opium and other psychotropic drugs were popular ingredients because of their effective analgesic properties. Hector Aubergier developed two popular specialties, opium pills and a topical opium balm, using indigenous opium cultivated in Clermont-Ferrand.[118] In early nineteenth-century France, debates over the legality of "secret remedies," the precursors to pharmaceutical specialties, brought property rights into conflict with the right to health.[119] However, the 3 May 1850 decree on secret remedies and the 1857 law on trademarks facilitated the legalization of pharmaceutical specialties.[120]

The spectacular rise of pharmaceutical "specialties" went hand in hand with the rise of industrial pharmaceutical production.[121] Entrepreneurs could mass produce and distribute their specialties in pharmacies across France. Production expanded rapidly. By the end of the century, domestic consumption of specialties approached 100 million francs.[122] On the eve of World War I, pharmaceutical specialties like Bonjean Elixir, an ether-based digestion remedy, comprised a quarter of the total revenues for one Lyon pharmacy.[123]

Although specialties were advertised and sold as uniquely efficacious remedies, many were merely modifications of remedies from the Codex.[124] For example, "Gallard's White Drops," a mixture of morphine hydrochloride and cherry laurel water, appear to be a morphine-based version of the "English Black Drops" listed in the Codex, whose active ingredient was opium.[125] Other remedies became popular because they

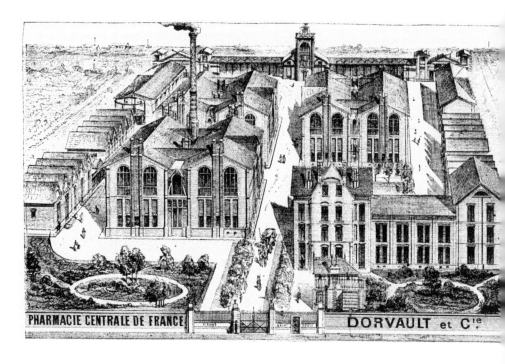

1.3 The Saint-Denis factory of the Pharmacie Centrale de France.

took on new forms that standardized doses and facilitated consumption. For example, Dr Clertan's "Ether Pearls" consisted of several drops of ether encased in a small hollow ball of supple transparent gelatin, a method of consumption that enabled patients to take a standard dose of this highly volatile substance without it evaporating.[126] French pharmacies offered a considerable variety of specialties. The PCF price catalogue included a sixty-page list of the thousands of different specialties it sold.[127] Beginning at the end of the nineteenth century, specialty labels contained the name and inventor of the remedy and a list of its active ingredients. This encouraged copying, which further diversified the variety of products on offer.[128] By 1900, France had become a major exporter of pharmaceutical specialties, which comprised almost 97 per cent of its total medicine exports by value.[129] Industrial production, standardized formulas, and the expansion of pharmaceutical specialties offered patients at the turn of the twentieth century a wider array of remedies than ever before.

The scientific techniques of modern pharmacy worked to standard-ize opium and other pharmaceutical remedies. Simplified formulas, laboratory testing, and industrial production transformed capricious botanical substances and volatile gases into steadfast technologies of modern medicine. Increasingly, pharmacists supplied their pharmacies with mass-produced drugs purchased wholesale from industrial manu-facturers like the PCF. As they did so, their role as commercial vendors of psychotropic medicines eclipsed their role as artisanal producers. As a result, for pharmacists, control over the distribution of medicines became a crucial marker of professional status.

REGULATING POISONS

Doctors and pharmacists positioned themselves as gatekeepers of psycho-tropic drugs to enhance their own professional authority. The 1803 laws of 21 Germinal and 19 Ventôse had created a system of legal monopolies that structured the practice of medicine and the circulation of psycho-tropic drugs within French society.[130] In theory, these monopolies over the prescription and retail sale of medicines were absolute. In practice, however, they were seldom strictly enforced. Patients seeking psychotropic remedies for their ailments could visit a litany of illegal practitioners and suppliers. Within this dynamic pharmaceutical marketplace, patients had more access to psychotropic medicines than ever before.

Opium, morphine, and chloroform were essential pharmaceutical remedies. However, they could also be dangerous poisons. The distinction depended entirely upon the dose administered. For example, injecting a few centigrams of morphine could easily dispel stomach pains, while injecting a whole gram of morphine would almost certainly cause a fatal accident. Therefore, medical expertise was key. In the twentieth and twenty-first centuries, debates over psychotropic drug regulation have concentrated on protecting the public from the dangers of addiction, but in the nineteenth century addiction was not the primary factor mo-tivating regulation. Early nineteenth-century pharmaceutical legislation classified these substances as potentially harmful poisons and regulated them alongside arsenic and strychnine. It was poisoning, not addiction, that drove these early attempts to regulate and restrict access to these substances in the name of public welfare.

By the July Monarchy, French pharmacists had been responsible for controlling and documenting the sale of poisonous substances for centuries.[131] However, they lacked clear criteria for determining which substances qualified as poisons. While the Germinal Law of 1803 required pharmacists to carefully record the sale of "poisonous substances," it did not provide a clear definition of what those were.[132] Instead, it merely provided a few examples of poisons, including arsenic, realgar, and corrosive sublimate (mercury chloride). In the 1840s, after the scandalous Lafarge Affair in which a young woman was found guilty of murdering her husband with arsenic, French legislators determined that clearer specifications were needed.[133] They passed the Poisonous Substances Law on 19 July 1845. The ordinance that followed on 29 October 1846 included a long list of seventy-two poisonous substances that were now restricted.[134] The new legislation officially categorized opium as a poisonous substance under French law and required pharmacists to regulate its distribution.

Pharmacists could only dispense these substances by the specific written prescription of a doctor, surgeon, *officier de santé*, or veterinarian. One pharmacist found this out the hard way, when the Royal Court of Rouen sentenced him to a 3,000-franc fine for selling 10 centilitres of Sydenham's Laudanum to a client without a doctor's prescription.[135] The ordinance required pharmacists to copy the exact details of the prescription into a special register, along with the name, date, and address of the individual purchasing the substance and the quantity supplied.[136] It also required that pharmacists store the listed poisonous substances in a designated poisons cabinet, to be kept locked at all times.[137] The Prefecture of Police, in cooperation with the Mairie, was responsible for inspecting pharmacies to ensure compliance with the laws. These measures were designed not only to prevent would-be poisoners from accessing dangerous substances but also to protect the public against the possibility of accidentally poisoning themselves if these substances were left lying around.

The 1846 ordinance met with staunch opposition from the pharmaceutical profession. While controlling access to pharmaceutical remedies was essential to their privileged professional status, pharmacists wanted to dictate the terms of the regulations. They found the law's restrictions to be unnecessarily invasive and nearly impossible to follow within the everyday practice of running a pharmacy. Shortly after the ordinance was issued, a commission representing the Pharmacy Society of Paris drafted a long report to the Minister of Commerce opposing the details of the ordinance.[138] The Pharmacy Society commission defined a "poisonous substance" as any substance that could cause death when administered at low doses and that could be consumed "without being perceived by the senses."[139] The report systematically rejected over fifty of the poisonous substances listed in the ordinance, conserving only thirteen substances in a revised list.

Although the Pharmacy Society appreciated the need to safeguard public well-being by restricting the sale of poisons that could accidentally be consumed without one's knowledge, the commission argued that substances easily detected by their noxious taste or strong colour should not be restricted, as these substances were less likely to cause accidents.[140] The commission also rejected substances that had no recorded cases of poisoning, such as digitalis, or that were widely available in people's gardens. By contrast, alkaloids and salts of opium were difficult to detect and poisonous in relatively low doses; therefore, the commission agreed with the government that they should be regulated. It proposed that the revised poisons list should include the category "alkaloids and salts of opium," which would cover morphine acetate and morphine hydrochloride along with codeine and opium's other alkaloids.

While it acknowledged the need to regulate highly toxic alkaloids, the Pharmacy Society commission believed that a restriction on opium itself was unnecessary. The report acknowledged that some mothers abused opium and laudanum and gave these substances to their children in irresponsible doses; however, it framed the problem as an English one. The commission claimed that in France, where these medicines could be administered and prescribed only under the supervision of a doctor, cases of abuse were much rarer.[141] As opium and laudanum had a very apparent colour and flavour, the commission argued, they could not be unwittingly consumed and therefore should not be included in the list of poisonous substances.[142] Furthermore, opium and laudanum were much less concentrated than pure alkaloids, so the risk of death from accidental overdose was far lower.

The Pharmacy Society's secondary argument for removing opium and its preparations from the poisonous substances list was an issue of practicality. If one included the derivatives of the items listed in the 1846 ordinance, the actual list of restricted products encompassed no fewer than two hundred substances. For reasons of space, it was impractical to attempt to keep such a large number of products under lock and key in a special cabinet. Furthermore, the pharmacists argued, a great number of these substances – including cantharides, opium, and laudanum in various preparations – were in almost constant demand from clients.[143] Practically speaking, the commission argued, it was actually more dangerous to require that a large variety of commonly used substances be kept locked up among powerful poisons. The poisons cabinet would be opened constantly to retrieve popular medicines like laudanum, undermining the goal of keeping poisons locked in the first place.

Despite several revisions, ambiguities persisted in French poisonous substances legislation throughout the nineteenth century. A decree of 8 July 1850 established a revised poisonous substances list to replace the sixty-eight-item list from 1846.[144] The new list included only nineteen items, among them "opium and its extract" as well as "poisonous plant alkaloids and their salts." The chapter on plant alkaloids in the 1837 Codex, the most recent version at the time of the 1850 decree, listed morphine and codeine, along with quinine, cinchonine, strychnine, brucine, veratridine, and emetine. However, the label "poisonous" left some room for interpretation.[145] Chloroform first appeared on the list of poisonous substances in 1850. Ether, however, was never included. Although the poisonous substances legislation theoretically restricted the supply of opium and other drugs to patients with specific written prescriptions, in practice, commercial logic and a high demand for these products ensured that pharmacists did not necessarily follow these legal prescriptions to the letter.

Pharmacists were not the only medical professionals invested in psychotropic drugs as mechanisms of professional legitimacy. Doctors also found them useful for establishing their reputations with patients.[146] In the 1840s, doctors in Paris and other major cities were constantly complaining that they had to compete for patients in an oversaturated medical job market.[147] Medicine had become a popular career choice for young bourgeois men anxious to solidify their privileged position within the post-Revolutionary social order.[148] The French Revolution had eliminated noble privilege and corporate control over admission to the medical faculties, yet the expense of four years of study for a medical doctorate made it an unrealistic path for most members of the popular classes. However, the 1803 Ventôse Law, which established doctors' medical monopoly in France, also created a second tier of medical practitioners known as *officiers de santé*, or "health officers."[149]

The position of *officier de santé* was established in response to the scarcity of physicians practising in rural areas. *Officiers de santé* took a less expensive and less rigorous examination and they were licensed to practise only within a particular *département*. Their qualifications varied dramatically, to the great chagrin of doctors. *Officers de santé* could be qualified through a six-year apprenticeship, service as a military surgeon, five years assisting at a hospital, or three years of studying in a medical faculty. Furthermore, various irregular practitioners who had practised medicine before the Revolution could be "grandfathered in" without having to submit to an examination at all.[150] Doctors resented what they viewed as unfair competition from unqualified practitioners who devalued their services by charging lower fees.[151]

Despite doctors' incessant grumbling, France did not, in fact, have too many medical practitioners. In 1847, France had 11,117 doctors and 7,532 *officiers de santé* to serve a population of 35.4 million. The problem was that they were not evenly distributed among the population. Medical expertise was concentrated in urban areas. Ambitious young doctors tended to establish practices in major cities, where they faced stiff competition for patients with sufficient means to afford their fees.[152] However, country doctors also struggled to make ends meet as liberal professionals. In 1854, Dr Jégo, a physician from Muzillac, a small commune in Bretagne, lamented, "We would be in a precarious state if we only had medical practice to survive."[153] For doctors who lacked independent wealth or a secondary occupation, establishing a reliable clientele was essential.

One of the most powerful ways in which doctors enhanced their own authority as medical professionals was to efficiently relieve their patients' suffering. When doctors prescribed swift and effective opiate remedies like laudanum or morphine, patients could feel these drugs soothing their ailing bodies. In the process, doctors gained credibility in the eyes of their patients, who would be more likely to consult them again for a future illness. Doctors appreciated the convenience and rapid action of hypodermic morphine injections. One country physician wielding his syringe exclaimed, "With this you can perform miracles and it's a remedy that you can bring with you everywhere and always."[154] Opiates also empowered doctors to treat chronic pain and terminal illness. They could relieve the chronic pain of gout, rheumatism, and neuralgia and enable patients to grow accustomed to living with these conditions. For cancer patients, opium provided unparalleled relief of suffering when doctors were powerless to provide anything other than palliative care.[155] Indeed, opium offered doctors a way to alleviate suffering even when they did not fully understand how to treat a patient's affliction. According to an 1843 report to the Academy of Sciences, "Even in cases where its direct involvement in the healing of illnesses is uncertain, opium can still render great services to humanity, by helping [patients] to endure pains that its precious calming properties partially mask."[156] Opium filled the void of medical ignorance. It enabled the doctor to project an image of competence to his patients by alleviating their symptoms of pain, even if it did not ultimately treat their underlying problem.

The popularity of prescriptions highlighted the transactional dimensions of the doctor-patient relationship. This, in turn, opened doctors up to criticism. As doctors jostled with one another to attract patients, did they truly have their patients' best interests at heart? An 1892 lithograph by Charles Maurin uses satire to highlight the economic stakes of medical prescriptions for doctors (Figure 1.4). Dedicated to his friend Dr Paulin, it depicts Asclepius, the Greek god of medicine, standing between a doctor and his patient.[157] He is giving "Truffles to the doctor … and drugs to the client." Identifying the patient as a "client" emphasizes her status as a consumer in a financial transaction. The image highlights distinctions of class and gender between the wealthy bourgeois doctor, dressed in his evening coat and tails, and his vulnerable female patient, who lies nude, languishing in bed. The doctor has a human bone nonchalantly tucked under his arm. He focuses his attention not on his patient's pain but on his own pleasure as he inhales the delectable aroma of the plate of truffles Asclepius holds out to him. The patient, on the other hand, strains to reach out for the drug that might bring her relief. Yet the god of medicine holds up the small bottle, tantalizingly and frustratingly out of reach. In this image, Maurin pokes fun at his friend for the mercenary prescription practices of doctors, suggesting that relieving their patients' suffering is a means to indulge in the finer things in life.[158] At the same time, it illustrates the cultural salience of drug prescriptions in France's increasingly medicalized society.

As psychotropic drugs had such a manifest impact on patients' pain, controlling access to them became a battleground for demarcating professional boundaries between the pharmacists who supplied the drugs and the doctors who prescribed them. In theory, doctors controlled access to psychotropic drugs through the practice of prescription. The doctor specified the dose required, and then a pharmacist supplied the required medicines to the patient based on the doctor's prescription. This distinction between doctor as prescriber and pharmacist as distributor theoretically served as a balance of power. However, given the uneven distribution of medical professionals across the French countryside, in practice there was significant overlap between these roles.

When it came to rural medical care, practicality trumped professional turf wars. In areas that lacked a pharmacy or dispensary, doctors had the right to supply medicines to patients directly without using a pharmacist as an intermediary.[159] However, rural patients often lived at a considerable distance from the closest medical practitioner. In 1865, over 81 per cent of France's communes reported that they had neither a doctor nor an *officier de santé*.[160] Patients in these areas relied on pharmacists (when available), herbalists, folk healers, midwives, and members of religious orders for medical advice and treatment.[161] Therefore, although the poisonous substances legislation technically filtered access to opiates and other drugs through the pharmacy, in reality patients had more options.

Despite their legal monopoly, pharmacists faced competition in the distribution of drugs from other suppliers, both licit and illicit. Druggists were wholesale suppliers who had the right to sell "simple drugs" in bulk quantities. Herbalists were licensed to supply fresh and dried indigenous medicinal plants after passing an examination before a medical jury certifying their knowledge of medicinal plant substances. The Germinal Law limited the scope of these licit suppliers. It prohibited druggists and herbalists from selling drugs or plant medicines in "medicinal quantities," that is, amounts designed to cater to individual medical needs. It also prohibited them from selling pharmaceutical preparations.[162] However, in practice many bent the rules. Pharmacists frequently accused druggists and herbalists of overstepping their professional boundaries and violating the provisions of the Germinal Law.[163] In 1873, the Société de prévoyance

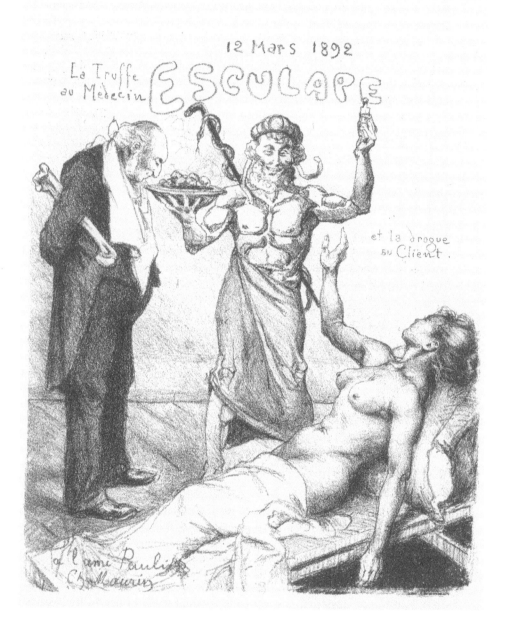

1.4 Charles Maurin's lithograph pokes fun at medical greed.
It depicts Asclepius, the Greek god of medicine, holding out
"Truffles to the Doctor" and "Drugs to the Client."

des Pharmaciens de la Seine in Paris prosecuted two men running illegal dispensaries, three women herbalists, and one herbalist-midwife for the illegal practice of pharmacy in a single month.[164] Occasionally, inspectors of herbalists' shops confiscated whole dispensaries hidden in back rooms. More often, though, violations of the Germinal Law involved the sale of particular products. These ranged from simple medicinal syrups and other typical pharmaceutical preparations to illegal secret remedies to more dangerous dispensary preparations, including opium pills, laudanum, acetate of morphine, and tincture of ipecacuanha.[165]

Competition from illegal sales continued to vex pharmacists into the twentieth century. In 1910, the Correctional Court of Lille prosecuted a grocer from Roubaix for illegally selling white poppy capsules in medicinal quantities to be used in a poppy infusion that was popular in the Nord as a sleeping draft for children.[166] Inspectors who investigated these kinds of illegal sales most often discovered secret remedies, purgatives, and powerful remedies like opium pills, laudanum, morphine, and ipecac, suggesting that these might have been the most lucrative and most frequently requested substances. Despite legislative restrictions, supply catered to demand. Druggists, grocers, and herbalists continued to supply medicines as long as there were customers willing to buy them. So, in addition to pharmacists, the presence of these other medicinal suppliers buttressed France's mid-century "pharmaceutical explosion."[167]

While herbalists with small shops likely had to rely on the sale of some medicinal remedies in order to survive, larger corporations seem to have supplied medicines to the public as well. The price catalogue for the Pharmacie Centrale de France includes two price columns for pharmaceutical specialties, or patent medicines. The first column contains a lower wholesale price charged to pharmacists, who would then resell them as retail commodities, and the second shows a higher price listed as "public," presumably the cost for a member of the public to purchase the medicines from the PCF directly.[168] For example, in 1877 the PCF sold five-litre flasks of extract for Mariani coca wine to pharmacists for 7.5 francs, while the public price was 10 francs.[169]

Poor and rural populations may have acquired medicines more often from members of religious orders than from licensed pharmacists.[170] In spite of religious prohibitions against clergy practising pharmacy, codified in the Synod of Milan in 1565, religious orders associated with hospitals often supplied the public with medicines.[171] Nuns provided medicines free of charge to the local poor. To finance this charitable service, they also sold medicines out of hospital pharmacies at lower prices than those offered by private dispensaries.[172] Furthermore, nuns often ran illegal dispensaries in rural areas to supply medicines to meet the needs of local populations. For example, as the number of medical practitioners declined between 1861 and 1884 in the *département* of Morbihan in western France, the number of illegal dispensaries run by nuns increased from 89 to 166.[173]

Doctors and medical syndicates frequently complained about religious orders overstepping their authority in the practice of medicine and pharmacy. In 1874, Amédée-Eugène Bataille, the pharmacy and grocery inspector in the *département* of Seine-et-Oise, criticized this practice. "Under the guise of charity and humanity," he complained, "these women keep a veritable pharmacy, not just first aid remedies, which, after all, are acceptable, but medicines of all varieties and strengths, even ones that are so toxic that pharmacists themselves keep them under lock and key."[174] Bataille criticized the nuns' disregard for the poisonous substances legislation in distributing opium and other "toxic" remedies to the needy. However, the nuns also performed a valuable social function by serving poor and rural populations. The charitable project of these religious hospitals and the fact that they were offering a public service to individuals for whom medicines would have been prohibitively expensive often caused people to look the other way. While the Germinal Law granted pharmacists a legal monopoly over the dispensation of remedies, and Article 8 of the Royal Decree of 25 April 1777 expressly prohibited clergy from selling "any simple or composite drugs," it was difficult to enforce such restrictions against nuns who provided such a useful public service.[175] Although Bataille was a pharmacy inspector, he continued to complain about nuns overstepping their boundaries in this manner for the next fifteen years – a testament to the hollow authority of France's poisonous substances legislation.[176]

Although nuns had no formal pharmacy training, they did have resources at their disposal to facilitate the appropriate preparation and prescription of medicinal substances. In 1877, the Sisters of Saint-André published a practical manual of medicines and basic ailments. Psychotropic drugs, including opium, laudanum, ether, chloroform, and, to a lesser extent, morphine, appear in the sisters' manual as both ingestible medicines and topical treatments. These substances combatted a remarkable range of ailments: quotidian discomforts including frostbite, burns, contusions, vomiting, and diarrhea; common illnesses including gastralgia, colic, bronchitis, rheumatism, and neuralgia; and life-threatening diseases including cholera, smallpox, and dysentery.

For the Sisters of Saint-André, relieving the suffering of the poor and afflicted took precedence over other considerations. Despite regulations imposed upon psychotropic substances through the French poisonous substances legislation, the nuns' manual rarely mentions recourse to a doctor's prescription for the administration of such remedies.[177] Indeed, its encyclopedic structure and detailed index actually facilitate the administration of medicines by non-specialists. The first of the manual's three sections, the "Medical Exposé," specifies that it is a "treatise on various maladies [and] their remedies taken from the best authors ... whose experience has proven their efficacy."[178] This appeal to the authority of outside specialists not only indicates a desire to establish the medical authority and effectiveness of the instructions in the manual but also implies that the manual could take the place of such authority. Its entries suggest that medical specialists were rarely involved in the actual interactions between the nuns and their patients. Entries for specific maladies often listed recipes for several effective remedies alongside basic instructions for their administration. For example, the entry on neuralgia lists two different recipes for anti-neuralgic pills; both contain opium extract, but the first recipe calls for quinine sulphate and marshmallow while the second calls for musk and digitalis.[179] Detailed recipes enabled anyone in possession of the manual and the right ingredients to produce the medicines described therein. Furthermore, listing the remedy alongside the condition it was used to treat would enable a nun to look up a patient's ailment in the manual and then take the appropriate course of action herself.

The manual's second section documents the most common pharmaceutical preparations. It lists detailed instructions for both preparation and administration. For example, the recipe for pectoral syrup calls for opium extract mixed with pectoral flowers, poppy flowers, arabic gum, and other fruits and herbs. The detailed instructions include only straightforward procedures such as decocting, infusing, boiling, and dissolving. The pectoral syrup was designed to sooth chronic bronchitis and dry cough when taken a spoonful at a time, four to five times per day.[180] The section also includes a recipe for "Calming Potion," which contains opium-based diacode syrup and was designed to be taken "by the spoonful every hour during an irritating cough and each time a sedative is needed."[181]

The third section of the manual, titled "Vocabulary of Medicines," includes the properties and uses of the most common medications along with their normal doses, presumably as a precaution to prevent accidental poisoning. Opium is listed as the nervous system's "sedative par excellence."[182] It was a widespread and flexible remedy for treating intense pains, insomnia, and general excitability. The manual lists the common doses for opium's different forms: 5 to 10 centigrams for powdered opium, 1 to 5 centigrams for opium extract, 5 to 30 grams for opium syrup, and 5 to 20 drops for opium tincture.[183] The inclusion of this detailed information on the appropriate dose for each form of opium suggests that the manual was designed for nuns to use without the supervision of medical or pharmaceutical experts. Like druggists and herbalists, nuns expanded the pool of pharmaceutical suppliers who made psychotropic substances available to a larger portion of the population.

Psychotropic drug regulation was incomplete and poorly enforced. Complaints about violations of the poisonous substances legislation in the mid-nineteenth century focused on the dangers of acute poisoning. Doctors and pharmacists were most concerned with policing their professional monopolies against the encroachment of illicit competition. However, in *fin-de-siècle* France, popular perceptions about what made psychotropic drugs dangerous began to shift.

In the 1880s, morphine addiction, or *morphinomanie* (literally "morphine mania"), became an increasingly visible and troubling social problem in France.[184] Medical professionals began to recognize that, in addition to being poisonous in high doses, morphine threatened the public with damaging physiological addiction. By then, however, they had been enthusiastically prescribing it for decades to treat countless physical and psychological ailments. In fact, while Charles Maurin did not explicitly specify the drug the patient was reaching for in his 1892 lithograph (Figure 1.4), he may have been alluding to morphine – particularly given what reliable customers addicts tended to be. Overprescription of this highly addictive alkaloid was probably the most significant factor in the spread of morphine addiction.[185] French physicians were acutely aware of their own role in the spread of this new social pathology and many were themselves morphine addicts.[186] However, eager to share the blame for this social crisis, doctors also denounced the negligence of pharmacists who "delivered morphine on the order of false prescriptions, previously filled [prescriptions], or even, sometimes, without a prescription."[187]

Pharmacists who freely offered drugs to their clients undermined doctors' attempts to control patients' access to medicines. Many doctors attributed this liberal attitude to the commercial logic that drove the pharmaceutical profession. Dr Casimir Degoix contended that "when it comes to pharmacists ... who deliver quite considerable quantities of this redoubtable poison many times on the same prescription ... they poison their client[s] to conserve their clientele."[188] On occasion, such behaviour landed pharmacists in court. The most famous case of the prosecution of a pharmacist for illegally supplying morphine was that of Gustave Armand-Vassy. Between May 1881 and October 1882, Armand-Vassy delivered successive instalments of 10, 15, 20, 40, 45, 50, 60, 100, and 110 packets, each containing 20 centigrams of morphine hydrochloride, until he reached a total of 693 grams at a cost of 1,650 francs.[189] Assuming a consistent dose, his client, Mme J, consumed over a gram of morphine per day. However, as addicts frequently need to increase their dose to maintain the desired effect, it is likely that her initial doses were much lower than a gram and her later doses much higher.[190] Mme J's husband took Armand-Vassy to court for continuing to provide morphine to his wife without a prescription. In May of 1883 the Tribunal de la Seine found Armand-Vassy guilty and sentenced him to eight days in prison and 3,000 francs in reparations.[191] The Armand-Vassy case offered doctors an extreme example of the profit-hungry pharmacist that they could hold up as a scapegoat for the rapid spread of *morphinomanie*. It also demonstrated the considerable profits involved if a pharmacist was willing to flout the provisions of the poisonous substances laws to sell morphine to an addict. Although the courts punished Armand-Vassy, many other suppliers remained undetected and unpunished.

Enforcement of the poisonous substances legislation was weak. Nevertheless, its provisions remained the only legislation restricting the distribution of psychotropic substances from 1846 until the beginning of the twentieth century.[192] In the *fin de siècle*, the increased visibility of morphine and cocaine addiction in French society provoked a shift in the logic of psychotropic drug regulation. Amid growing international concerns over addiction and drug smuggling in the early twentieth century, France participated in a series of international meetings to discuss the regulation of psychotropic drugs.[193] Facing pressure from abroad, France issued a decree on 1 October 1908 that targeted opium smoking and public opium dens. However, it was not until the Law of 12 July 1916 – "concerning the importation, commerce, possession and use of poisonous substances, notably opium, morphine, and cocaine" – that these substances were regulated specifically as *stupéfiants* (narcotics) rather than poisons.[194] For most of the nineteenth century, psychotropic substances were exchanged as critical therapeutic products in the pharmaceutical marketplace and were restricted primarily to prevent accidental death rather than addiction.

EXPANDING CONSUMPTION

Patients' everyday encounters with drugs and increasing popular knowledge about their effects played a key role in the normalization of psychotropic consumption. While many patients encountered drugs in hospital or via medical prescription, others sought out drugs on their own. Often, sick patients would try self-medication before consulting a medical practitioner, even after the introduction of public assistance programs for medical care made consulting a professional more affordable for the poorest segments of French society. Despite the best efforts of doctors and pharmacists to police the boundaries of drug consumption, popular medical manuals and portable pharmacies enabled patients to consume psychotropic commodities on their own terms. From hospital medicine to self-medication and family pharmacy, patients became increasingly familiar with an ever-expanding array of psychotropic medicines.

Many people would have encountered opiates and other psychotropic pain remedies while in hospital. The rise of a new clinical medicine in Paris hospitals in the first half of the nineteenth century enhanced the reputation of French physicians internationally.[195] Foreign doctors and medical students travelled to the French capital to experience the practical, hands-on clinical approach to the study and treatment of disease in its numerous modern hospitals. Unlike the smaller British and German hospitals, Paris hospitals had a centralized administration and were owned by the state. These large modern institutions catered to tens of thousands of patients each year.[196] In 1795, the French government established a single, centralized pharmacy to produce all of the medicines used in Paris hospitals in order to standardize and economize pharmaceutical production.[197] The Pharmacie Centrale des Hôpitaux de Paris supplied high-quality pharmaceutical remedies for hospital use throughout the nineteenth century.

Statistics from the Pharmacie Centrale demonstrate that hospital consumption of psychotropic drugs increased markedly after mid-century. For example, in 1855, hospitals in Paris consumed only 272 grams of morphine. By 1875, several years after the introduction of subcutaneous injections, the yearly morphine consumption of the city's hospitals had risen to 10,335 grams.[198] Morphine consumption continued to rise, and in 1882 hospital consumption in Paris reached the astronomical figure of 20,320 grams (Figure 1.5). Despite this dramatic increase in morphine consumption, as well as the consumption of other analgesics such as chloral and bromides, opium did not lose its popularity. Opium consumption remained consistent, at around 200 kilograms per year, with minor fluctuations through the 1880s (Figure 1.6).[199] The consumption of opium and laudanum gradually began to decline in the early decades of the twentieth century. However, the popularity of pain-relieving alkaloids continued unabated. Even after popular concerns emerged over the rise of morphine addiction in the *fin de siècle*, Paris hospitals continued to consume 20 kilograms of morphine, 30 to 40 kilograms of codeine, another alkaloid of opium, and 10 kilograms of cocaine every year through World War I.[200]

As France's consumption of medical care and pharmaceutical products increased in the late nineteenth century, these became more accessible to even the poorest citizens. In the early 1790s, during the French Revolution, the Committees on Health and Poverty had attempted to establish a system of free medical care for the poor, viewing the "citizen-patient's" right to health as a way of realizing the ideals of *égalité* and *fraternité*.[201] However, revolutionary contingencies and deficient funding prevented these plans for a system of social medicine

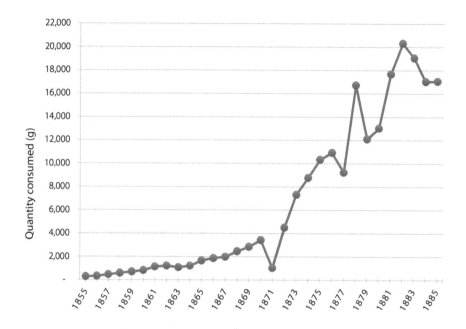

1.5 Morphine consumed in Paris hospitals between 1855 and
1885 from the Pharmacie Centrale des Hôpitaux de Paris.
Source: Morphine statistics from 1855 to 1875 cited in Charles
Lasègue and Jules Regnauld, "La thérapeutique jugée par les
chiffres," *Archives générales de médecine* (1877): 14; statistics
from 1876 to 1885 cited in Bourgoin and Beurmann,
"La thérapeutique jugée par les chiffres," *Bulletin général
de thérapeutique médicale et chirurgicale* 115 (1888): 160.

from being enacted, leaving the health care of the poor to the charity
of religious orders. Nevertheless, the idea that health should be considered a fundamental individual right persisted. By mid-century the
government began to accept responsibility for the health of the poor
and indigent.[202] In the wake of the Revolution of 1848 and the cholera
epidemic of 1849, increased fears of social revolution and contagion
provoked the government of the Second Empire to take a more active
interest in supervising the health of citizens.[203] In 1854 and 1855, the
Ministry of the Interior encouraged France's *départements* to establish
and finance local programs for free medical assistance, with the hope
that improved medical care in the countryside would discourage urban

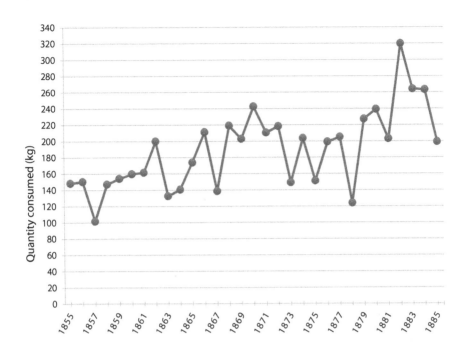

1.6 Opium consumed in Paris hospitals between 1855 and 1885 from the Pharmacie Centrale des Hôpitaux de Paris. *Source:* Opium statistics from 1855 to 1875 cited in Charles Lasègue and Jules Regnauld, "La thérapeutique jugée par les chiffres," *Archives générales de médecine* (1877): 14; statistics from 1876 to 1885 cited in Bourgoin and Beurmann, "La thérapeutique jugée par les chiffres," *Bulletin général de thérapeutique médicale et chirurgicale* 115 (1888): 160.

migration and prevent revolutionary insurrection.[204] However, as they were financed locally, these health programs relied heavily upon the charitable labour of nuns.[205]

While these local efforts to provide health care to the poor and homeless met with limited success in the mid-nineteenth century, they highlighted the enormous demand for such care and established almost universal support for the merits of organizing a system of free health care for those in need.[206] Under the Third Republic, this system was finally realized. On 15 July 1893, France passed the Free Medical Assistance Law, which established the principle that access to medical care was a fundamental right.[207] The law declared that "every ill Frenchman, deprived of resources, will receive from the commune, *département*, or state, according to his residency, free medical care at home, or if it is impossible to effectively care for him at home, in a hospital establishment."[208] Outside of Paris, the free medical assistance programs served between 5 per cent and 6 per cent of the population.[209] Furthermore, the increase in mutual aid societies in the *départements* at the turn of the twentieth century made medical care and pharmaceutical consumption increasingly affordable to individuals who did not qualify for free medical assistance under the 1893 law.[210]

In the years leading up to World War I, French citizens had greater access to pharmaceutical remedies than ever before. In 1876, France had 6,200 dispensaries; by 1911, it had 11,500 dispensaries – an increase of over 85 per cent.[211] France's consumption of pharmaceutical products increased accordingly. Based on the average annual sales figures reported in the *Union Pharmaceutique* between 1895 and 1899, France's total annual production of pharmaceuticals might have been as much as 150 to 200 million francs.[212]

At the same time, psychotropic remedies were becoming more affordable. Between 1896 and 1906, the wholesale price of raw opium dropped to 22 francs per kilogram, a significant decline from its high point of 100 francs per kilogram in 1868 (Figure 1.7). The PCF monitored the international opium market carefully and adjusted wholesale prices of opium derivatives and alkaloids accordingly. So, for example, while the PCF's wholesale price of morphine hydrochloride was 75 centimes per gram in 1873, by 1899 the price had dropped over 50 per cent to between 26 centimes and 35 centimes per gram, depending on the amount the pharmacist purchased.[213] Given that a gram was about one hundred times the typical dose for pain relief, morphine would have been affordable for the average consumer, even factoring in a considerable retail markup.

Furthermore, workers' wages had increased relative to the cost of medical care over the course of the nineteenth century. While doctors used a sliding scale to determine their fees based on their patients' socio-economic status, in the early nineteenth century even a 1- or 2-franc consultation might have easily exceeded an agricultural labourer's daily wages. However, by the *fin de siècle*, wages had increased such that agricultural labourers could make 3 francs per day, making medical treatment a less significant financial sacrifice.[214] Doctors also occasionally

accepted payment in kind based on their patients' economic circumstances. Dr V.F. (1828–1918) from La Roche-sur-Yon in the Vendée, for
instance, "did not charge many families but he often returned from his
visits with butter and chickens."[215] In rural areas in particular, the medical
marketplace was more flexible depending on a patient's ability to pay.

While urban areas tended to have higher percentages of doctors and
pharmacists per capita than rural areas, anecdotal evidence suggests
that the proliferation of psychotropic drug use extended into the French
countryside. In 1888 a man from a small town in southern France wrote
to a journalist in Paris, complaining that "the custom of [consuming]
remedies that are supposed to eliminate suffering has spread univer-
sally. Everyone uses and abuses them."[216] As rural patients often lived
a considerable distance from the nearest doctor or pharmacist, they
frequently turned to self-medication as an initial course of action.[217] For
example, they might brew a poppyhead tea to ease the pain of a toothache or purchase laudanum from a local unofficial purveyor of drugs.
Self-medication and family pharmacy empowered patients to treat their
own pain. Through these practices, patients solidified the consumption
of psychotropic drugs as a routine and essential part of everyday life.

Pharmaceutical manufacturers developed first aid kits, known as
"portable pharmacies," to facilitate self-medication in cases where a physician was unavailable. These emergency medical kits contained bandages,
basic medical tools, and the most useful medicines, with psychotropic
pain remedies featuring prominently. In the nineteenth century, the
capitalist logic of France's industrializing economy encouraged fast-
paced production that precipitated workplace injuries.[218] In the case of
serious accidents, patients who remained untreated risked succumbing
to their injuries before a doctor was able to arrive on the scene. In 1845,
the Ménier Company offered three models of large portable pharmacies
designed for business and agricultural use, which contained numerous
psychotropic pharmaceuticals including morphine syrup, ether syrup,
acetic ether, sulfuric ether, Sydenham's Laudanum, Rousseau's Laudanum,
cynoglosse pills, opium pills, morphine hydrochloride, theriac, diascordium, and opium extract.[219] The Pharmacie Rogé sold a kit that it
had originally designed for the Railroad Company of Southern Italy,
containing laudanum, chloroform, sulfuric ether, ipecac (an emetic),
quinine (for fevers), and diascordium, an opiate mixture used to treat

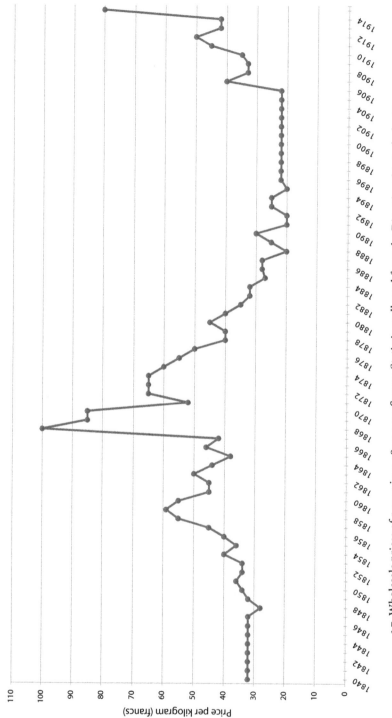

1.7 Wholesale prices of raw opium, 1840–1915. *Source:* Statistics collected from the Direction Générale des Douanes, *Tableau général du commerce* (Paris: Imprimerie Nationale, 1840–1915).

mild diarrhea.[220] The wide variety of psychotropic remedies in these kits enabled first responders to spare injured workers from additional pain and to treat them for minor ailments they might experience on the job

Portable pharmacies came in a variety of sizes, tailored to both individual and industrial use. The pharmaceutical manufacturer Le Perdriel of Paris offered over twenty varieties, from pocket pharmacies designed for hunters, fishermen, members of the clergy, and soldiers to much larger first aid chests intended for use on ships or in factories, schools, farms, or large families.[221] For customers' convenience, Le Perdriel offered a catalogue of all of the models it sold, accompanied by prices and descriptions, which were available in France's major pharmacies. These portable pharmacies put psychotropic pharmaceuticals at citizens' fingertips.

To facilitate self-medication, Prosper Cavaillès, a Paris pharmacist, published a practical guide for the use of portable pharmacies. The guide provided instructions for the safe and proper use of these kits, which had become a vital necessity for individuals travelling or living in the French countryside. It also served as a marketing tool to sell the Pharmacie Rogé's range of portable pharmacies. The smallest models were called "pocket pharmacies." The most basic model cost 12 francs and contained tweezers, scissors, a small role of bandages, a list of instructions, and three flasks that contained arnica solution, ammonia, and sulfuric ether.[222] Despite the small number of medicines included, the kit offered patients remedies for a wide range of maladies. Arnica solution was commonly used in cases of bruising or cerebral trouble. Ammonia could be used topically as a caustic in cases of poisonous animal or insect bites, inhaled carefully in the case of fainting, and taken in minuscule quantities internally to combat drunkenness. Finally, sulfuric ether was an antispasmodic and analgesic that could be consumed by placing a few drops on a sugar cube or in a tepid herbal tea to treat stomach cramps, spasms, nervous episodes, and neuralgia.[223] The larger pocket pharmacies built upon the items included in this basic kit, suggesting that sulfuric ether was considered one of the most useful analgesic medicines that individuals could be trusted to use on themselves or their families without immediate medical supervision.

Portable pharmacies and popular medical guides enabled French citizens to treat themselves for reasons of practicality and economy. Doctors and pharmacists distinguished themselves as medical specialists with a body of knowledge acquired through years of rigorous study. However, with these resources individual citizens could treat the minor ailments of daily life from the comfort of their own homes. The manuals, which provided instruction to the layman on the basics of self-medication, were written explicitly for a popular audience, eschewing topics that would be difficult to understand or remedies that required medical expertise. Therefore, these manuals provide a window through which it is possible to examine how French citizens might have interacted with psychotropic substances on a daily basis. Popular medical guides' recommendations for the use of psychotropic drugs reveal how essential and commonplace these substances had become in everyday life in the nineteenth century.

Parisian pharmacist Félix Dehaut published a popular medical guide, *Manual of Domestic Medicine, Hygiene, Surgery, and Pharmacy*. It enjoyed surprising longevity; by 1863 the manual was already in its tenth edition, and Dehaut published the twenty-ninth edition in 1925. He advertised the manual as being "within reach of everyone and indispensable to all families."[224] Furthermore, in 1878 he published an abbreviated version of the manual in dictionary format, specifically designed for people who did not read very well. This version, titled *Small Guide to Health*, included several illustrations to facilitate comprehension.[225] Dehaut designed the book as a reference guide to enable the average person to treat common illnesses, chronic conditions, and, for injuries and accidents, to provide emergency care while awaiting the arrival of a doctor.

Dehaut's goal was to extend limited practical medical knowledge to the average citizen to supplement consultations with medical professionals like himself. In other cases, popular medical authors had no connection to the medical profession whatsoever. For example, in 1884 François Lescure, a landowner from Auch in southwestern France, published *The People's Medicine*. He designed this guide for the poor, the labouring classes, and those who were far from health services, so that they could treat themselves with one of the guide's remedies without a doctor or while waiting for a doctor to arrive.[226] Lescure's guide worked through accretion. Instead of listing a single remedy to treat each malady, it included several formulas for different remedies that Lescure had compiled from medical journals, popular medicine, and the recommendations of specific medical practitioners, as well as his own personal remedies. Therefore, patients could choose from among several different remedies. The recipes for remedies recommended in both Lescure's and Dehaut's popular medical manuals include opium, laudanum, morphine, chloroform, and ether in various forms. Both manuals assumed that these psychotropic substances – although restricted by law to a doctor's prescription and a pharmacist's dispensation – were, in fact, accessible to the average individual.

Opium and its derivatives were included in a wide variety of different remedies for conditions ranging from uterine pains and inflammation to toothache, earache, and insomnia. Both Lescure and Dehaut found laudanum to be a useful and effective remedy for all manners of belly pain, including intestinal inflammation, gastralgia, colic, menstrual cramps, and painful diarrhea.[227] Administered either internally in the form of an enema or externally in the form of a cataplasm or a liniment, laudanum solved these digestive crises.[228] Additionally, topical laudanum offered relief for lumbago, torticollis (stiff neck), toothache, and contusions.[229] Lescure's guide also included numerous recipes for opiate-based syrups and potions. These included a remedy for whooping cough that included opium syrup; a potion designed to treat diabetes that contained opium extract and theriac; and an anti-asthmatic potion that contained morphine hydrochloride.[230] Dehaut recommended opium-based cynoglosse pills for intestinal troubles and insomnia. He explained that, "usually, these pills only need to be taken for a few days, and only need to be ordered from the pharmacist ten at a time."[231] Dehaut made no mention of visiting a doctor for a prescription and even instructed his readers on how much to order themselves. Cavaillès also described the uses for cynoglosse pills in his guide to portable pharmacies, which suggests they would have been easily accessible to the average consumer. However, being more cautious of the pills than Dehaut, Cavaillès recommended that patients should seek the advice of a doctor, as their consumption could sometimes be dangerous.[232] Significantly, though, Cavaillès presented a medical consultation as a recommendation, not a necessity. Despite the opium they contained, cynoglosse pills were a commonplace remedy for a common irritation. As such they fit well within the purview of family medicine.

Although the guides described many opiates as quite common pharmaceutical commodities that people could easily acquire at their local pharmacy, Dehaut argued that morphine was different. He explained, "this valuable, but dangerous, remedy cannot be handled except by doctors, who obtain marvellous results from it, as soon as it acts to calm violent pains on which other remedies have no effect."[233] For treating excruciating pain, morphine had no match. It could relieve the acute torture of passing gallstones and also offer a palliative treatment for the prolonged agony of cancer.[234] In the wake of the debates over *morphinomanie* in the 1880s, Dehaut's 1893 guide recommended consulting a professional. As only physicians were technically authorized to prescribe and administer morphine, Dehaut encouraged "people who suffer from intolerable pain to ask their doctor to administer these *injections* of morphine, which do not impede the course of the disease, but which allow [the patient] to await cure without useless suffering."[235] Although the guide deferred to the physician to actually administer the injections, it also encouraged the patient to advocate for his or her own course of treatment.

Opiates were not the only psychotropic remedies of family pharmacy. While ether and chloroform achieved widespread popularity as surgical anesthetics, they were also consumed in a more quotidian manner as treatments for common maladies. As everyday pharmaceuticals, ether and chloroform took many forms. With both substances, a patient could inhale them, drink them in a mixture, swallow them on a soaked sugar cube, or administer them topically in the form of a liniment, cataplasm, or soaked cotton tampon. Dehaut recommended ether for various types of nervous troubles, "indispositions," gastralgia, toothache, and morning sickness.[236] Given that it was a powerful antispasmodic, he also recommended taking ether orally to combat particularly tenacious cases of the hiccups.[237] Dr Clertan's specialty ether and chloroform "pearls" were relatively inexpensive and convenient remedies for stomach cramps, excessive yawning, nervous troubles, and morning sickness.[238]

Psychotropic drugs did not always pass through pharmaceutical commerce and industry to reach consumers. Popular medical guides also included simple home remedies for pain relief using basic ingredients. Chloroform liniments, oil-based preparations designed to be rubbed on the afflicted area, were used to sooth the violent pains of rheumatism and neuralgia.[239] Dehaut included a simple formula for "calming chloroform liniment" – 10 grams of chloroform mixed with 30 grams of olive or poppyseed oil – so that individuals could prepare it themselves.[240] Poppy capsules also featured prominently in these manuals as simple remedies for everyday pain. Poppy heads boiled with marshmallow root produced a soothing gargle for mouth pain and inflammation.[241] Lescure recommended using a poppy decoction in a topical wash to treat hemorrhoids, earaches, and abscesses and a poppy cataplasm to treat gout.[242] In this manner, an individual who lived in the countryside far from a dispensary could produce a home remedy from local botanical ingredients without needing to visit a medical professional. Although the consumption of mass-produced pharmaceutical medicines increased significantly during the second half of the nineteenth century, simple home remedies continued to provide inexpensive alternatives to professional care. Despite the efforts of doctors, pharmacists, and the state to control and regulate access to psychotropic drugs, through self-medication and family pharmacy individual consumers took pain relief into their own hands.

Opium and other psychotropic drugs became an integral part of everyday life in the nineteenth century. Through indigenous cultivation schemes, opium became part of the agricultural fabric of France and its colonies. Pharmacists and entrepreneurs sought to reduce France's dependence on foreign powers while producing a high-quality product that would not only increase domestic revenues for small farmers but also provide a reliable base ingredient for the pharmaceutical industry. With increasingly precise formulas and mechanized production techniques, psychotropic commodities became progressively more reliable for everyday consumption.

Psychotropic medicines fundamentally altered patients' lived experiences by enabling them to transcend pain and suffering in powerful new ways over the course of the nineteenth century, offering relief for acute pain and prolonged agony alike. Agriculturalists, druggists, pharmacists, doctors, and consumers tried to harness the tremendous commercial and therapeutic power of psychotropic drugs, for profit, for professional legitimacy, and for the relief of suffering. In so doing, they normalized psychotropic consumption. Within this new psychotropic society, psychotropic commodities empowered French citizens to relieve their own pain.

{ 2 }

SELF-
EXPERIMENTATION

*The observer listens to nature; the experimenter
interrogates it and forces it to reveal itself.*
– Georges Cuvier

*The experiment is something personal; it is difficult
to convey through teaching or books.*
– entry on experimentation, from Dechambre's
Encyclopedic Dictionary of Medical Sciences

Doctors needed to understand drugs in order to prescribe them. Experiments to determine the specific physiological effects of drugs on the human body depended on securing reliable research subjects. Presuming that no one's testimony was more reliable than their own, doctors decided to experiment on themselves. Self-experimentation enabled doctors to experiment on human subjects in an ethical manner.[1] Yet this research involved overlapping motivations of scientific and hedonistic curiosity. Doctors who offered their minds and bodies as the sites of psychotropic self-experimentation demonstrated remarkable vulnerability, their bodies exposed to the probing, stabbing tests of their colleagues and their minds subjected to chemical invasion that could lead to violent shifts in mood, emotion, and even a temporary state of madness. However, many of them were excited to experience the sensory distortions of ether or the bizarre hallucinations of hashish. Self-experimenters tried to produce generalizable knowledge to help advance therapeutic medicine even as they gained individual knowledge tied to the unique sensations of their own bodies and minds. In seeking medical knowledge, these researchers also sought the self.

In the mid-nineteenth century, self-experimenters had to contend with both new ideals of scientific knowledge production and new understandings of the self. During the Enlightenment, sensationalist philosophers had understood the self as a collection of mental faculties including memory, reason, and imagination held together by individual consciousness. They viewed the mind as a blank slate bombarded with sensations from the outside world that were inscribed onto the self like a seal onto softened wax.[2] However, after the French Revolution, amid anxieties over the breakdown of corporate society, French intellectuals turned away from sensationalist philosophy's passive, fragmented self, which they blamed for political turmoil. Instead, they embraced a new vision of a robust, unified self driven by individual will, which they hoped would promote social and political stability.[3] In the post-Revolutionary era, this vision of the autonomous, willful self served both the political aspirations of bourgeois men and their professional ambitions in the competitive climate of France's industrializing economy.[4]

While individual free will was essential to political citizenship in nineteenth-century France, it presented new challenges for the scientist. For centuries, scientists had embraced experimentation as a way to acquire knowledge about the natural world.[5] During the Enlightenment, scientists believed that imposing the self on the experiment – that is, using judgment and reason to select the most relevant data – was necessary to reveal essential truths about the object of inquiry. However, as Lorraine Daston and Peter Galison have demonstrated, in the early nineteenth century the goals, methods, and values of scientific experimentation began to shift toward a new ideal of "objectivity."[6] Objectivity emphasized the importance of producing knowledge in a mechanical, unprejudiced manner. Unlike contemporary Romantic artists, who actively worked to cultivate and express their own subjectivity in their work, scientists began to worry that a willful self would impose its own subjective theories and hypotheses on experiments, compromising their integrity.[7] Objective knowledge rejected subjective interference. Therefore, scientists engaged in new "technologies of the self" to excise the self from their experiments, separating their own subjective thoughts and feelings from the objective practices of data gathering.[8] Within this new scientific climate, the willful self had become a liability. For drug researchers in particular, self-experimentation made the question of individual free will even more challenging.

The following case studies examine self-experimentation in two senses: experimentation *on* oneself, the transformation of the body of the experimenter into the medium for knowledge production; and experimentation *with* the self, seeking enhanced self-knowledge through the manipulation of one's state of consciousness. First, the pneumatic self-experiments that French *académiciens* conducted upon themselves in 1847 enabled them to practice corporeal mutilation independent of sensory agony. Second, psychologists, artists, and other curious individuals consumed hashish paste as a method of exploring new levels of consciousness and expressions of self unfettered by the dictates of judgment and reason. Finally, prolonged self-experimentation with morphine exposed the incredible psychosomatic power of a material drug over the human organism as addiction gradually came to dominate the user's thoughts and actions.

As a research methodology, self-experimentation made it difficult to isolate subject from object. This was particularly the case for drug research, which depended upon exploring the mind-body connection. As researchers tested the power of the mind over the body – attempting to exercise free will to resist the effects of the drugs they consumed – they revealed the extraordinary physiological power of the body over the mind. In so doing, they exposed the human mind and body as fundamentally interconnected. While individual self-experiments resist clear categorization, they all reveal a shifting power dynamic between a material drug and the individual will of the experimenter. Self-experimenters struggled to maintain control over their own minds and bodies in order to be able to witness the experience of gradually losing control. However, they soon discovered how challenging it was to attempt to impose the strictures of objective scientific experimentation onto an experience that was, by its very nature, profoundly subjective.

INHALING (UN)CONSCIOUSNESS

From the very beginning of the nineteenth century, self-experimentation defined medical research on anesthetic gases. In 1800, English chemist Humphry Davy (1778–1829) conducted pioneering self-experiments at the Medical Pneumatic Institution in Bristol on the inhalation of nitrous oxide, or "laughing gas," which caused a commotion across the European scientific community.[9] Inhaling nitrous oxide, Davy experienced manifest pleasure, laughing and sometimes dancing about the room. However, he found that he could not inhale the gas for longer than five minutes, at which point the pleasure diminished as "vivid ideas passed rapidly through the mind and voluntary power was altogether destroyed."[10]

Fascinated by Davy's descriptions of the effects of the gas on the human body, in the summer of 1802 the renowned French chemist Antoine François Fourcroy (1755–1809) invited a group of interested individuals to observe the remarkable effects of nitrous oxide for themselves. Assembled in the open air of Fourcroy's garden, the group observed a young English painter named Underwoldt inhale the gas. After thirty seconds, Underwoldt launched himself from his chair and pirouetted around before flinging himself on the grass in violent convulsions to the great alarm of those assembled. His face took on a deathly pallor and Fourcroy later noted, "Certainly, if we had not been warned in advance, according to M. Underwoldt's own admission, that all these phenomena were the signs of the most delightful enjoyment, we would have thought he was in the grip of the most burning pain."[11] After a few minutes, a giddy Underwoldt came to and asserted that he had experienced the sweetest and liveliest sensations.

The dramatic shift from violent convulsions to tranquil calm provoked skepticism. Some suspected Underwoldt of simulating the effects, particularly given that two other men present had inhaled just as much nitrous oxide as Underwoldt but hardly experienced any effects at all. The distinguished chemist Louis Vauquelin had observed Underwoldt's convulsions carefully and concluded that they must have been caused by the gas, "but the sole means that he had of judging … was to submit himself to its effects." After a few deep breaths of nitrous oxide, Vauquelin felt discomfort and constriction in his chest that prevented him from breathing deeply. He turned pale and felt a buzzing in his head as though someone was beating a drum next to his ear. Soon his strength abandoned him and "he fell from his chair, sprawled on the ground. There, his eyes blurry and directed toward the sky, he could neither speak, nor breathe, nor make any movement."[12] Terrified and feeling faint, Vauquelin listened in horror as several onlookers prevented anyone from coming to his aid, as they believed that he was enjoying a state of ecstasy similar to Underwoldt's.

After a few minutes of almost complete immobility, Vauquelin took a huge breath, his speech faculties returned, and he was able to get up; however, his legs trembled and his head remained fuzzy for several hours. The following day he observed several trickles of blood in his spittle.

This alarming incident illustrates the obstacles and dangers of self-experimentation as a research methodology. First, the knowledge to be gained was experiential: it depended upon the testimony of the experimental subject. However, psychotropic self-experimentation influenced consciousness, sensation, and motor control, inhibiting the subject's ability to communicate in the moment. The radical disparity between the viewers' perceptions of what was occurring and what Underwoldt and Vauquelin actually experienced as experimental subjects reveals the limitations of mere observation as a method of knowledge production in such cases. Second, the human body could not be standardized. Other scientists' inability to perfectly reproduce the initial experiment's results to confirm their accuracy was a particular challenge of human experimentation.[13] While Underwoldt and Vauquelin both had strong visceral reactions to the inhalations, their subjective experiences were radically different. Third, and perhaps most importantly, unlike apparatuses constructed from glass, metal, and rubber, the human body is a highly fragile piece of organic equipment. As Vauquelin very nearly demonstrated, interrupting even one of the body's vital processes could lead to dangerous or even fatal consequences.

After Vauquelin's harrowing experience with nitrous oxide, French enthusiasm for pneumatic experimentation waned, although a few curious individuals replicated the experiment. One of these, Dr Mathieu Orfila, experienced a crisis similar to Vauquelin's, claiming, "I experienced such sharp chest pains and such a suffocation, that I remained convinced that if I had continued the experiment, I would not have returned."[14] Dangerous or unpleasant experiences while inhaling nitrous oxide may account for the fact that the medical community in France and abroad did not introduce such gases into therapeutic practice, despite the fact that Davy had observed the power of nitrous oxide to relieve pain in 1800.[15] French doctors' interest in inhalation experiments was only rekindled decades later, in January 1847, when the ether research of a few of American dentists and surgeons reached the French Academies.

Although several individuals fiercely battled over credit for the first discovery of ether's anesthetic properties, the medical community most commonly credits American dentist William Morton. On 16 October 1846, Morton successfully anesthetized a young man about to undergo an operation to remove a jaw tumour at the Massachusetts General Hospital in Boston. After the operation, the patient declared that he had experienced no pain.[16] On 7 December, Morton published his extraordinary findings on the effects of ether in the *Boston Medical and Surgical Journal*, and news of his discovery spread at a precipitous pace.[17] Morton's dramatic demonstration of ether's anesthetic power captivated the medical community. The success of this surgical feat rested largely upon knowledge that Morton and other practitioners had acquired through self-experimentation.

Morton and his rivals for the original discovery of ether anesthesia all used themselves as guinea pigs for their research. One of these rivals, Dr William Crawford Long, had performed a painless tumour removal operation using ether in 1842 but did not publish his results at that time. Long originally discovered ether's anesthetic potential by inhaling it as a form of amusement with friends. While on ether, they noticed that they felt no pain when they fell or bruised themselves.[18] Another rival, a Connecticut dentist named Horace Wells, had experimented on himself with ether and nitrous oxide in 1844.[19] While both substances acted to desensitize the body to pain, Wells found nitrous oxide "more agreeable." So, he anesthetized himself with nitrous oxide and had a friend of his, Dr John Riggs, extract one of his upper molars to prove that it could be done painlessly.[20] Morton himself began his ether research with animal experimentation on insects, cats, and even his family's black spaniel, but he soon turned to humans. His first experiments anesthetizing his two assistants had failed because he had used a poor-quality ether. However, his wife recalled that one night, after he had procured a supply of pure ether, Morton was so impatient to test it that he "shut himself up in his office, and tested it upon himself, with such success that for several minutes he lay there unconscious."[21] Morton and other early experimenters disregarded potential dangers to gain personal experience inhaling these gases so they could be confident in their ability to relieve the pain of surgery.

It was not long before news of Morton's success crossed the Atlantic.[22] On 13 November 1846, Charles Jackson, who had worked with Morton on the ether experiments, wrote a letter to the French Academy of Sciences, which at the time was the pre-eminent scientific institution for registering scientific discoveries from both France and abroad.[23] He requested that the Academy appoint a commission "responsible for conducting the necessary experiments to certify the accuracy of [his] assertions … about the marvellous effects of the inhalation of ether vapours."[24] Jackson submitted the letter, still sealed, to the Academy on 28 December; however, the Academy of Sciences did not unseal it and discuss it openly until the meeting on 18 January 1847, by which point Morton and Jackson's discovery had become widely known. The previous week, Joseph François Malgaigne, a surgeon at Saint-Louis Hospital, had drawn attention to this remarkable new use for ether in general anesthesia at the Academy of Medicine. Curious to discover whether Morton's claims held up, Malgaigne ran five trials on patients. In three cases the ether inhalations resulted in pain-free surgeries, in the fourth case the ether produced a diminution of pain, and in the fifth case inhalation for ten minutes produced no effect at all.[25]

Malgaigne's trials piqued the interest of his colleagues.[26] The new ether anesthesia elicited mixed responses of both intense excitement and marked apprehension. The novelty of the procedure and its momentous potential for transforming surgical practice prompted doctors, dentists, surgeons, and veterinarians to experiment with it before several crucial questions had been answered, including the appropriate dose and apparatus, the length of anesthesia, and the potential dangers of prolonged use.[27] While animal experimentation and clinical observation supplied valuable information, self-experimentation was a crucial part of the process of knowledge production. Doctors used themselves as experimental subjects and objects in order to invoke the authority of personal experience.[28]

A veritable frenzy of self-experimentation dominated the sessions of the Academy of Sciences and the Academy of Medicine between mid-January and February of 1847. All over Paris, from private sitting rooms to public lecture halls, doctors congregated with colleagues and medical students and took turns serving as experimental subjects. On 26 January, just two weeks after Malgaigne's experiments, the subject of ether anesthesia consumed almost the entire session of the Academy of Medicine.[29] During a session of the Academy of Sciences on 1 February, renowned surgeon and anatomist Alfred Velpeau claimed, "there are now several hundred doctors or students in Paris who have experimented or who experiment daily on themselves with the inhalation of ether. All prudence, every precaution one might want to recommend to us, we have, of course, followed."[30] Self-experimentation endowed surgeons with the authority of personal experience, yet this authority rested upon the experimenter's ability to ensure the safety of the experiment and the accuracy of its results.

The Society of German Doctors in Paris organized one of the earliest and most exhaustive experiments during its meeting on 15 January 1847 to determine the exact conditions under which ether anesthesia was successful. The society strove to be as precise as possible with the experiments, establishing scientific credibility by carefully recording their procedures, noting the temperature and conditions of the room, and measuring and documenting their subjects' vital signs throughout the experiment. To regulate the amount of ether administered, they used M. Lüer's simple inhalation apparatus, which consisted of a flask with three openings: one to let the ether in, one to let outside air in, and one connected to a mask through which the subject breathed the etherized air.[31] The subject's nose was left uncovered, but each time observers saw him breathing through his nose they would use their fingers or surgical pliers to close it.

The society's report painstakingly documented the experiences of a dozen different experimental subjects, some of whom had conducted several experiments in succession. A table documented their ages, the duration of their ether inhalations (ranging from just over one minute to thirteen minutes), the exact number of inhalations, and notes on any irregularities observed during the experiment. The table also included measurements of the subjects' breathing and pulse before the experiment, as well as several measurements taken over the course of their inhalations.[32] These experiments enabled the members of the society to conduct careful observations of the impact of ether inhalations on the body's major physiological processes.[33] In recognition of their meticulous scientific process, when the *Gazette médicale de Paris* published the report it lauded their research: "Among the numerous studies and experiments attempted everywhere on ether inhalation, we are happy to distinguish those that were instituted by the Society of German Doctors of Paris. They bear the stamp of genuine scientific experiments."[34] This warm praise of the society's methods reflected the scientific community's increasing emphasis on objectivity and empiricism in the mid-nineteenth century.[35]

True objectivity required the scientist to suppress subjectivity.[36] However, self-experimentation inherently blurred the boundaries between subject and object. During the eighteenth century, electrical researchers who subjected their own bodies to powerful electric shocks had struggled to separate their intellectual judgment from the physical pain of electrocution to maintain their authority as researchers capable of rational observation and analysis.[37] Asserting what Simon Schaffer has called the "Cartesianism of the genteel," these elite men of science distinguished themselves from women and members of the lower classes by claiming to be uniquely "capable of separating their disorderly bodies from the cool deliverances of their intellectual judgment."[38] Nineteenth-century ether experimenters similarly emphasized their superior judgment and free will as markers of social and scientific authority. All of the experimental subjects from the Society of German Doctors were healthy, young, male doctors "endowed with a good and strong will to know what to expect from the results." Furthermore, they needed to have "the necessary training to analyze their impressions and to communicate them to others."[39] The success of the experiments depended on the reliable testimony of young men willing and able to restrain the self in order to accurately convey their impressions of ether's effects.

Through targeted, small-scale mutilations, the society's experiments demonstrated that for the majority of subjects, ether inhalations could eliminate the sensation of pain. With each case, they tested the subjects' sensibility by jabbing their fingers, hands, ears, head, and face with pins and by cutting their arms with a scalpel. Frequently, they also conducted more invasive tests. In addition to pokes and prods, in most cases they also applied burning tinder or hot wax to the subjects' arms "to make deep sores" and yet "insensibility was always complete." In one case, a subject experienced no pain from the burn but rather an "agreeable feeling of warmth."[40] Incisions and burns of this nature would likely leave lasting marks on the bodies of the experimental subjects. The fact that, after inhaling ether, they could feel little to no pain from such corporeal mutilation indicated that the gas was disrupting the normal sensory connections between the mind and the body, preventing the nerves from translating the cuts and burns on the body into the perception of pain in the mind.

While the experiments relied upon the subjects' testimonies of their own subjective experience, the report published in the *Gazette médicale* excised their voices and transformed their impressions into a table of quantified data. The *Gazette médicale* highlighted the objectivity of the Society of German Doctors' experiments, recording how they meticulously measured and quantified the body's physiological changes under the influence of ether. In so doing, however, it glossed over some of the uncomfortably erratic effects of ether on the mind. Dr Philibert Joseph Roux had been invited to witness one of the experiments. He reported back to the Academy of Sciences describing psychological side effects that were downplayed in the report published in the *Gazette médicale*. After a few minutes of torpor from the ether, almost all of the subjects Roux observed experienced an "expansion of noisy hilarity."[41] This in itself was not alarming. The *Gazette médicale* report noted that two subjects experienced "joyous dreams" that they did not remember and awoke laughing inexplicably.[42] However, according to Roux, one individual whose breathing had seemed short during the inhalations "was seized, after the drowsiness had finished, by a sort of furious delirium: he upturned the chairs that surrounded him, violently launched himself on a table, hurling piercing screams." Roux confessed that "we could hardly contain him for a few minutes, in truth, a very short time, that this state lasted."[43] Far from the rational man of science, this subject appeared swept up in a violent, mad delirium. Unruly and recalcitrant, he demonstrated the dangers and risks associated with permitting a psychotropic substance to invade one's mind and take over the body's sensory perceptions and motor functions. In this case, ether seized operative control over the experimental subject in a complex upheaval of the typical power dynamics between human subject and material object.

The subjects' sometimes extreme reactions in the experiments demonstrated just how unfamiliar the scientists were with anesthetic gases. One of the crucial goals of these early acts of self-experimentation was to determine the optimal conditions for ether inhalations. One young doctor at Charité Hospital conducted regular experiments on himself each morning to differentiate between ether's two stages – excitement and collapse – to determine precisely when he became insensitive to pain. At first, during the excitement stage, the doctor turned red, but he became pale at the moment of collapse, during which time insensibility was complete and surgery could be performed. Several other young men observed similar phenomena on themselves.[44] Another doctor wanted to find a way to avoid the uncomfortable constriction of the bronchial tubes during ether inhalation. Through repeated self-experimentation, Dr Hutin developed a technique he called the "education of the airways." By introducing ether vapours gradually by opening the valve of the apparatus a little at a time over the course of five inhalations, he could alleviate the discomfort of the initial ether inhalations for his patients.[45]

For some doctors, self-experimentation with ether was an ethical way to produce knowledge about this new anesthetic technique without compromising patient welfare. One such doctor was Pierre Nicolas Gerdy, professor of surgical pathology at the Paris Faculty of Medicine. During the debates at the Academy of Medicine in late January, he argued, "Before conducting any experiment on patients, I wanted to study the influence of ether on myself."[46] Many of his colleagues had no such reservations. They had engaged in both clinical experimentation on patients and self-experimentation immediately following ether's meteoric rise in popularity. In contrast, Gerdy prioritized patient welfare in his experiments, offering his own body to repeated trials in order to expand medical knowledge. Once he had determined that ether was safe for surgical use generally, he took additional steps to protect individual patients. The day before a surgery, he submitted each patient to ether as a sort of trial run, "to teach them how to use it appropriately, and to observe its influence on each of them."[47]

Despite Gerdy's professed focus on patient welfare, he also used his self-experimentation as a platform for flaunting his own courage and strength as a medical researcher. Bodily sacrifice played an integral role in demonstrating the self-experimenter's authority and commitment to the pursuit of knowledge.[48] Gerdy's research revealed numerous potential side effects of ether inhalations, including "irritation, chest soreness, a nasty mouth, disgust for ether, discomfort, and head pain." He claimed, "I experienced all of these effects for ten to twelve days, after twenty-five experiments practised over two days."[49] At a time when the concentration of ether was not standardized and doctors debated how long they could continue to administer it without causing negative side effects, Gerdy ran numerous, even excessive, trials on his own body. He risked potential asphyxiation and suffered the discomforts of such experimentation for the advancement of medical knowledge.

Gerdy conducted experiments on himself using ether-soaked sponges in a flask, which he breathed through a straw. While the ether-charged air initially tickled his throat and caused him to cough, he explained, "being very determined to resist it, I promptly triumphed over this little obstacle." As the ether vapours soothed the prickling sensation in his throat and calmed his cough, he began to feel a warm inebriating numbness engulfing his brain, which then spread all over his body from his toes to his legs and arms and then to his kidneys and genitals. "It increased rapidly with each inhalation," he recalled; "in the sensitive organs it was accompanied by an agreeable warm sensation and a tingling sensation, a quivering or vibration similar to that one experiences when touching a vibrating body, a large bell that resonates."[50] Gerdy experienced the ether spreading and reverberating through his body as it gradually took hold of him.

Ether enabled Gerdy to master bodily pain. To test its anesthetic properties, he declared with bravado, "after making myself numb, I pierced through the skin of my hand with a needle from the outside in, then from the inside out; I only felt a slight pain."[51] Gerdy enthusiastically offered his body to be mangled in the service of scientific knowledge. In a gesture that was as much self-aggrandizing as self-sacrificing, he stabbed through his own hand, as though inflicting the stigmata of modern science.

The pursuit of scientific objectivity would normally dictate that the researcher avoid imposing his will on the experiment.[52] However, Gerdy had to deploy his will to resist the effects of the ether. Losing consciousness would have rendered him unable to remember and communicate his experiences. He felt his eyelids getting heavier, but he claimed that "because I wanted to observe myself up until the last moment, I did not allow myself to indulge in any temptation, to abandon myself to the seductions that charmed me, and I did not fall asleep."[53] Gerdy's struggle to retain consciousness against the alluring prospect of ethereal sleep demonstrates the difficulty of maintaining control over his mind and body when these were the objects of his psychotropic experimentation.

Ironically, the only way to be able to testify to the anesthetic effects of ether was to resist the ultimate effect being tested: the loss of consciousness.

The question of free will dominated Gerdy's account of his self-experimentation. The image of the doctor martyring himself in the name of scientific knowledge and medical progress depended upon his intellectual freedom as an autonomous, rational subject. However, psychotropic self-experimentation destabilized the privileged position of the mind as the controlling force of the human organism. Despite the effects of the ether, Gerdy attested, "my thoughts were very clear and my intelligence perfectly free. My attention was also very active, my will always firm, so firm that I wanted to walk and that I walked, in fact, to observe the state of my locomotion."[54] In any other state, the mind commanding the body to walk around would be an unremarkable occurrence rather than an indicator of one's "firm" will. However, as ether gradually severed the sensory communications between Gerdy's mind and his body, he emphasized his free will to reassert control and to highlight his status as a bourgeois man of science.

Free will was the essential mark of bourgeois selfhood in nineteenth-century France.[55] Following the violence and political turmoil of the French revolutions of 1789 and 1830, the July Monarchy promoted bourgeois interests to maintain the social order. French intellectuals had come to believe that the passive, fragmented self of sensationalist philosophy – which viewed the mind as a blank slate inscribed with external impressions – had left the individual vulnerable to the kind of excesses of imagination that could lead to revolutionary violence. To counteract the dangers of this type of passive selfhood, they instead embraced a new vision of a unified self guided by individual free will.[56] In 1832, philosopher Victor Cousin institutionalized this new unified vision of the self in France's *lycée* philosophy curriculum, where it maintained prominence throughout the nineteenth century. In the *lycée*, young bourgeois men learned to cultivate a robust, active self to distinguish themselves from women and from men of the lower classes.[57] The free-willing Cousinian self became a tenet of bourgeois masculinity used to justify their social dominance.

For Gerdy, free will was an indication of not only his professional commitment but his status as a bourgeois male. Following his own experiences, Gerdy noted that eight or ten other people, both men and women, had repeated the experiment with similar results, but "not absolutely similar ... as some of them, as in sleep, lost consciousness of themselves."[58] Gerdy appealed to the collective authority of multiple test subjects to corroborate his assessment of ether's effects on sensation. Yet he distinguished himself from these other, lesser experimenters through the strength of his will. Unlike women, who could be expected to lose consciousness, or other men with less robust wills, Gerdy remained aware of himself and resisted the impulse to give in to sleep. In this manner, he elevated his own authority as a self-experimenter who, while exploring ether's psychotropic power, could simultaneously overcome it.

While Gerdy tested ether on himself in the name of patient welfare, another physician placed himself in actual surgical conditions to report on ether's effects. B.J.F. Horteloup, a hospital physician in Paris, acted as an expert witness to the experience of ether anesthesia while King Louis Philippe's dentist, Jean-Étienne Oudet, extracted his tooth.[59] After coughing through his initial inhalations, Horteloup gradually lost consciousness. "I do not know what period of time had passed," he recalled, "when I was fully awakened by two or three strong pinches on the wrist; I was dreaming that you wanted me to get up in spite of myself, and I resisted." In this moment of semi-consciousness, Horteloup recognized Oudet's office and heard voices. He called out to them, but Oudet immediately reapplied the inhalation apparatus. With a few deep breaths, Horteloup "fell once more into a deep coma."[60]

While the experience of waking up mid-anesthesia might have been alarming, Horteloup affirmed that he did not suffer despite moving in and out of consciousness. "I was awakened," he explained, "as if someone had vigorously shaken me in the middle of a restorative sleep ... I have a vague memory of having let out groans to complain of the barbarity that was disturbing my rest; it was the removal of my tooth that had produced this result, but I did *not suffer at all*."[61] Horteloup's bottom molar had been "solidly implanted" in his jaw by two strong roots, one of which had adhered to the bone.[62] In any other circumstance, the procedure would have been excruciating. That Horteloup could endure the extraction in the absence of suffering, remembering only the "barbarity" of disturbed sleep, was practically miraculous.

Unlike the self-experimenting doctors who were pricked with pins and jabbed with scalpels, Horteloup had undergone an actual surgical procedure, with all of its associated anxieties. Although his knowledge of the recent ether research conducted by his colleagues likely would have given him a degree of confidence beforehand, Horteloup's experience came close to that of an average patient. The next time, Horteloup urged, "I would not hesitate to submit myself to ether inhalations for a similar operation; and I especially recommend it to those who are nervous … [because] I did *not feel anything painful* at the moment when *my tooth was removed.*" In fact, other than some nausea in the carriage home after the procedure, he experienced no ill side effects and attested that, later that night, "I was perfectly restored to my natural state."[63] Most accounts of clinical observations include only a brief few words describing whether the patient experienced pain during surgery. Horteloup's privileged position as a doctor and the fact that he moved in and out of consciousness enabled him to describe his experiences as a surgical patient in great detail and endowed him with the valuable authority of personal experience.

While most ether research in 1847 focused on its potential as a surgical anesthetic, one doctor, Jean-Joseph Sauvet, engaged in self-experimentation in order to explore its disruption of the mind's normal cognitive functions.[64] Determined to experience this "artificial madness" for himself, Sauvet inhaled ether in front of two witnesses, the prefect of Meuse and another doctor, François-Émile Renaudin, who assisted him with the experiment. Like other self-experimenters, Sauvet struggled to maintain control over himself as an experimental subject, even as he felt his self-control diminishing under the power of ether's vapours. "Hardly had I inhaled a bit of ethered air," he explained, "when a shudder of gentle warmth travelled down all of my limbs." Soon he found it difficult to maintain the ether apparatus on his lips as his left hand became limp, so "on a signal, a servant positioned near me seized the apparatus and placed it firmly on my mouth."[65] Ether's physiological modifications prevented Sauvet from maintaining control over his own body. Despite Sauvet's role as a "self-experimenter," his ability to continue the experiment hinged upon the servant's force.

Ether made Sauvet an unruly experimental subject. He gave in to an overpowering desire to dance around. This movement suspended his ether inhalations, causing him to regain consciousness to find himself struggling with his "operator."[66] Only two minutes had passed. When he breathed ether in again, his delirium quickly returned. Someone asked Sauvet whether he could feel what they were doing to him, to which he replied, "I feel that I am being pinched; but this sensation is nothing painful." In fact, they were stabbing him rather hard in the hand with a needle, but he experienced no pain and did not attempt to pull his hand away. In addition to testing the degree of etherization, Renaudin and the others helped to monitor Sauvet's vital signs during the experiment as a safeguard against asphyxiation. This was no easy task, as ether made Sauvet intractable. When offered a glass of water, he kicked the tray out of the servant's hands. When Renaudin tried to check his pulse and the dilation of his pupils, Sauvet recalled, "without respect for his scientific examination, I began to repeat his gestures by exaggerating them."[67] Sauvet's mockery of Renaudin's scientific process demonstrates the impossibility of maintaining strict scientific objectivity in the face of such a subjective self-experiment, particularly one specifically designed to disturb the mental faculties.

In a prolonged state of ether-induced "delirium," Sauvet felt himself "irresistibly drawn" to waltz around the room with an armchair as his dancing partner. His companions chased him around trying to get him to sit down again. Then he saw a tiny woman, twenty centimetres tall, dancing a polka on the keys of a piano. He sang along with her, only to realize it was not a polka he was singing but "La Marseillaise."[68] While some individuals experienced unpleasant initial moments of delirium under the influence of ether, Sauvet attributed this to their apprehension about the anesthesia. Rather than inhaling ether out of surgical necessity, he explained, "I lent myself spontaneously, voluntarily and with pleasure; I submitted myself to etherization, quite convinced that it presented no danger; I wanted to study it on myself, in a word, I was impatient to see myself in this new state."[69] While Gerdy and others had tried to exercise their will to remain conscious and in control of their experiments, Sauvet deliberately relinquished control to experience a state of mental fragmentation in which his memory remained but his reason and judgment ceased to exist. He emphasized the self as the object of the experimental transformation. With pleasure and impatience, he offered his own self, driven by both personal and scientific curiosity, to seek this altered state.

Sauvet believed madness, immensely complex and difficult to understand, could be experienced with the aid of psychotropic substances.

Using ether, he experienced irresistible impulses and vivid hallucinations in the absence of judgment and reflection. In this manner, he empathized with mental patients. He had found the hallucination of the tiny woman dancing on the piano so clear and detailed that, he explained, "I understand now, more than ever, the obstinacy of the hallucinating madmen who persist in saying *I saw* when we want to persuade them that they have not seen, but that they *believed to have seen*." Sauvet was highly aware of the stigma attached to an experimenter who abandoned himself to the "artificial madness" of ether, even temporarily, in an age that lauded reason and scientific objectivity. Thus, he explained that he had acted out of a sense of duty to humanity to produce knowledge that might assist doctors in the treatment of mental illness. In this context, he challenged, "anyone among you who can guarantee that he has never ceased to be reasonable a single moment in his life, come and throw the first stone!"[70] Earlier, Sauvet had expressed his own pleasure, willingness, and desire to see himself in a state of madness; here, he defends the value of such personal experience for scientific research. For Sauvet, the experiment wedded scientific inquiry and personal curiosity. He did not view these motives as mutually exclusive and embraced his irrational self for both research and pleasure.

Most accounts of research on ether conducted through self-experimentation appeared in the first few months of 1847, when excitement over its anesthetic power swept the medical community in France and abroad. However, a new anesthetic gas ultimately surpassed ether as France's surgical anesthetic par excellence. In March 1847, physiologist Marie-Jean-Pierre Flourens reported to the Academy of Sciences that chloroform could be used to anesthetize animals.[71] In November of that year, Edinburgh obstetrician James Young Simpson conducted the first human experiments with chloroform anesthesia. Naturally, Simpson and his colleagues began by experimenting on themselves.[72] Then they proceeded to observe its beneficial anesthetic effects in surgery and childbirth. Professor Jean-Baptiste Dumas of the École Polytechnique happened to be in Edinburgh to witness Simpson's initial surgical experiments with ether, and when he returned to Paris the following week he shared the details of his observations with his colleague, Dr Roux, who immediately began experiments of his own.[73]

In Paris, demand for purified chloroform surged as surgeons rushed to confirm Simpson's findings.[74] Once again, anesthetic researchers used chloroform in the clinic and engaged in self-experimentation with the gas simultaneously. Once again, Pierre Nicolas Gerdy insisted on experimenting on himself before giving chloroform to patients. In November 1847, Gerdy performed an initial, rudimentary experiment on himself and found chloroform to be very similar to ether. He had read Simpson's accounts of chloroform anesthesias performed in Scotland, and he decided to try it the next day on a patient during an operation for a spinal fistula.[75] While the patient was generally satisfied with the relative comfort of the operation, Gerdy observed sores around her nose and mouth the day after the surgery. Allowing his clinical practice to inform further self-experiments in order to research chloroform's side effects, he went home and inhaled chloroform again on a sponge. As in the case of his patient, he felt the chloroform burn his nose and mouth. It made him numb, like ether, but he did not lose consciousness.

After the effects wore off, Gerdy decided to administer chloroform again using an ether inhalation apparatus to try to avoid burning his nose and mouth, but this time he lost consciousness for five or six minutes. After dreaming and talking a bit, he woke up vomiting. The numbness from the chloroform lasted for about thirty minutes after he woke up, but he felt nauseated for several hours afterward and continued to experience throat and chest irritation.[76] As with his ether experiments, Gerdy subjected his body to physical discomfort and danger in the service of improved patient care. Gone, however, was the scientific heroism of his previous experiments. During the ether experiments, Gerdy had presented himself as a strong-willed scientific researcher, valiantly resisting ether's effects to remain conscious. Yet his strong will was no match for the anesthetic effects of chloroform. Nothing offered a starker contrast to his previous experience than losing consciousness and waking up vomiting.

Individual reactions to chloroform varied widely, possibly as a result of the questionable quality of the substance that researchers used in their initial experiments. Like Gerdy, one medical student who only inhaled chloroform for a minute felt nauseated at its sickly sweet taste and smell.[77] However, at the Hôtel-Dieu Hospital in Paris, Dr Armand Gaide and another medical student both experimented with chloroform and in less than thirty seconds they experienced complete insensibility and an ecstasy that was the expression of "indescribable happiness."[78] Most self-experimenters experienced insensibility and lost conscious quickly. Three student interns at the Hôtel-Dieu Hospital in Reims who experimented with chloroform all fell rapidly into a state of complete anesthesia. When a pharmacist's assistant tried it, though, it produced a violent rage.[79] Despite some initial setbacks, chloroform researchers eventually concluded that chloroform had several advantages over ether: first, it acted more rapidly than ether did; second, less of it was required to produce a deeper anesthesia; and third, patients would return to consciousness more rapidly after surgery. Yet researchers were not blind to its potential dangers. Animal research had demonstrated that while ether would kill a guinea pig in eight to twelve minutes, chloroform would only take two or three minutes.[80] While chloroform soon supplanted ether in France as the preferred anesthetic of surgeons, researchers advocated using great caution with that "marvellous and terrible agent."[81]

While researchers employed self-experimentation to produce knowledge about the effects of chloroform on the human mind and body, as they had done with ether earlier that year, the published accounts of this chloroform self-experimentation were generally less detailed. Given chloroform's rapid action over consciousness, it is possible that self-experimenters were unable to resist this effect long enough to remember or describe their experiences. Or perhaps after publishing on the frenzied anesthesia research that took place in the first few months of 1847, the medical press was growing tired of the subject. Anesthesia revolutionized surgical practice. Ether and chloroform appeared to be evidence of the progress of medical science. However, anesthesia researchers struggled to embody the emerging ideals of scientific objectivity as the subjective experience of self-experimentation connected and distorted subject and object, mind and body.

HASHISH, MADNESS, AND THE SELF

Hashish research reflected a different set of priorities than research into ether and chloroform. Instead of seeking knowledge about surgical anesthesia, hashish researchers embarked on a more nebulous exploration of the mind, consciousness, and indeed sanity itself. Self-experimentation with hashish facilitated a process of psychotropic introspection. Hashish researchers were captivated by the mental distortions the drug produced, which resembled a state of artificial madness. The alluring prospect of experiencing bizarre dreams, fantastic visions, and vivid sensory distortions led curious individuals to consume hashish as an act of self-exploration. Eager to discover what hashish might uncover in the depths of their consciousness, they readily relinquished reason and free will. Self-experimentation with hashish appealed to Romantic artists and men of science alike. While the "artificial madness" of hashish appealed to asylum doctors searching for new therapeutic remedies, it also invited philosophical reflections on the nature of selfhood and the relationship between the mind and the body.

One of the earliest French physicians to engage in self-experimentation with hashish was Dr Louis Aubert-Roche. Stationed in Alexandria, Egypt, in the mid-1830s, he became intimately acquainted with the drug while searching for an effective treatment for the plague.[82] After trying anti-inflammatories, stimulants, and revulsives to no avail, Aubert-Roche thought of hashish, a substance "that the Arabs use like opium to plunge themselves into a distinct space of ecstasy and contemplation. Curiosity brought me to use it myself ... to understand the action of this substance that had astonished me. So I resolved to try it."[83] By fulfilling his own desire to experience this "distinct space of ecstasy," Aubert-Roche inadvertently stumbled across a potential treatment for the plague.[84]

Like most Frenchmen who experimented with hashish in the nineteenth century, Aubert-Roche's introduction to the substance was through the myths propagated by the famous French Orientalist Silvestre de Sacy (1758–1838).[85] In 1809, Sacy gave a speech at the Institut de France in which he recounted the legend of the Assassins, initially popularized in Marco Polo's thirteenth-century travel writings.[86] A product of various erroneous myths about the Nizari Isma'ilis of Syria, the legend describes a sect of medieval Islamic assassins.[87] According to Sacy, a sheik known as the Old Man of the Mountain possessed the secret recipe for a potion that he used to secure his subjects' fierce devotion. Without fear or hesitation, they executed his orders, no matter how violent or dangerous, in order to experience the delights of the sheik's pleasure garden, fantastically enhanced with the aid of this mysterious potion.[88] Sacy claimed that the mysterious potion that spurred the assassins to violence was in fact hashish. Modern scholars have exposed this conclusion to be false.[89] However, Sacy's status as France's pre-eminent Orientalist scholar lent credence to this association of hashish consumption and Oriental violence.[90] The Assassins legend appears in most nineteenth-century writings on hashish. Fascination with it motivated numerous experiments with hashish as users sought to take an artificial journey to an imagined Orient.

Aubert-Roche took hashish in part because the reality of the "Orient" did not live up to his expectations. Instead of the exotic charms portrayed in *A Thousand and One Nights*, upon his arrival in Egypt he found that "unfortunately the Orient is a bit like the fable of the floating sticks. The illusion passes quickly to give way to the sad reality."[91] In small green tablets of hashish flavoured with pistachio, rose, and jasmine, Aubert-Roche hoped to discover the wonders of his imagined Orient, using the material substance to excite his imagination to new depths. Prudent at first with his dose of this unfamiliar substance, he felt tempered effects but still experienced surprising gaiety and bizarre ideas swirling though his head. He resolved to experiment further. A few days later, he doubled his dose, elongated himself on a divan, and drank coffee to hasten the effects. After experiencing peculiar sensory distortions, he later recalled, "the strangest and most diverse ideas pass[ed] through my head with astonishing rapidity, from time to time reason mastered the effects of the substance; but soon they had the upper hand. Moreover, I felt a perfect [sense of] well-being; not a single painful sensation, the past, the present, the future no longer existed."[92] Aubert-Roche felt transcendent bliss under the influence of hashish, escaping temporal and corporeal reality to experience something pleasantly unfamiliar. While his rational mind struggled against the hashish, the drug soon took hold, immersing him in a passive state of ethereality where the self could experience and enjoy but not control.

Following this vivid description of allowing his mind to be swept up in the altered state of consciousness produced by hashish, Aubert-Roche noted that when he awoke the next day, he did not experience the heavy-headedness or sour taste that typically followed a night of bacchanalian indulgence. Additionally, he retained a vivid memory of all that had occurred the previous evening. He then admitted,

"I continued to take this substance with my friends, willingly examining the effect it produced on us; still, I was amazed at the active manner with which it affected the nervous system."[93] Aubert-Roche recounted his self-experimentation in a lengthy monograph on the treatment of typhus and the plague and followed his account with clinical observations of cases in which he used hashish to treat plague victims.[94] This juxtaposition illustrates how his self-experimentation merged research and pleasure, subjectivity and objectivity, rationality and sensuality. Aubert-Roche's research intrigued his colleagues in Paris, who called for further research on hashish.[95]

In 1841, Aubert-Roche took hashish with a friend and colleague, Dr Jacques-Joseph Moreau de Tours (1804–1884), who would become France's foremost advocate of self-experimentation with the substance.[96] Moreau was a prominent clinical researcher who worked at Bicêtre, the large public asylum for men in Paris, and at Jean-Étienne-Dominique Esquirol's private asylum in Ivry, just outside the city.[97] He saw hashish as a subjective vehicle he could use to access the alienated mental states of his patients. For the next few years, Moreau experimented extensively with hashish on himself, his friends, and his colleagues before publishing his 1845 monograph, *Hashish and Mental Illness*. "The only way to fully understand this effect," he claimed, "is personal experience. But we are scared of it and we do not find that the results ... are worth the effort of running the risk of being poisoned ... So, we abstain and we make do with the experience of others."[98] Refraining from hashish, Moreau implied, was not only bad science but contemptible cowardice. He firmly believed that personal experience was the "criterion of truth." He contended, "I challenge the right of anyone to discuss the effects of hashish if he is not speaking for himself and if he has not been in a position to evaluate them in light of sufficient repeated use." Instead of approaching madness as an outsider, Moreau argued, "hashish gives to whoever submits to its influence the power to study in himself the mental disorders that characterize insanity, or at least the intellectual modifications that are the beginning of all forms of mental illness."[99] He claimed that by using hashish the psychological researcher could artificially create the experience of madness within his own brain, but this process required the researcher to "submit" to hashish's influence and allow himself to be led into unknown levels of consciousness.

Moreau disconcertingly suggested that madness might lie dormant in sane individuals, waiting for hashish to awaken it.

For an experimental researcher, deliberately provoking a kind of madness in one's own brain would seem to compromise the experiment by incapacitating the intellectual faculties normally deployed to observe and analyze it. However, Moreau sidestepped this issue. Although hashish produced intellectual disorders that reached "quite a great intensity," he asserted, "nevertheless I had not lost consciousness of myself for a single moment; I always kept the power to assess, to analyze the strange situation in which I had placed myself voluntarily."[100] Moreau insisted that he continued to be a credible observer of his own experiences. He also emphasized the voluntarism of his experiment. In contrast to the mental patients he was trying to emulate, Moreau willfully produced in himself a temporary state of madness, which would dissipate after a time, leaving his mental faculties intact.

Even when hashish took control of the mind, Moreau asserted, an underlying self-awareness remained. Hashish's disturbance of the moral faculties "can be supported to a high degree without the *self* being destroyed, without the conscience being shaken, without ceasing to suitably judge one's position … as though it concerned someone completely other than ourselves."[101] He suggested that the hashish researcher could call up a state of madness at will, while simultaneously maintaining the ability to discern and assess his experiences. He evoked a kind of splitting, in which the analytical self separates from the mad self engaged in the hashish experience. In such a manner, the self-experimenter could both observe and experience madness.

While Napoleon's occupation of Egypt between 1798 and 1801 ignited France's fascination with hashish, the colonization of Algeria precipitated its popularity.[102] In the 1840s, North African cannabis preparations became more readily available in France.[103] In Paris at this time, while Aubert-Roche and Moreau were conducting their research, hashish soirées became popular venues for those who were curious about the possibilities of altering one's consciousness with psychotropic substances. Neither purely social nor purely scientific, these salons facilitated an intimate form of self-experimentation.

Art and science collided at the hashish soirées. While Romanticism has traditionally been portrayed as a turn away from Enlightenment rationalism and the prominence of science in the post-Revolutionary industrial order, as John Tresch has demonstrated, there were significant ties between science and Romanticism in the 1830s and 1840s.[104] In May 1840, Dr Alexandre Brière de Boismont received an invitation from writer Stéphane Ajasson de Grandsagne to attend a singular meeting of about thirty people, gathered to consume hashish and experience "all the phenomena that were observed among the followers of the Old Man of the Mountain."[105] Several notables of the medical community attended, including pre-eminent asylum doctors like Esquirol and Guillaume Ferrus; Professor Bussy of the Pharmacy School; and many other men of letters, savants, and artists. Brière de Boismont claimed that the presence of such esteemed witnesses would ensure "a good observation and the certainty that the experience would be real."[106] Three men took the "liqueur": A.K., a famous novelist (probably Alphonse Karr); D., a lawyer; and B., a painter and musician. For safety, the others observed and monitored the three experimental subjects closely during the experiment, took their pulses at various points, and followed the development of their symptoms.

The experimental subjects found it quite difficult to express what they experienced. B. claimed to experience "voluptuous sensations" and ecstasy, but observers noted that "he cannot find the terms to express what he feels."[107] Hashish inhibited the user's ability to communicate, making it somewhat problematic as a research tool. The difficulty of adequately describing the hashish experience was one reason why Moreau and others advocated for self-experimentation as the most effective means of understanding its physiological and psychosomatic effects. Proponents also believed that the hashish experience was unique to each individual, in a particular time and context. One's state of mind, attitude toward the experiment, and sensory perceptions during the experiment all contributed to the unique state of altered consciousness the drug produced. Experimenters believed these hashish experiences to be as contingent upon the stuff of self as they were on the chemical action of the drug. Therefore, hashish became a popular vehicle for the exploration of selfhood.

During the July Monarchy, introspection was an important "technology of the self" for bourgeois men of science and Romantic artists alike.[108] Cousin's *lycée* philosophy curriculum trained the bourgeois male to hone his selfhood through the conscious process of introspection, which required isolation from the senses and the exterior world and self-reflection directed by the will. While women and working-class men had a unified, a priori self in theory, the state-educated elite distinguished themselves by claiming to have a superior capacity for reflection that enabled them to fully cultivate the robust, free-willing self. Within the individualistic and theoretically meritocratic post-Revolutionary social order, introspection enabled the state-educated elite to justify their own elevated social position.[109] For the Romantic artist, however, introspection afforded an opportunity to explore the self, to penetrate the interiors of individual consciousness for artistic inspiration. Unlike eighteenth-century neoclassical aesthetics, in which the artist was supposed to reflect reality like a mirror, the Romantic artist acted as a lamp, projecting the self onto his work. Through introspection, the Romantic artist cultivated imagination and emotion, which he then used to transform his perceptions of the world to produce art that reflected the self.[110]

Writer and critic Théophile Gautier vividly documented his extensive self-experimentation with hashish in his quest to achieve a state of *kif*, an Arabic term that referred to the state of bliss the drug produced.[111] In an 1843 *La Presse* article, Gautier described his first experience with hashish paste as the fulfillment of the universal human urge to experience the self unfettered by material conditions. "The desire for the ideal is so strong in man," Gautier explained, that he tries with all his might "to release the ties that bind the soul to the body and, as ecstasy is not within the reach of all dispositions, he drinks happiness, smokes forgetfulness, and eats madness in the form of wine, tobacco, and hashish."[112] Paradoxically, the act of consuming a material, psychotropic substance to alter his mental state actually reaffirmed and accentuated the mind-body connection he was attempting to transcend.

Gautier experienced his intoxication in waves, punctuated by moments of rational consciousness. He explained, "What is strange about the hashish intoxication is that it is not continuous; it takes you and leaves you, elevates you to heaven and returns you to earth without transition – as in madness, one has moments of lucidity." This comparison of the hashish experience to madness reappears throughout Gautier's writings on hashish.[113] After he returned to lucidity following his first hashish experience, he remarked that "a half-hour had hardly passed when I fell under the empire of hashish once again."[114] Using the language of imperialism to describe hashish, Gautier upended expected power dynamics. Rather than behaving as an active human subject, he relinquished his free will to a material commodity, adopting a passive form of subjectivity. The power dynamics of imperialism were also over-turned: Gautier, the Western subject, was subordinated to the "empire" of an Eastern material substance.

These vivid descriptions of hashish's influence on the senses de-picted the experience as larger and wilder than life. A new sensory plane sprang forth from Gautier's own consciousness, awakened with the aid of hashish. When hashish took hold the second time, he found himself amid billions of butterflies, watching as gigantic flowers made of gold, silver, and crystal bloomed all around him, making crackling sounds like "bouquets of fireworks." He explained, "My hearing was prodigiously developed; I heard the noise of colours. The green, red, blue, [and] yellow tones came to me in perfectly distinct waves." Sensory distortions – the fantastic images of motion and colour and the melding together of the senses of sight and sound – governed this experience of altered consciousness. Gautier later noted that his second experience had lasted fifteen minutes and described his third as "the last and the most bizarre, [which] ended my oriental evening."[115] Experiencing a discon-tinuous hashish state punctuated by moments of lucidity emphasized the psychotropic power of hashish. During these lucid interstices, Gautier never fully regained possession of his will, and he had no choice but to let himself be swept away by hashish once again.

Three years after his first experience with hashish, Gautier published another, lengthier account of self-experimentation in the *Revue des deux mondes*. This account of his experiences with hashish at the Hôtel Pimodan immortalized that peculiar group of bohemian artists and intellectuals who became known as "the Hashish Eaters' Club."[116] The Hashish Eaters gathered in the apartments of artist Fernand Boissard (1813–1866) to consume *dawamesk*, an edible hashish paste from North Africa known as the "paste of paradise."[117] *Dawamesk* allowed them to experience a temporary state of mental alienation while facilitating a deep investigation of the self. In addition to conducting experiments with colleagues at Charenton Asylum, Moreau experimented with ha-shish socially at the Hôtel Pimodan. There, both he and Aubert-Roche continued their research in a social setting.[118] Under their direction, the Hashish Eaters' Club acted simultaneously as a controlled experiment in pursuit of scientific knowledge and a sensuous exercise in pursuit of self-understanding. Eschewing contemporary bourgeois ideals, which advocated an active, unified, and rational self, the Hashish Eaters instead adopted a passive, sensuous form of experiential self-knowledge that allowed them to revel in its fragmentations.[119] By embracing a substance that brought out the exotic, dangerous, and irrational elements buried beneath the mental surface, the Hashish Eaters pursued madness as the path to individual enlightenment.

Many of the Hashish Eaters were Romantic artists and writers, for whom an opportunity to access one's "inner life" unadulterated by external reality held significant appeal. Some believed that hashish had the power to stimulate creativity and artistic genius by unlocking previously undiscovered imaginative faculties. Others were skeptical. Yet curiosity and the desire for experiential knowledge were powerful forces. The Hashish Eaters negotiated a desire to remain in control of their mental faculties with an eagerness to experience a wild, unthinking, feeling self. Two famous literary figures, Charles Baudelaire and Honoré de Balzac, claimed to have participated as mere observers, although both men tried hashish at least once. Their discussion of the merits and dangers of hashish use reveals a struggle between curiosity about experiencing unrefined, unfiltered selfhood and anxiety over the idea of relinquishing free will and reason to the caprices of a psychotropic substance.

Balzac relished self-control. He used sexual abstention and copious amounts of strong coffee to fuel his late-night writing binges.[120] In fact, he boasted about the strength of his will. Gautier recalled that Balzac felt it would be useless for him to participate; "the hashish, he was sure, would not have any effect on his brain."[121] Baudelaire claimed that Balzac abstained at the Pimodan. When offered the *dawamesk* paste, Balzac sniffed it but returned it untouched.[122] Nevertheless, in his private correspondence with Mme Hanska, his future wife, Balzac admitted that he had tried hashish at the Pimodan with Gautier on 22 December 1845. He claimed, "I resisted the hashish and I did not experience all the phenomena; my brain is so strong, that it would require a stronger dose than that which I took."[123] Balzac found the idea of allowing a material substance to take control of his consciousness disconcerting. Yet, despite his "strong brain" and force of will, he admitted that he heard celestial voices, saw visions of "unprecedented splendour," and experienced a distorted perception of time in which it seemed to take twenty years to descend a single staircase.

To justify his self-experimentation, Balzac framed it as a mental exercise, emphasizing his curiosity and free will. He insisted that Gautier had not persuaded him to take hashish. Instead, he claimed, he did it of his own accord because he was interested in the psychological study of the "quite extraordinary phenomenon" on himself. This concept of self-study needed to be experienced first-hand. Citing Humphry Davy's self-experimentation with nitrous oxide, Balzac contemplated, "it's so strange that we should deny those effects as long as we have not experienced them [for ourselves]."[124] The knowledge attained through this experiment and the satisfaction of his curiosity could be gained not from the study of something external but rather though the *experience* of something internal, achieved by ingesting a material, state-altering substance with the power to harness the senses and reveal the underlying essence of the self.

As Gautier later recalled, Baudelaire came to the Pimodan rarely and as a simple observer while others consumed *dawamesk*. However, Gautier thought it likely that Baudelaire had tried it once or twice for the physiological experience.[125] Like Balzac, Baudelaire had ambivalent feelings about self-experimentation. Although Baudelaire's famous 1860 book *Les Paradis Artificiels* contains some quintessential examples of self-experimentation with drugs, it demonstrates ambivalence and even hostility toward drug consumption.[126] In "On Wine and Hashish," Baudelaire passionately condemns hashish and its detrimental effects, not on the consumer's physical well-being but on his free will.[127] In "The Poem of Hashish," he refutes claims that hashish could produce artistic genius, arguing that "hashish reveals nothing to the individual but himself." Instead, the desire to use it to expand one's creative faculties is a vicious circle because "it is the nature of hashish to diminish the will, and thus it gives with one hand what it takes with the other, that is to say, imagination without the ability to make use of it."[128] Baudelaire's laudanum addiction might have contributed to his reservations about hashish, as he had already experienced first-hand the pernicious effects of drug addiction on productivity and the will.[129] Both he and Balzac viewed hashish's subordination of their free will with a mixture of curiosity and apprehension.

To alleviate users' concerns about potential dangers, the Hashish Eaters' Club introduced protective measures to contain and manage the social experience of collective hashish use. While each individual Hashish Eater relinquished his rational will to the *dawamesk*, one member, known as *le voyant*, or "the seer," abstained from the "voluptuous intoxication" so he could direct their experiences from the outside. According to Gautier, this individual's job was "to oversee the fantasia and prevent those among us who would have believed they [had] wings from leaping out the windows."[130] As Moreau enthusiastically participated in the hashish experience, the Hashish Eaters likely took turns acting as *voyant*.[131]

In addition to his role as designated anti-defenestrator, the *voyant* took charge of the group's mental well-being by conducting the Hashish Eaters through the experience and asserting control over their "madness" by using music to alter the mood. After one particularly frightening episode of collective disturbance, the *voyant* went over to the piano, his fingers "sinking into the ivory of the keyboard, and a glorious chord, resonating with force, silenced the rumours and changed the direction of the *ivresse*."[132] While the Hashish Eaters described their experience as one of internal discovery, the senses acted as conduits from the external world. The tremendous sound of the piano reached Gautier while under the influence of hashish. "The notes vibrated with such power," he proclaimed, "that they entered my chest like brilliant arrows; soon the melodious air seemed to emanate from within me; my fingers moved across an absent keyboard; the sounds burst forth blue and red and electric sparks; the soul of Weber was embodied in me."[133] Music held particular sway over the Hashish Eaters' heightened senses and proved an effective means of controlling the "experiment."

The Hashish Eaters explored the self through an Orientalist lens. Describing his journey to the Ile Saint-Louis, Gautier highlighted the disparity between external life and internal life. He claimed, "Nothing in my perfectly bourgeois appearance could have made one suspect me of this excess of orientalism." He added, "I had more the air of a nephew going to dine at his old aunt's house than a believer on the verge of tasting the joys of Mohammed's heaven in the company of twelve surprisingly French 'Arabs.'"[134] Juxtaposing his bourgeois exterior with his internalized Orientalism, Gautier flaunted his evasion of bourgeois social propriety. He and the other Hashish Eaters adopted an "Arab" identity, if only for the evening, to commit "excesses of orientalism" in order to explore their own subjectivities in a topsy-turvy world in which object dominated subject and East dominated West.

By framing the hashish state as a form of artificial madness, Moreau and the Hashish Eaters evoked a common imperialist trope. Nineteenth-century French psychiatrists maintained that the high temperatures and excessive sunlight of exotic climates were hazardous to European minds. They feared that prolonged exposure to these environments would produce madness in Europeans who were accustomed to temperate climates, a phenomenon Richard Keller has labelled "the psychological menace of colonial space."[135] Although physically the Hashish Eaters remained in modern Paris, mentally they journeyed to an imagined Orient in which they could escape the shackles of reason and access an unfettered inner self. They embraced the alienation of an imagined Oriental identity and reconstructed themselves through it in an act of Orientalist fantasy that upended, yet ultimately reaffirmed, the power dynamics of French imperialism.[136]

In Gautier's account of the Hashish Eaters' Club, the meeting took on a reverent ritualistic form. A doctor, most likely Moreau, presided over the session.[137] "The doctor stood before the buffet, which held a tray laden with small Japanese porcelain saucers. He used a spatula to take a dollop of greenish paste or jam the size of one's thumb from a crystal vase and placed it next to a silver gilt spoon on each saucer," Gautier recounted. "The doctor's face shone with enthusiasm ... 'This will be deducted from your share of paradise.'" The doctor presided over the ritual distribution of the *dawamesk* among the members of the club with a physicalized and fervent enthusiasm, "eyes sparkling, cheeks flushed, the veins on his temples bulging, and nostrils flaring."[138] The doctor's performance evoked the mythical Assassins legend, emulating the Old Man of the Mountain as he bestowed access to paradise on his illuminated subjects. The ceremonial elements of the distribution of the hashish mimicked Catholic communion, yet the spiritual sentiment behind these actions evoked ties to an Orientalist vision of Islam, manipulating and subverting expected notions of French religiosity. The religious undertones of the ritualistic experience suggest a desire to achieve some form of spiritual transcendence.

Midway through the evening, following the whirling euphoria of the "fantasia," Gautier plunged into "that blissful period of hashish that the Orientals call *kif.*" In a Cartesian separation of the mind and the body, Gautier experienced a state of bliss divorced from worldly materialism or sensuality. He explained, "I no longer felt my body, the connections between mind and matter were released; I moved by my own will in an atmosphere that offered no resistance."[139] *Kif* offered the perfect conditions for indulging in an exploration of self, allowing the will to act without resistance, independent of material reality. Ironically, however, it was *dawamesk*, a decidedly material substance, that produced this state of otherworldly "immaterial" bliss. As a result, Gautier's ability to move willfully through the immaterial reality of *kif* was fleeting. The hashish soon came to dominate his will and he lost control of the experience. Vivid hallucinations terrified him as he struggled to escape from this new state of madness that distorted time and space

Following the swirling madness, profound ethereal bliss, grotesque visions, and sensory distortions, Gautier ended his story of the Hashish Eaters' Club on an enigmatic note, claiming, "My reason had returned, or at least that which I call [reason], through lack of another term. I was coherent enough to give a report on a pantomime or a vaudeville, or to writing three-letter rhyming poetry."[140] After the liberating madness of the hashish experience, "reason" had become something of an empty term – sufficient for mundane tasks but hollow in comparison with the enlightened madness of the hashish state. Recalling his earlier commentary on the Assassins legend, he lamented that those who took hashish, "when they awoke from their intoxication, found life so sad and so faded, that they would gladly make sacrifices to return to the paradise of their dreams."[141] By penetrating the depths of his own imagination in the pursuit of self-discovery, pushing psychological fragmentation to the very limits of madness, Gautier experienced a chaotic bombardment of vibrant emotions, sensations, and perceptions. Despite his fears of the monstrous possibilities lying dormant within his own mind, the thrill of letting go, of allowing himself to take a passive role within his own psyche, revealed his own disillusionment with normative consciousness directed by reason and individual will.

Later in life, Gautier claimed that "after ten or so experiences, we renounced the intoxicating drug forever, not because it did us physical harm, but the true *littérateur* does not need anything but his own natural dreams, and does not like his mind to be subjected to the influence of any [outside] agent."[142] While Gautier eventually renounced the artificiality of the hashish experience, the power that this material agent held over the will continued to both plague and fascinate hashish experimenters. Doctors, artists, writers, and other intellectuals continued to experiment with hashish throughout the nineteenth century and marvel at its ability to reveal inner life.[143]

In the medical community, Moreau passed his fascination with hashish on to a new generation of doctors. While teaching at Bicêtre and Salpêtrière Hospitals, he invited his interns to engage in self-experimentation.[144] He also deployed pharmacy interns to produce hashish from cannabis samples he cultivated in the Bicêtre garden in Paris and at the Ivry asylum. In April of 1848, in a lull between the political turmoil of the February Revolution and the June Days, a pharmacy student Moreau had mentored, Edmond de Courtive, defended his thesis on the chemical and physiological properties of hashish.[145] After observing the remarkable effects of hashish at Bicêtre in 1846, Courtive expressed a great desire to "study them more intimately" on himself. In 1847, Dr Foley, a colleague at the Civil Hospital of Algiers, sent him some hashish from Algeria and Courtive began his self-experimentation. Since then, he explained, "I have not stopped experimenting on men, animals, and also on myself."[146] Courtive's account of his self-experimentation with hashish exposed the tensions and disjunctures between objective experimentation and subjective experience.

Like many of his contemporaries, Courtive viewed hashish through the Assassins legend, as a dangerous exotic substance. However, he was convinced that he could use Western science to isolate the active properties of cannabis to transform it into a reliable therapeutic medicine. The first part of Courtive's thesis was devoted to chemical experimentation with refining various samples of cannabis grown in different regions of France – including a sample that Moreau grew in Ivry – and Algeria.[147] Even in this more empirical section on the results of his chemical analysis of the samples his self-experimental focus is apparent. He described each sample, noting the dose required to experience cerebral effects, which he determined through extensive self-experimentation. "What I did for one Cannabis, I did for another," he explained. "I can say that I swallowed hundreds of pills, and all of my [refined] products, like a true test machine [*machine à l'épreuve*]."[148] He also saved part of each sample, which he shared with Moreau so that Moreau could test them himself.[149]

By evoking the steady, standardized, and mechanical processes of a machine to describe his exhaustive experimental consumption of the hashish samples, Courtive presented himself as an objective analyst. Processing "hundreds" of samples by consuming them, he constructed his own body as an experimental instrument. Yet the psychotropic action of the hashish over his mind and body, its power to distort and transform each, compromised this premise of an objective analyst documenting data collected from a test machine. Courtive qualified the body-as-machine metaphor, explaining, "truthfully, I should say that I was sometimes reckless, because I have neither the stomach nor the nervous system of Vaucanson's ducks. But I had no other purpose than to seek to know the effects of this extraordinary Hashish, in order to enlist masters of the art to occupy themselves more seriously with it."[150] Unlike eighteenth-century inventor Jacques de Vaucanson's famous digesting mechanical duck, Courtive's body was vulnerable to the potential dangers of overconsumption.[151] To determine which hashish preparation and dose had the least dangerous and most potent effect, Courtive exposed himself to the dangers and discomforts of a wide variety of remedies.

While Courtive sought to produce objective research about the effects and potency of numerous different hashish samples, he was also profoundly interested in the subjective experience of the drug. In the acknowledgments of his thesis he thanked Moreau de Tours for his "affectionate interest" and encouragement of his research. Courtive recounted several of the "fantasias" he experienced during his extensive self-experimentation. After taking 15 grams of Algerian *madjoun* dissolved in water with another pharmacy intern, Courtive felt a bizarre distortion of his mental faculties. He struggled between, on the one hand, the desire to continue to exercise his free will and restrain himself and, on the other, the desire to give in to impulsive urges "to let myself go, to be happy."[152] He found his body acting independent of his will, as thoughts pummelled his mind, distracting from his self-observation.

Courtive's second hashish fantasia closely resembled a graduate student's nightmare. On 14 April 1847, a whole year before his thesis defence at the Pharmacy School, Courtive took three 5-centigram pills containing alcoholic hashish extract, followed by a cup of coffee. While eating breakfast he felt disoriented; he perceived himself to be sitting still and moving around simultaneously. Then, he experienced a doubled self as though he were multiplied.[153] Although he could see himself eating breakfast, he simultaneously perceived himself at the Pharmacy School awaiting his professors' judgment during his thesis defence.

Believing that he was standing before his thesis committee under the influence of hashish, he boasted, "I am triumphant; I took hashish so that my judges could better judge this marvellous philter of the mental patient. And as I took it, I hashished them with a look, at a distance, as if magnetized. Then the amphitheatre presented one of the most amusing spectacles. *MM. les professeurs* abandon themselves to a charming hilarity." Laughter and madness seized the room and the experience took on grandiose proportions. "Science finally triumphed," Courtive recounted, "and I saw the delegations of English, Russians, Americans, etc. arrive, who came to congratulate France for having discovered the *nec plus ultra* of earthly happiness, the essence of the soul, that from now on we could analyze, isolate, [and] combine in a thousand ways."[154] The spectacle became even more astonishing, as his professors assumed different forms. Monsieur O. transformed into a huge rattlesnake and called the jury to order. Monsieur D. turned into a malicious chameleon, Monsieur C. into an enormous crocodile, and Monsieur L. into a giant pneumatic machine. The madness continued as more people, including Moreau and Aubert-Roche, flooded into the amphitheatre. Then, suddenly, the school spontaneously caught fire.[155]

While this bizarre scene unfolded at the Pharmacy School, Courtive simultaneously saw himself back at home eating breakfast. Then, all of a sudden, there were two selves sitting across the table from each other. He watched as his other self ate breakfast while laughing and mocking him. Describing this strange doubling, or rather tripling, of self, Courtive wrote, "But, as I recognized that it was really me, by a visual illusion, I told myself, we joined together and we laughed to see my ⅓ self, who believed he had duped us." The two selves sitting at the breakfast table revelled at the downfall of his third self at the Pharmacy School, who was "bound, garroted, and straddled atop an enormous glass syringe, that threatens to reduce him to cinders, because it's a fire-coloured liquid material that boils in his flanks."[156] After this last vision, the "charm disappeared in an instant" and Courtive found himself alone at the breakfast table grasping a piece of bread. In this fantasia, Courtive's self was fragmented and the three pieces operated independently of one another, the two at the breakfast table taking pleasure in the demise of the third self at the thesis defence.

Courtive recounted two additional hashish fantasias: one was an Orientalist fantasy of epic proportions and the other a bizarre scene where he played the violin and encountered a strange green man made of cooked spinach.[157] Courtive tried to record his own impressions as they came to him, which was quite a challenge under the influence of hashish. He explained that with "all these capricious and surprising visions … many run together, because our mind, our self, or our individuality, if you like, sometimes multiplies itself to infinity."[158] For Courtive, by incorporating hashish into the body, the self could be unhinged, split into fragments and indefinitely multiplied, undermining the Cousinian vision of the self as unified and immutable.

Courtive, like Moreau and Aubert-Roche before him, enthusiastically believed that hashish had the potential to transform medical therapeutics, but it never reached a level of therapeutic significance comparable to that of opium, morphine, ether, or chloroform in the nineteenth century. While hashish enjoyed a period of popularity in medical research and therapeutics in the late 1830s and 1840s, its popularity declined during the Second Empire.[159] There were several reasons for this. Hashish's decline as a therapeutic medicine occurred, in part, because chemists and pharmacists found it difficult to produce medicines that contained a standard dose of its active properties.[160] Furthermore, medical enthusiasm for the drug waned after an ill-fated attempt to use hashish to treat the victims of the 1848–49 cholera epidemic in Paris.[161] Finally, as David Guba has demonstrated, France's imperial expansion in Algeria in the 1840s and 1850s magnified the Orientalist associations of hashish with madness, religious fanaticism, violence, and disorder, which further delegitimized hashish as a rational remedy of Western science.[162]

Although hashish's career as a therapeutic medicine was relatively short lived, individuals continued to experiment with it to explore the unconscious forces of their minds. In 1877, physiologist Charles Richet (1850–1935), another one of Moreau's interns, published an article in *Revue des deux mondes* titled "The Poisons of the Intellect." In it, he explored the influence of alcohol, chloroform, hashish, opium, and coffee on the human intellectual faculties. Richet sought to understand the "phenomena of life" by exploring how these various substances disrupted the body's organic functions.[163] As with the Hashish Eaters' Club, Richet's self-experimentation blended individual curiosity with the pursuit of knowledge. Like Gautier, Richet recognized a universal impulse to stimulate the mind with toxic substances.[164] The Hashish Eaters' Club fascinated Richet, because its gatherings "were experiments that not only had the attraction of the unknown but also all the charm of a purely psychological inebriation, even more spiritual and more active than wine."[165] He had read Moreau's and Gautier's writings on hashish and freely admitted, "I have frequently taken it myself at various doses and I have administered it to many of my friends."[166]

Pleasure, madness, and the surrender of control characterized Richet's hashish experiences. The dizzying rapidity of ideas bursting forth from the brain under the influence of hashish indicated a loss of self-control. In a normal state, Richet argued, individual free will directed all of the faculties, from judgment and memory to the imagination and the association of ideas.[167] The will was the essential mark of the Cousinian self: the autonomous command centre that exercised control over mind and body. Richet, by experimenting with hashish, sought to incapacitate the will to experience his own inner self unrestrained by its influence.

Richet compared hashish inebriation to the mental state of a hysterical woman, whose intelligence "is defective for two main reasons, the exaggeration of the emotions and the absence of the will." For Richet, as for many other hashish experimenters, relinquishing control and letting the hashish envelop his consciousness had a certain allure. The desire to embrace the "defective" mental state of a hysterical woman, defined by a lack of self-restraint and emotional control, destabilized the image of the rational, calculating man of science. With hashish, as with hysteria, "this power over yourself has also completely disappeared. You can no longer master yourself, you are out of control, and you are abandoned without restraint to the more or less reasonable conceptions of your mind."[168] By disabling his capacity for self-mastery, the man of science voluntarily abandoned his masculine rationality and embraced the volatility of a pathological mental state gendered female. With a small pill or a bit of green paste, the self-experimenter could indulge in the exploration of a new, uninhibited state of consciousness.

While this loss of control appealed to Richet's experimental curiosity, it could cause embarrassment in social settings. One night, Richet took hashish and then went to an evening party before it took effect. Listening intently to a serious conversation, he recalled, "I began to leap for joy and to express my enthusiasm for the originality of the thought that had just been put forward." He had not realized that hashish had overpowered his will until he could no longer control himself. "My idea was not absurd," he explained, "it was only exaggerated, and I had hardly conceived it when it manifested in spite of myself, *without the self,* so to speak, as an outward gesture."[169] After the hashish wore off, he came to his senses again and felt deeply ashamed. Richet, the hashish eater, stood apart from the other partygoers. While their actions were dictated by reason and free will, his were dictated by impulse and emotion, magnified by the drug he consumed.

By relinquishing judgment and volition, the hashish eater, like the dreamer, could experience the unrestrained flow of his unconscious impressions. In this manner, Richet used hashish to observe the very mechanisms through which thoughts were constructed. "This mysterious and silent birth, which in a normal state produces our thoughts and our judgments, is no longer mysterious or silent," Richet explained, because "we see how everything is related and everything is linked, we are witnesses to the formation of our ideas; [but] unfortunately we are no longer masters of them, and we are forced to follow their disorganized course." Like Moreau before him, Richet observed the striking similarities between dreams, madness, and the hashish state. In all three states, "external impressions become all-powerful, and the mind is subjected without restraint to the stimulation of the senses." In a normal waking state, individuals were only aware of a fraction of the ideas transformed and provoked by external stimuli. As Richet explained, "the attention and the will cover all of this unconscious work with a thick veil, and, in the middle of the confused activity of intellectual operations, the intellect only sees what it wants to see."[170] Hashish enabled Richet to passively witness his own intellectual process without conscious intervention, peering beyond the "thick veil" that shrouded these "mysterious" and "silent" faculties in a normal state. He thus gained experiential knowledge of his thinking self by relinquishing control, stepping back, and allowing his mind to work without him.

While Richet's incapacitated will during his hashish experiments enabled him to engage in deep metaphysical contemplation of the nature of the mind, he ended his study by reasserting the importance of individual free will. He believed that man had an obligation to cultivate an active, willful self. Yet he acknowledged that introspection was a complex process. "Man is neither angel nor beast," he explained, so "he should keep his will intact and not destroy it with poisons; but he should also respect and cultivate these unconscious, almost instinctive, faculties which are another part of himself ... the feelings, the passions, all these spontaneous movements of the soul, all these brilliant conceptive faculties that sleep in a corner of the mind ... that the will can awaken."[171] Although free will ultimately prevailed, drugs had offered Richet a tantalizing glimpse into the unfiltered stuff of selfhood.

Avid self-experimenters who were similarly captivated by hashish as a way to delve into the sensual and emotional depths of their own consciousness published guides for novices. These guides recommended practices for safe experimentation and tricks to enhance one's experience. In 1881, pharmacist Jules Giraud published an article titled "The Art of Varying the Effects of Hashish" in Professor Benjamin Ball's new journal of mental maladies, *L'Encéphale*.[172] Experiential curiosity motivated Giraud. Yet he published his article in a psychological journal, suggesting that he intended his practical advice to be consumed primarily by medical professionals.[173] "Disengage yourself as much as possible from any external preoccupation," he instructed. For those not searching for a "medical effect," who instead hoped to "enjoy that voluptuous stupor so sought after by amateurs of *kif*," he made the following recommendation: "You should keep yourself in that degree of somnolence where you are still conscious of what is happening in the imagination. Some musical tunes [and] a sufficient dose of coffee is enough to prevent the encroachment of sleep."[174] Giraud provided his medical audience with explicit instructions for experiencing the "voluptuous stupor" of amateurs instead of any particular medical effect. While pleasure seeking and individual curiosity had always been part of the motivation for even the most scientific of self-experimenters, Giraud focused explicitly on how to create and sustain a pleasurable experience.

He also advised his readers on the appropriate type and dose of hashish to consume. For his own experiments he preferred to use *haschichine* resin, purchased from either the Maison Dausse or the Pharmacie Centrale, which he found to be the most active. However, the quantity of *cannabine* could vary widely among different batches of resin, so for novices he recommended hashish in pill form. Users could achieve the maximum effect by consuming hashish one hour before a meal. Giraud reassured his readers that the only negative side effect he experienced was throat irritation, to which he was predisposed anyway. Moreover, one student, who had taken twenty times more hashish than Giraud had, experienced no adverse effects at all. Another student took 1.5 grams of *haschichine*, which "simply provoked spermatorrhea," or spontaneous, involuntary ejaculation.[175] Apparently, in Giraud's estimation, this was a relatively minor side effect.

For Giraud, hashish was an internal and highly individualized experience that existed in delicate balance with the self. He explained, "It seems that at the threshold of this unknown world a genie appears who is ready to give you the key on the condition that you first divest yourself of your human personality." While at first glance this might appear to be a journey into oblivion, leaving the individual self behind, it was actually more complex than that. In order to experience the effects of "this psychological dynamite," the hashish eater needed to know how to conjure things, as "you will have a rough or delightful *ivresse*, average or rich in discoveries, depending on the direction that you let your imagination take by the things you look at and, especially, the sounds you hear."[176] So, while hashish had fantastic properties for expanding consciousness, the nature of the experience depended upon the individual and his surroundings.

Sensory stimuli like music or coffee could expand and shape the experience. However, with a bit of effort and internal focus, hashish could serve as a vehicle for an intensely intimate exploration of the self. "If you have no music, or if you prefer to draw from your own depths" to shape your experience, Giraud recommended, "plunge yourself into the most complete silence; if necessary, stuff your ears with cotton and there, alone with your thoughts, use what remains of your will to turn your attention to the preferred subjects." Giraud believed the images and ideas an individual conjured up during a hashish state were a product of the self. Immersed in complete silence, the experimenter could experience his self in its raw state without the influence of external sensation. Initially, the will could act to provide a general direction for the hashish experience through focused thought, but during the hashish state the individual could not willfully control or anticipate what would happen next. Rather, he had no choice but to passively experience the state of *kif* in "magnificent panoramas that unfold on the screen of [the] brain."[177] While Richet had equated the self with the will, Giraud argued that it was only by incapacitating the will that one could experience one's true self.

The issue of control was a complex one for Giraud. Although he had to sit back and wait for the effects of hashish to take hold, as a scientific observer he was reluctant to lose control over the situation entirely. During a hashish experience in Rambouillet Forest, near Paris, Giraud recalled, "I suffered a lot to feel my will surrender in the face of so many ideas that I could no longer master." While he sought an altered state of consciousness, Giraud found the inability to master his own ideas disconcerting and attempted to control his experience through intellectual focus. "As I had submitted my brain to the test of an intellectual operation," he explained, "I had fewer hallucinations than if I had gazed carelessly into the gaps between the trees." Nevertheless, he still experienced some illusions, noting that "the object on which I fixed my eyes became one of those question-cards where in a drawing, one ends up distinguishing a cat, a shepherdess, a Prussian, etc."[178] As hashish distorted perceptions, maintaining a rational, intellectual focus proved to be an impossible task. He struggled to maintain self-control while searching for the deeper self-knowledge that he believed hashish had the power to reveal.

Giraud's work on how to vary the effects of hashish targeted individuals who wanted to enhance their experiences with the drug. There were other guides focused on ensuring that neophytes could experiment with hashish without harming themselves. An architect by profession, Ernest Bosc (1838–1913) was an enthusiastic supporter of self-experimentation with psychotropic drugs. In 1895, he published a study, *Theoretical and Practical Treatise on Hashish and Other Psychic Substances*, which enjoyed enough popularity for him to publish a second edition ten years later.[179] The study vacillates between encouraging readers to seek out the experiential wonders and pleasures of drug experimentation and cautioning users to avoid excess.

Bosc began his preface with the Latin epigraph *Uti et non abuti*, or "To use and not abuse." He acknowledged the dangers of abusing any drug to the point of addiction, of destroying one's mind in the insatiable pursuit of "artificial pleasures." However, he had no intention of preaching or moralizing to his readers. "It is impossible to halt the violent human passions," he explained, "so, we leave man at liberty to use drugs, but we give him recipes and practical advice to enable him to satisfy his favourite passion, without danger to his health." Bosc designed the book to serve as a practical guide to facilitate self-experimentation in relative safety, as "inexperienced smoker[s] commit great blunders."[180] Far from discouraging new users from experimenting with psychotropic drugs, his guide sought to facilitate the pursuit of artificial pleasures.

While Bosc intended the treatise to be useful to others, he candidly admitted that it would be "pure hypocrisy" to claim he had experimented with so many drugs solely with the interests of his readers in mind. "In truth," he wrote, "I began out of curiosity, to please a friend, then I indulged in the pleasure of my beautiful discoveries, and finally I used it out of taste, [I] admit it ... out of passion."[181] Bosc was not alone. Self-experimentation with hashish continued to entice doctors, artists, and intellectuals well into the twentieth century. In 1913, Jules Claretie, director of the Comédie Française, engaged in a hashish soirée with three friends that imitated the structure of the Hashish Eaters' Club.[182] Walter Benjamin first experimented with hashish in a Marseille hotel room in 1927 and for the next few years continued to experiment with it and document his impressions. His writings on the subject were published posthumously in a collection called *On Hashish*.[183] Diverse though their experiences were, self-experimenters used hashish to explore the complex contours of their own "inner life," as mind and body, will and reason, were divorced, fragmented, and distorted.

ADDICTION AND THE WILL

The allure of the sensory distortion and emotional expansion of the hashish fantasia or the opium dream was a double-edged sword. On the one hand, these psychotropic states produced the pleasure and excitement of expanded consciousness. On the other hand, with such

intense intellectual and sensory distortion many users feared a permanent loss of self or reason. In *Artificial Paradises*, Baudelaire wrote, "He
who would resort to a poison in order to think would soon be incapable
of thinking *without* the poison. Can you imagine this awful sort of
man whose paralyzed imagination can no longer function without the
benefit of hashish or opium?"[184] A laudanum addict for much of his life,
Baudelaire was better equipped than many to discuss the dangers of an
intellect dominated by a psychotropic substance.[185]

As numerous scholars have demonstrated, opium, like hashish, offered artists and intellectuals a vehicle to a sort of expanded consciousness,
which many believed could grant them access to a higher state of artistic
and intellectual production.[186] The privileged experiential knowledge to be
gleaned from an intimate encounter with a psychotropic substance could
unveil fantastic sights, sounds, and feelings that rational consciousness
normally suppressed. Yet opium, laudanum, and morphine were highly
addictive substances that did not yield their miraculous visions without a
price. For many, the seductive charms of an opium reverie soon gave way
to the prolonged agonies of physiological addiction. If free will was the
ultimate marker of robust Cousinian selfhood, morphine demonstrated
how tenuous and contingent that will actually was.

Self-experimentation was entangled with morphine research from the
very beginning. In 1817, Friedrich Wilhelm Sertürner, a German chemist
from Einbeck, published an article on morphine that led the medical
community to appreciate its therapeutic value. First he described the
chemical process by which he had isolated the crystal alkaloid. Then,
in a section titled "The Effects of Morphine on the Human Body," he
recounted the experiments he had conducted on himself and three
seventeen-year-olds in order to determine morphine's physiological
effects.[187] Initially, each of them, Sertürner included, took half a grain of
morphine (roughly 26.5 milligrams) dissolved in alcohol and distilled
water.[188] Sertürner noticed a general redness that spread over the faces
of his companions and even appeared in their eyes. He felt as though
his own vital forces had been exalted.

After thirty minutes, they all took another half grain of morphine.
They felt light-headed and experienced a passing desire to vomit.
"Without waiting for the effect," Sertürner admitted, "after a quarter
of an hour, we swallowed another half grain of morphine in a coarse

powder with several drops of alcohol and a half-ounce of water. The effect was sudden for the three young people; they felt a sharp pain in the stomach, a weakness, and a general numbness, and they were ready to faint." This experiment was extremely dangerous. Sertürner was researching a new, highly potent alkaloid and had no concept of what an appropriate dose might be. Jumping in headfirst with three unsuspecting youths, Sertürner had foolhardily consumed 1.5 grains of morphine (almost 80 milligrams) in less than an hour. After realizing that he had likely poisoned himself and his companions, Sertürner swallowed vinegar and made the others do the same. This elicited violent vomiting, clearing out the morphine remaining in their stomachs. For at least one of his subjects, "the lack of appetite, constipation, numbness and the head and stomach pain did not disappear until several days later." Sertürner's account of his morphine experiments demonstrates the danger of self-experimentation as a research methodology. He determined that "morphine is a violent poison, even in small doses," but only at the price of acute bodily crisis.[189] Consuming a substance many times more potent than opium, Sertürner very nearly martyred himself and three young men in the name of scientific research.

While Sertürner and his unsuspecting guinea pigs narrowly escaped death from acute morphine poisoning, morphine posed an additional danger to unwitting consumers in the form of slow, long-drawn-out addiction. A highly potent alkaloid, morphine has a nearly instantaneous effect when injected. Doctors only began to understand and research the pathological nature of morphine addiction in the late 1870s and early 1880s, by which point they had already been prescribing the drug for decades.[190] For experimenters fascinated by the idea of control – over pain, over their experiments, and over their own minds – morphine posed a formidable challenge.

For self-experimentation with opiates, researchers had to be careful to avoid slipping from controlled experimentation into unbridled addiction. Richet condemned the ease with which substances like opium and alcohol could entrap their users in a dangerous cycle of overuse.[191] Nevertheless, he took opium himself and, and as with hashish intoxication, he found the acute state of opium reverie appealing in its ethereal passivity. About an hour after taking opium and passing into a dream state, "you feel a certain pleasure in surrendering, and you let yourself be engulfed by a sweet torpor."[192] Richet described how ideas transformed into images and flowed rapidly without control. At first, during the pseudo-dream state, the user could still perceive the sounds from outside, but soon he retreated into an interior world. "The active, conscious, voluntary self no longer exists," explained Richet, "and you imagine that another individual has come to replace it. Little by little all becomes vaguer, ideas lose themselves in a confused haze, you have become entirely immaterial, you no longer feel your body, you are all mind."[193] Through this psychotropic Cartesian separation, Richet was able to explore his underlying mental substance in an appealingly cerebral space.

In 1893, Dr Ernest Chambard published a lengthy monograph on morphine addiction, in which he reproduced Richet's account of his opium reverie. Chambard described Richet as a researcher who "joined the gifts of a brilliant imagination to the most rigorous scientific mind." Richet experimented with opium in the stage "before dependence dispelled its mysterious and fleeting charm."[194] Thus, although he temporarily abandoned his "active, conscious, voluntary" self to the experiment, he did not suffer the lasting torments of opium addiction. Chambard and other early addiction researchers acknowledged the very real dangers of addiction; however, this did not prevent them from engaging in self-experimentation. Echoing his old mentor, Moreau de Tours, Chambard claimed that "in order to truly appreciate the euphoric properties of a morphine injection to their full extent and intensity, one must practice on oneself." He described the simultaneous calming and exciting influence of the drug that stimulated the intellectual faculties and allowed for the elaboration and association of ideas so that "a few moments after the injection, it seems as though a bright ray of sunshine finally pierces the dark clouds and illuminates all existence."[195] Like Richet, Chambard acknowledged only the personal experience of the acute euphoric state of morphine intoxication, not the prolonged condition of morphine addiction. In this manner, he distinguished himself from his addicted patients, constructing himself as a scientific researcher rather than a slave to addiction. Once again, free will and self-control were deployed to legitimize self-experimentation. Some of his colleagues were less fortunate. Georges Pichon, one of the leading experts on *morphinomanie*, was also one of morphine's harshest critics.[196] Nevertheless, Pichon died in 1893, at the age of thirty-two, as a result of his entrenched morphine addiction.[197] For him at least, free will was unable to overcome the overpowering need for morphine.

For many unfortunate individuals, self-experimentation led to a chronicle of morphine addiction. The diary of Dr X, a French physician based in colonial Indochina, elucidates the unequal power dynamics between a morphine addict and the drug that became the primary focus of his entire existence.[198] In 1896, the Lyons review *Archives d'anthropologie criminelle, médecine légale et de psychologie normale et pathologique* published long extracts of the late Dr X's diary, as transcribed by Dr Gouzer, the senior naval doctor who attended to the deceased morphine addict during the last weeks of his life. The diary covered fifteen years of Dr X's life, between October 1880 and March 1894, during which time morphine steadily and relentlessly seized control of his body and mind.[199]

Dr X's diary documented a lengthy and agonizing experiment in addiction. It served simultaneously as a repository for his subjective impressions and a log of empirical data he collected about himself. He used it to measure himself, recording his doses of morphine, his withdrawal symptoms, and his mental and physical states. At times, it resembles a medical case file more than a personal journal. The intense emotions of frustration, fear, and longing Dr X experienced on a daily basis and the physical miseries of withdrawal when he missed an injection demonstrate morphine's incredible dominance over him. Throughout his fifteen-year addiction, morphine regulated his daily routine, his thoughts, his actions, his health, his bodily functions, and ultimately his sense of self. Yet by measuring and recording these things, the diary served, however imperfectly, as a technology of self-discipline. Dr X was both the subject and the object of the diary, the physician who was also his own patient.

In the opening entry from 2 October 1880, Dr X wrote, "I am truly used to this morphine and I have nothing but thanks for it. I am paler, but much more active and content, almost never in bad mood now. I will continue until I clearly see a harmful effect."[200] Unfortunately, he either did not observe or refused to acknowledge morphine's "harmful effects" until addiction held him tightly in its grip. During its early stages, Dr X found morphine to be intellectually stimulating and liberating, claiming, "I have never worked with such great ease."[201] However, morphine imposed a regulatory time that increasingly began to shape his daily routine. Soon his syringe was the first thing he reached for in the morning. "How can you resist," he lamented, "when, suffering terribly, being half-dead, unable to move or even speak, you know that a new dose of poison suffices to put you back on your feet[?]"[202] The need to inject morphine at specific times made it difficult for Dr X to work. He used morphine while on duty, but it was often difficult to balance his dosage. Too much morphine made it difficult to focus.[203] Yet without a maintenance dose of morphine it was impossible for him to function at all. For nine years, Dr X admitted, "I have been a real patient, an invalid, a slave to the most tyrannical mania, in the end, not at all a man like other men. The marvellous thing is that I was able to hide it."[204]

As an addict, Dr X constantly worried about securing an adequate supply of morphine. In colonial Indochina, opium for smoking was readily available, but morphine was often in short supply and had to be shipped from Europe.[205] Dr X seemed to receive regular shipments of morphine via courier.[206] In the earlier years of his addiction, he received shipments of 5 to 10 grams of morphine at a time, but by the summer of 1884 he began to receive shipments of 60 grams. Unfortunately, the relatively slow pace of colonial shipping networks, with sometimes unforeseen delays, clashed with Dr X's urgent need to satisfy his addiction. While he occasionally supplemented these shipments with small amounts of morphine from a local pharmacy, doing so made him nervous because he feared his addiction would be discovered.[207] Dr X was constantly plagued by the frustrations of mediating a metropolitan addiction in a colonial space.

Dr X's physiological dependence on morphine caused him to obsess over securing his next dose. When a shipment was late he panicked, afraid of the physical and mental consequences of morphine withdrawal on his person. After receiving a shipment he felt relief, but frequent binges plunged him into fear and despair. Every time he resolved to reduce his dose, morphine tightened its grip on him. During a short trip in January 1885, Dr X exclaimed in anguish, "What did I forget? My little trunk where all my morphine is!!! And I won't be able to have it for eight days. It's terrible, what am I going to do? I am frightened!"[208] He often tried to view periods of scarcity as an opportunity to overcome his addiction. Yet, agonizing withdrawal always led him to seek out alternatives, including laudanum, opium pills, opium extract – which he found disgusting – and, in desperation, the occasional opium pipe.[209]

Dr X occasionally acquired morphine duplicitously by exploiting his status as a colonial physician. In April 1885, he wrote, "Undreamed of good luck! I found 12 grams of morphine sulphate at the sisters' hospice that they willingly gave me. This time I promise to get better by reducing slowly but without relapses. Can I do it?"[210] Another time he wrote, "Found morphine. I will be able to give it back again in exactly a month. But don't want to return to abuse any more as I have done formerly."[211] Whether deceiving nursing sisters or "borrowing" morphine to tide him over when his supplies ran short, Dr X's moral flexibility in these cases demonstrates morphine's inexorable power over him. For over fifteen years, morphine consumed his thoughts as he exercised all of his mental energy securing his next dose.

Morphine consumed Dr X's body as well as his mind. Extensive morphine injections cause considerable physical damage. The morphine addict's skin hardens at the injection site. According to Benjamin Ball, one of Moreau's former interns and a leading morphine researcher, "patients wear out their needles rapidly and are constantly obliged to replace them" because the points of the needles become so dull that they "can no longer penetrate this thickened leather … the arms of certain subjects resemble slotted spoons."[212] The body's natural defences produce this hardening and pocking of the skin. Abscesses – collections of pus that form on the skin at the site of an injection – serve as a defence mechanism against infection by drawing white blood cells to the afflicted area and forming an abscess wall to separate the infected tissue from the healthy skin surrounding it. With prolonged use, abscesses become more and more common, making it difficult for the addict to find a place to inject that has not already been damaged. In 1882, after an abdominal abscess had bothered him for ten days, Dr X wrote, "Yesterday after supper I applied Vienna paste [to the abscess]. This afternoon, I opened the abscess with a lancet. 83 grams of thick pus came out of it. I felt relieved immediately; but I am anemic, exhausted, I still had a fever during the night."[213] His grotesquely specific measurement of the pus from his abscess is indicative of the kind of quantitative measurements he kept on himself in his journal. These measurements, which could be controlled and documented with absolute precision, served as a counterpoint to the addiction itself, which he could neither fully understand nor overcome.

In October 1892, ten years after he documented his first abscess, Dr X bemoaned his frightful physical condition. He had two enormous abscesses on his sides, one on his right side that extended down to his waist where another was threatening to form, a smaller one on his belly, another near his groin, and a final abscess on his right buttock, all of which were extremely painful and limited his movement. Although Dr X spent the whole morning tending to his wounds, "nevertheless I did my duty [at the hospital] as I am afraid people will come to know. What misery! Poor me!" Two days later he described that it was painful to get into bed as the abscesses had still not opened. He wondered, "Will I be able to get dressed tomorrow and go to work, still hiding the truth?"[214] A few days later the large abscess on his side was weighing him down "like a ball of lead." After garnering his courage, he punctured it: "What a relief!!!"[215] Dr X's journal is filled with descriptions, measurements, and complaints of the abscesses that painfully inscribed the history of his addiction onto his body.

The physical transformations that Dr X considered side effects of his morphine addiction were intimately connected to his sense of self. He viewed himself as different from other men, connecting his morphine use to his perceived loss of masculinity. He blamed morphine for his persistent sexual indifference.[216] He also believed it was responsible for his hair loss and rapidly aging appearance. In 1884, after many half-hearted and unsuccessful attempts to cure his addiction, he wrote, "Two large considerations have made me decide to renounce morphine: 1) regaining vigour and hair; 2) becoming a man like other men once more, full of energy every day and at every hour, which I am not now and of which I am ashamed."[217] Dr X believed morphine was draining the youthful vitality he believed he should have had at the age of thirty-five. He was acutely aware of its degenerative impact on his appearance and sense of self. He complained constantly of his misery and his lack of control. When he reduced his morphine consumption, he observed his hair regrowing darker.[218] Still, he could never fully extricate himself from the grip of that "adored and dreadful morphine."[219]

In December 1887, after fixing his only remaining syringe, which had broken, he was almost sorry to have succeeded. He explained,

"I wanted finally to cure this disease that for seven-and-a-half years has poisoned my animal life while sometimes consoling my intellectual life. But the advantage is not in proportion to the disadvantage and I will not believe myself to be a complete and robust man except at such time as I shall be cured." Morphine transformed Dr X's very conceptualization of himself as a man. The physical misery and weakness of his poisoned animal life sullied his perceptions of self. "This mania would never have seized me," he complained, "or I would not have become undone so quickly if my life was not so abnormal, if my faculties had real and active employment. All the damage comes from there. I was made for a very different life than that which my position and circumstances have accorded me. It's the slavery that made me vicious."[220] His miseries were forcefully connected to his inability to exercise control over his own body and actions, let alone factors outside of his control. Morphine had made him a slave to the caprices of his unruly addicted body.

Dr X returned to France permanently in 1891. Over the next three years he continued to struggle with his addiction, his loneliness, and his isolation, still hopeful of curing himself. He began to lose more and more weight and his journal entries became more frequent. He seems to have been aware that the end was near. As Dr X repeatedly injected morphine it increasingly regulated his life, reframing his self-perceptions and reshaping the contours of his body. His morphine habit was self-destructive in the most literal sense of the term, for through his chronic morphine abuse he felt his human essence slipping away from him. Mentally consumed by the desperate need to secure his next dose and physically consumed by the abscesses that cratered his skin, he was no longer himself. He was altered physically, mentally, and emotionally, a decrepit fossil of the vibrant youth he had once been.

Tragic examples like the case of Dr X were often not enough to dissuade individual curiosity. In 1909, three decades after French doctors began to seriously research and document the dangers of morphine addiction, Louis Fauchier began his research for a remarkable medical thesis, *Contribution to the Study of the Morphine Dream and Morphinomania*. Acknowledging that many magisterial studies on *morphinomanie* had already been published, Fauchier explained that the originality of his work lay in his experimentation with morphine on himself. He wanted to provide a scrupulous and honest account of the state of "morphine delirium."[221] Maintaining professional credibility while gaining first-hand knowledge of the "delirium" produced by a highly addictive substance was challenging. Fauchier explained, "I won't have the nerve to claim that I was driven to my experiment only out of scientific curiosity; there is always something unhealthy in the heart of man. However, I can say that in advance, I sorted out the conditions of my attempt; I did want to *morphinise* myself, but I was just as resolved to not intoxicate myself irreversibly."[222] To avoid an entrenched addiction, Fauchier decided to perform two rounds of experiments spaced fifteen days apart. In each round he administered an injection, the amount of which increased each day for six days.

Fauchier began his first round of experiments by injecting 1 centigram of morphine hydrochloride into his outer thigh. At first, he felt minor discomforts, including vague joint pain, stomach cramps, and an acute sensitivity to light and sound. Once he extinguished his lamp, plunging the room into darkness, he "began to understand morphine's euphoria." He experienced no hallucinations or illusions, but, he explained, "The night was sweet to me; I can hardly express the bliss I experienced in any other way." Ease and satisfaction defined the experience. In this state of bliss he felt powerful. "Everything that was once difficult appeared easy to me," Fauchier noted, "certain problems of real life presented themselves to me in a new form [and] provided me with ready-made solutions. I was there, motionless, frozen, sprawled on my back, eyes closed, arms alongside my body, satisfied, wanting nothing."[223] Eventually, he fell asleep around five o'clock in the morning and woke up without somatic troubles.

On the second day of the experiment, Fauchier injected the same dose of morphine and experienced the same preliminary symptoms of discomfort. His description of his experience that night was brief: "Same euphoria, same complete satisfaction after exactly twenty minutes. However, this time, the serenity didn't last as long." Afterward, he experienced agitation and irritating insomnia. The third evening, he doubled his dose to 2 centigrams of morphine. After fifteen minutes he experienced a distressing sensation of vertigo, followed by "a veiled harmony, vague, distant, but delightful." After observing that a higher dose extended his feeling of well-being, Fauchier took an even higher dose the following day: 2.5 centigrams. This time, his body reacted badly.

Instead of ethereal calm and satisfaction, he spent the night in discomfort. After fifteen minutes of painful vomiting, he drank a litre of tepid water to try to absorb the morphine. An hour later he fell asleep, exhausted. In the morning he woke very pale and without appetite. Nevertheless, he rallied his energies during the day and by the evening, he noted, "I was ready to do it again. Besides, I wanted my injection more than ever. The habit had taken hold. I could not have slept."[224]

After four short days of experiments, Fauchier already felt the siren call of *morphinomanie*. In spite of this, he continued to increase his doses – to 3 centigrams and then 3.5 centigrams – to finish out his first series of injections. In less than a week, he had gone from waking up with a good appetite and functioning well during the day to experiencing frustrating insomnia, being unable to eat breakfast, vomiting in the morning, and experiencing "great weariness and irresistible sleep" in the afternoon after his fifth injection. On the last of six nights, with 3.5 centigrams of morphine coursing through his body, Fauchier wrote, "The euphoria came on cue. However, it was crossed through with frights."[225] The fire in his room cast terrifying shadows. He hallucinated the sounds of furniture moving and cats meowing. The hallucinations were so vivid that when he felt the touching melody of a song envelop him, he found himself crying without understanding why.

Although Fauchier claimed that he would provide a "true description" of morphine's dream state, he found the task exceedingly difficult. Instead, his thesis documented his struggle to resist addiction. His narrative focused more on his body's physiological experiences of dependence and withdrawal than any specific knowledge gleaned from his "morphine dreams." Perhaps in an effort to reassert his status as an objective medical professional in the face of the outpouring of emotion and loss of control over his body's desires, Fauchier clarified his experimental process. He noted that "all my solutions were prepared by myself, in the most aseptic way and rigorously dosed."[226] After re-establishing his scientific credibility through an appeal to hygiene and precision, Fauchier launched into his account of the auditory hallucinations of that final night.

Fauchier's body, accustomed to the drug after the gradually increasing injections, rebelled against his sudden abstinence. After the fifth injection, when he had lost much of his appetite, he experienced "persistent constipation," which he treated with laxatives. The day after his final injection, he anticipated that he would experience the desire to inject at his normal hour. He dreaded the agonies of withdrawal, so he took precautions to distract himself. He dined out in the city, went drinking with friends, and attended a spectacle, but he found everything tedious. Nevertheless, the diversions kept him out late, and when he returned at daybreak he was able to sleep a bit. The following night, he medicated himself with 50 centigrams of Véronal, a barbiturate sleep aid. However, he noted, "The following days at the critical hour, I invariably thought of my injection, I wanted it. I was able to restrain myself." By acknowledging the abiding desire for an injection, Fauchier cited his own self-control even as he exposed that his body's desires were attempting to overrule those of his mind. Yet, that self-control was tenuous. "I was very proud of not having yielded to the acquired inclination," he admitted. "However, if I had examined myself harshly, I would have noticed with what impatience I awaited the licit time to fall back into my habit."[227] Fauchier felt the chemical yearnings of morphine addiction. Within the structured environment of the experiment, he tried to establish and maintain his self-control as morphine gradually eroded it.

Fauchier began his second round of injections with an initial dose of 2 centigrams and increased it by 1 centigram per day until he reached a maximum dose of 7 centigrams. Rather than documenting his experiments each night in this second round, he described more general sensations and experiences under the influence of morphine. One of these, which he had not previously experienced, was a "conscious delirium" in which his personality was completely doubled. His "reasonable self" retired to the shadows, leaving only his "delusional self," to think, speculate, and imagine things. "This portion of the intelligence is developed to the highest degree," he explained. "It is extraordinarily enhanced."[228] Fauchier's two selves operated independently. While the "delusional self" took charge, the reasonable self faded into the background, observing and admiring the "delusional self," which was amplified during the morphine reverie.

Morphine was a formidable drug. The seductive charms of the cerebral experiences it promised lured users into the chemical entrenchment of addiction. Fauchier claimed that he consumed only twelve injections, totalling less than 40 centigrams of morphine. Yet these few injections revealed "on a small scale" how powerful an addict's state of need could be. Enticed by the morphine dreams, he "glimpsed the imminence of a frightful danger."[229] Fauchier and other self-experimenters experienced physiological disturbances brought on by morphine withdrawal. They witnessed the very real limitations of their own free will when faced with the material necessity of continuing to inject.

Doctors, pharmacists, and other men of science engaged in self-experimentation to produce essential knowledge about precisely how psychotropic drugs affected the human mind and body. Self-experimentation endowed them with the incomparable authority of personal experience. However, as a research method it was dangerous. Researchers imposed structures and safeguards on their experiments to reduce the risk of accidents. Nevertheless, they risked possible asphyxiation, mutilation, death, madness, and addiction. Doctors emphasized their willingness to sacrifice themselves in the name of science. For many self-experimenters, though, their professional commitment to scientific inquiry was bound to a more personal curiosity to explore the self by using drugs to expose the unconscious faculties hidden in the corners of their minds.

Self-experimentation involved a power struggle between the will of the experimenter and the psychotropic action of the drug. In the ether experiments of 1847, experimenters strove to exercise their own free will as objective men of science, even as they undermined it with a material substance that transformed their consciousness. While willing to objectify their bodies as experimental tools, these ether experimenters were uneasy about doing the same to their minds. For others, however, this mental subjugation became the goal of their experimentation. The Hashish Eaters, for example, revelled in the lack of free will that characterized the experience. Through hashish they could access a deeper level of consciousness without being constrained by will or reason. In this way, they sought to discover the stuff of selfhood. For morphine experimenters, the issue of the will was even more fraught. Over time, morphine's chemical action within the user's brain produced a physiological addiction that overpowered his will. The Cousinian vision of a unified self governed by individual free will became a crucial tenet of bourgeois society in the nineteenth century. However, self-experimentation with psychotropic drugs revealed the extent to which free will was subordinated to the body's chemical imperatives.

{ 3 }

DRUGGING
THE MIND

Morphine exerts such a dominating effect ...
that it takes the entire functioning of the
human machine under its control.
–Henri Guimbail (1891)

French doctors were intrigued by morphine's demonstrable power over the human mind. They hoped to harness this power to cure madness. In the mid-nineteenth century, doctors mobilized drugs in the asylums to regulate their patients' minds, intending to coax them back to a state of reason. Drugs regulated the duration and intensity of hysterical attacks. They calmed mania. In some cases, morphine appeared to be an elixir of sanity. Yet, by the mid-1880s, medical enthusiasm had waned as doctors observed a new pathology sweeping the asylums: *morphinomanie,* or "morphine mania."

Addiction as a concept developed slowly and tentatively. While doctors had long observed that patients could become accustomed to morphine with prolonged use, the medical community only began to recognize morphine addiction as a pathological condition in and of itself in the early 1880s. Addicts seemed to have an overpowering physiological dependence on morphine. Through clinical research, doctors began to realize the extent to which addiction was a disease of their own making.

However, in the 1880s it did not face quite the same stigma it would acquire in the twentieth century. Many addicts had become addicted in the course of medical treatment. Furthermore, there was a great deal of uncertainty about the nature of addiction as a mental pathology. This raised pressing questions about addiction and criminal responsibility when addicted defendants began to use the insanity defence to argue that morphine had led them to theft, blackmail, and murder. Medical-legal experts had to determine how morphine influenced intelligence, morality, and free will in order to classify addicted defendants on a spectrum from the legally sane to the criminally irresponsible.

This medico-legal question of responsibility was bound up with a larger exploration of the power of drugs over the mind. In the ostensibly meritocratic society of post-Revolutionary France, bourgeois men appealed to their own supposedly superior reason and self-control to justify their socio-political dominance.[1] However, drugs had the power to compromise both. With prolonged use, morphine upended the expected power dynamics between human subject and material object. Examining the action of psychotropic drugs over the human mind complicated the traditional view of the liberal self as autonomous, rational, and driven by free will. Instead, it invited a different view of the self – an embodied self in which reason and free will had to contend with the body's chemical imperatives.

A CURE FOR MADNESS?

For psychotropic drugs to become useful therapeutic tools in France's asylums, doctors first had to accept that the treatment of madness was not only possible but desirable. During the Old Regime, mental patients had been confined alongside other socially marginalized groups – the indigent poor, the aged, the criminal – within the large institutions that comprised Louis XIV's Hôpital Général. The misleadingly named Hôpital Général had no explicitly medical purpose and functioned as an institution of incarceration to protect society from undesirable elements.[2] However, the Enlightenment inspired French thinkers to interrogate the origins of madness. In his 1746 *Essay on the Origins of Human Knowledge*, Étienne Bonnot de Condillac defined insanity as a confused imagination that "associates ideas in an entirely disorderly fashion and sometimes influences our judgments or our conduct."[3] While everyone occasionally experienced "eccentricities of imagination," the madman had difficulty distinguishing imagination from reality. Condillac did not view madmen as fundamentally "other." Instead, they existed on a spectrum between reason and insanity.[4] Mental pathology was relative rather than absolute.[5] Therefore, by the late eighteenth century, medical writing assumed that curing insanity was at least theoretically possible, albeit unlikely.[6]

This idea of madness as a mental imbalance rather than an inherent pathology encouraged doctors to move beyond incarceration for its own sake to develop specialized institutions designed to treat mental patients. However, by 1818, France only had eight mental asylums that served 5,153 patients.[7] Alienists – as specialists in the treatment of mental illness were called in the nineteenth century – campaigned for almost two decades to create a national asylum system in France. Ultimately, they succeeded during the July Monarchy with the passage of the Asylum Law of 30 June 1838, which required each *département* to have a public mental asylum.[8] This law solidified the reputation of alienists as medical specialists and expanded their professional authority. By 1899, France had many private asylums that served wealthy patients and an extensive public asylum system, serving over 64,000 patients.[9] The isolation of mental patients in asylums served two purposes: it wed the goal of maintaining social order outside the asylums with the goal of curing mental illness within them.[10] Thus, during the nineteenth century, Salpêtrière and Bicêtre – the same hospitals that had served primarily as generalized institutions of incarceration during the Old Regime – were transformed into specialized centres for the research and treatment of mental illness. Psychotropic drugs would prove instrumental to this work.

The therapies employed to treat mental patients in the early nineteenth century reflected a reorientation of thinking about mental illness. The sensationalist philosophy of the Enlightenment – which held that an individual's physical and mental conditions influenced one another – had increased medical emphasis on the mental realm.[11] Philippe Pinel (1745–1826) concluded that insanity could exist independent of discernible brain lesions and that madness with moral causes could and should be treated with "moral remedies." As chief physician of the Salpêtrière Hospital, Pinel popularized a new method for curing madness known as the "moral treatment." Unlike treatments such as purging and bloodletting, which acted upon the patient's body, the "moral treatment" acted directly upon the mind by manipulating the patient's emotions and imagination using gentleness, curative "ruses," distraction, and diversion to restore calm and sanity.[12]

Historians of French psychiatry have emphasized the significance of the "moral treatment" in realizing the political ideals of the French Revolution. The moral treatment's emphasis on "gentleness" and methods that acted on the intellect provided a stark contrast to the "regime of chains" of previous centuries.[13] Although incarcerating mental patients deprived them of their fundamental right to liberty as citizens, using the moral treatment to attempt to cure them in a humane manner took into consideration their essential humanity and "capacity for freedom."[14] Nevertheless, despite its political salience, the moral treatment was only one of several methods used to treat mental illness. Clinical practitioners continued to use physical treatments including cold showers, bleeding, and purging in conjunction with treatments that acted upon the mind.[15] They also turned to drugs.

Even Pinel, the champion of the moral treatment, had recourse to opium in the most intractable cases. In his 1801 monograph on mental alienation, Pinel acknowledged that "it is when the attacks are exacerbated in duration and violence, and when periodic mania, regular or irregular, threatens to become fatal or to degenerate into continuous mania, that one should look for powerful assistance in the use of baths, showers, opium, camphor, and other antispasmodics."[16] He was cautious with the use of opium, prescribing it only in cases that "do not yield to moral remedies," including religious melancholia, delirium, regular intermittent mania, and maniac fury without delirium, a particularly intractable condition where the patient experienced "the most refined malice, or the horrible instinct of tigers and wild beasts." While it was useful in certain cases, Pinel cautioned, "until now I could only do imperfect tests on the use of opium ... and I am waiting for the establishment of a systematic treatment of the insane in asylums to make them more complete."[17] Despite the lack of sufficient clinical research, even the most reserved psychiatrists mobilized opium to combat particularly difficult cases.[18]

Early nineteenth-century psychiatry saw a growing interest in the use of drug therapies, not only to treat symptoms but to try to cure mental illness. In the 1840s, as the psychiatric profession was in the process of establishing itself as a legitimate specialty, efficient and effective remedies for mental illness were extremely limited. While the moral treatment had many proponents, the curative ruses and performative elements of this highly individualized treatment method required significant time and resources in an asylum system that was chronically underfunded and overcrowded.[19] Therefore, asylum doctors began to conduct clinical research on drug therapies, which were far simpler and less time consuming to administer.

Psychotropic drugs offered exciting therapeutic possibilities. Doctors were eager to test their efficacy as analgesics, anesthetics, and consciousness modifiers.[20] The effect of psychotropic drugs on the human mental apparatus varied widely, according to the dose administered and the particular nature of the patient's constitution and mental condition. As it was difficult to determine precisely *how* psychotropic drugs operated on the human mental apparatus, doctors began with the assumption that any substance that could provoke a change in a patient's mental state merited further clinical investigation.[21]

Historical scholarship on French asylums has focused disproportionately on the experiences of female patients.[22] During the nineteenth century, doctors believed that women were more vulnerable to mental illness than men because of their irrational, emotional natures and the pathological influence of their reproductive bodies.[23] Despite these biased assumptions about their inherent pathology, women were not a significant majority of the patients admitted to France's asylums.[24] Asylum doctors conducted clinical drug research on both male and female patients. While some worked at private *maisons de santé* or regional asylums, the vast majority of clinical research on drugs took place at two large public asylums in Paris: Bicêtre for men and Salpêtrière for women. These institutions served patients of modest means who could not afford to pay for private care in a *maison de santé*.[25] While doctors conducted clinical research on both men and women, the segregated nature of France's asylum wards meant that case studies of one sex tended to predominate in medical treatises on a particular drug.[26]

Doctors transformed their asylum wards into sites of medical experimentation. In France's large state-sponsored hospitals, doctors developed a new form of clinical medicine that cemented Paris's international reputation as the centre of medical science in the first half of the nineteenth century.[27] Doctors could observe thousands of patients in specialized hospital wards, which enabled them to create statistical analyses of particular medical conditions and conduct clinical research on possible treatments. However, while clinical research was central to Paris's scientific reputation, it was not always intentional or systematic. Early drug research at Bicêtre and Salpêtrière often began as a result of curiosity, hunches, or fortunate therapeutic accidents. Doctors developed new treatment protocols through trial and error. Through observation and experimentation, they developed various theories to account for the success of psychotropic drugs in treating certain kinds of mental pathologies. This research exposed the blurred boundaries between treatment and experimentation in Paris's new clinical medicine.

Dr Jacques-Joseph Moreau de Tours conducted groundbreaking research on hashish, opium, and datura stramonium to treat mental illness in the 1840s. He championed self-experimentation as a research methodology.[28] Moreau believed that personal experience of the artificial madness produced by hashish was crucial to the psychiatric researcher's understanding of the enigmatic condition known as "madness." He also believed that the very same properties that could provoke a temporary state of madness in a sane individual could be used therapeutically to return a madman to sanity.[29] Moreau adopted the theory that mental disorders were rooted in organic lesions of the nervous system.[30] However, he acknowledged that the organic lesion was only a mediate cause of mental alienation, and its immediate cause remained unknown. Even as late as 1869, by which point he had been studying and treating mental alienation for over forty years, Moreau admitted that the pathological basis of most forms of delirium was "more or less completely unknown and surpasses all our means of investigation."[31]

By self-experimenting with hashish the psychiatrist could become a madman temporarily, in order to observe the effects of this artificial madness on his own mind and body. After ingesting hashish, an individual "witnesses the rapid dissolution of his capacity to think; he feels his thoughts, his mental activity, carried away by the same whirlwind which agitates the cerebral molecules affected by the toxic action of hashish." Moreau noted, "I doubt that anyone who attempts this experiment and who thus temporarily becomes psychotic will ever be of the opinion that the body is of little importance in mental disturbance. Instinctively, through deep insight, the mind tends to identify with the organs in order to materialize."[32] For Moreau, madness was highly contingent upon the connections between mind and body. He hoped that hashish, a substance that could produce temporary madness in a healthy individual, could produce sanity in a madman.

Despite Moreau's enthusiasm for hashish, its success as a treatment for madness was limited. After having experimented extensively on himself and his friends and colleagues in the early 1840s, Moreau administered *dawamesk* (hashish paste) to patients on his service at Bicêtre, the large public asylum for men in Paris. He observed no change in mute psychotics or patients with dementia. Two of the depressives experienced "strong reactions" to the hashish, but when the excitement passed they returned to their previous states. Unwilling to admit utter defeat, he noted that he had only a small supply of hashish to administer and that using it to cure madness might work with a higher dose.[33]

Moreau did not give up. In 1856, Benjamin Ball, one of Moreau's interns at Bicêtre, published the case of a twenty-six-year-old man suffering from mental disturbances, which included auditory hallucinations of mewling kittens. After showers, quinine, and belladonna had all failed to cure him, Moreau treated him with hashish extract over the course of three days to produce a "complete disturbance of his ideas." After this heightened disturbance caused by the hashish had dissipated, the patient was cured of his hallucinations.[34] The patient was released from Bicêtre a few weeks later, fully cured. By exacerbating his patients' symptoms, Moreau used drugs to shock them back to sanity.[35]

Moreau's enthusiasm for hashish made an impression on his colleagues. In 1868, Pierre Berthier, the chief physician at Bicêtre, published a short essay on the hypnotic properties of hashish in treating mental illness. He had discovered the therapeutic virtues of hashish by accident, when an agitated insomniac patient experiencing continuous hallucinations fell into a deep twelve-hour sleep after swallowing all at once a mixture of hashish that was supposed to have been spread out over the course of the day. Through clinical experimentation, Berthier determined that doses of hashish under 5 centigrams produced excitement while doses over 5 centigrams had a sedative effect. Although Berthier acknowledged that the therapeutic use of hashish was generally quite limited in France, he claimed to have administered hashish to eighty-six of his patients at Bicêtre and noted that many among these had benefited from its hypnotic effects.[36] Whereas Moreau had treated hashish as a cure for madness, his colleague Berthier used it as a palliative treatment for its symptoms, particularly agitation and insomnia. Although psychiatrists periodically experimented with hashish over the course of the nineteenth century, outside of Moreau's circle at Bicêtre the drug never gained a widespread reputation as a cure for madness.[37]

Ether offered another possibility for treating mental illness. Beginning in 1847, members of the Academy of Medicine and the Academy of Sciences engaged in a veritable frenzy of research on the use of ether and chloroform for general anesthesia.[38] While enthusiastic surgeons and physicians peppered Parisian medical journals with accounts of their experiments with ether as an anesthetic, Moreau de Tours began researching its impact on the nervous system and motor functions. He hoped to use ether to treat the convulsions of epilepsy, a condition that many psychiatrists considered to be incurable as it was resistant to most medications.[39]

To determine whether administering ether could prevent epileptic attacks, Moreau conducted a clinical experiment at Bicêtre on a random sample of nine epileptic men. He compiled a chart of the number of attacks each patient experienced between August 1846 and January 1847 in the absence of treatment. Then, he added statistics for February and March 1847, when the patients were treated with ether every morning (Figure 3.1). Moreau's research was on the cutting edge. The two months during which he administered ether to his epileptic patients coincided with the initial wave of ether research at the Academy of Sciences and the Academy of Medicine.

The duration and action of ether varied incredibly between patients and even with the same patient over time. One day a patient might become insensible after three to five minutes of inhalations while the next day it might take more than twenty minutes. Moreau cautioned that if a doctor did not make sure to stop administering the ether immediately at the first signs of stupor, the patient was likely to experience a nervous

	Août.	Sept.	Oct.	Nov.	Déc.	Janv.	Févr.	Mars.
Moussard,	7	5	3	6	4	28	8	0
Laroche,	51	69	41	55	59	52	20	25
Gazou,	12	6	10	11	14	14	5	5
Thévenin,	18	19	18	29	14	22	21	13
Rouyer,	0	2	5	12	0	4	8	9
Maurice.	0	0	2	10	0	0	3	4
Petit,	0	0	2	6	2	1	1	3
Martin,	4	7	5	4	3	3	5	2
De Lanoy,	2	1	3	1	0	2	1	0

3.1 Moreau's table of the number of epileptic attacks patients
experienced each month from August 1846 to March 1847.
During the last two months (February and March 1847), patients
were treated with ether in an attempt to prevent their attacks.

accident very like his normal epileptic attacks.[40] Despite his high hopes
for a cure, however, Moreau observed that ether had only relieved the
epileptic attacks of a single patient.[41] Nevertheless, in 1848 the journal
Annales médico-psychologiques reprinted Moreau's observations on
epilepsy. Although his research indicated that in certain cases ether
could exacerbate a patient's epileptic attacks, the journal's editor noted
that "this is certainly no reason to give up any kind of experimentation;
but it must be done within certain limits."[42] While they recommended
caution, doctors seem to have had few qualms about using their mental
patients as guinea pigs in the name of medical progress.

While Moreau created distinct clinical experiments to test drugs'
therapeutic potential, most psychopharmacological research in the 1840s
was more piecemeal. Some observations were accidental. For example,
at Salpêtrière, the large public women's asylum in Paris, Jean-Pierre
Falret found that ether had no effect on a patient's delirium when he
administered it to her during an unrelated surgical procedure.[43] This
observation was a contingency of clinical practice rather than a deliberate
psychopharmacological experiment. More often, psychiatrists published
reports on isolated cases in which they used ether or chloroform to
treat mental illness. These treatments often had mixed results. At the
Academy of Sciences in June 1847, Dr Lemaitre presented the results of

two cases in which he used ether to treat epilepsy. For the first patient, ether served merely to make his epileptic attacks shorter and less severe. For the second patient, ether initially exacerbated the patient's intense delirium and agitation. After prolonged etherization over the course of three days, however, Lemaitre observed that the patient's delirium ceased and he returned to a perfect state of health.[44] Dr Achille Requin achieved a similar result using chloroform to treat a male hysteric in 1849. The patient, Charles M…, had experienced hysterical crises every four months since the age of fifteen. While chloroform inhalations had initially seemed to exacerbate his nervous symptoms, after a few seconds his hysterical attack ceased completely. Requin reported that the patient left the asylum two days later, fully cured.[45]

Although these and other isolated case studies inspired optimism among certain practitioners, ether and chloroform were only rarely used as curative remedies. Much more commonly, doctors and asylum staff used these gases as palliative remedies to treat and manage nervous attacks, agitation, and other symptoms of intractability among their patients. Despite their somewhat unsatisfactory results, these early nineteenth-century experiments with hashish, ether, and chloroform demonstrate that psychiatrists explored many different avenues in pursuit of a pharmacological cure for madness. By mid-century, however, one psychotropic remedy had emerged as a clear favourite.

Opium was one of the oldest remedies in the psychological pharmacopoeia. By the nineteenth century, it had already been used to treat madness in Europe for centuries. Paracelsus (1493–1541) and seventeenth-century Dutch physician Bernard Heute had both used opium's sedative properties to treat mania.[46] In the nineteenth century, opium's versatility and manifest psychotropic action made it the most popular pharmacological treatment for madness.

Around mid-century, reports of isolated cases suggested that opium could be used to cure mania and delirium.[47] Moreau de Tours, who saw therapeutic utility in any substance that acted directly upon the mind, experimented with opium as he had with ether and hashish. One patient, J. F…, a young Danish man suffering from manic agitation and delirium, had shown no improvement even after six months of therapeutic bombardment with the typical arsenal of mid-nineteenth-century psychiatry: bleedings, purges, cupping, and baths. So Moreau decided to administer a small dose of opium, which he steadily increased each day. After four days, the patient was calm and began to exhibit signs of recovery. He left the asylum fully cured a month later.[48]

Opium's action over the human mental apparatus was difficult to pin down. Dr Claude-François Michéa argued that opium produced two distinct, simultaneous modifications of the nervous system, as "it is at once sedative and stimulant."[49] For the purpose of treating *vésanies* – a nineteenth-century term used to describe mental disorders that did not have organic origins – Michéa argued that opium actually increased delirium and agitation. This, in turn, exacerbated the patient's symptoms to jolt them out of their mania or delirium.[50] Although some doctors used opium to exacerbate mania in order to cure it, others administered opium for its sedative action, using it to calm their patient's mania directly. For example, Dr Jules Baillarger successfully used opium to calm the intense manic agitation of a female patient, exacerbated every month during her menstrual period.[51] Nineteenth-century doctors believed that women were more vulnerable to mental disturbances during particular phases in their reproductive lives, including puberty, menstruation, childbirth, and menopause.[52] Opium's sedative effects restored calm and composure to a mind agitated by what Baillarger viewed to be the pathological caprices of the female body.

Before systemic clinical experimentation, doctors administered opium to their patients somewhat haphazardly. Over two years of treating manic patients, Baillarger explained, "I have often had recourse to opium at quite high doses, and if it is far from always bringing a rapid improvement, I have not seen, [even] in the least favourable cases, that the duration of the illness has increased."[53] This attitude is indicative of the state of psychopharmacological research at the time. Baillarger did not seem concerned with the long-term consequences of prolonged opium exposure. In fact, he considered opium, even in high doses, to be less dangerous to a patient's health than prolonged baths.[54] Nor was he alone. Both Moreau and Michéa recommended increasing daily doses of opium over time. However, Michéa advised suspending treatment after ten to fifteen days without results, because longer exposure risked the possibility of cerebral congestion – the swelling of the brain produced by increased arterial blood flow – or veinous congestion, which could lead to death or a stroke.[55] In the 1840s, doctors understood the risks of excessive opium use in terms of the immediate dangers of overdose, rather than the longer-term effects of addiction.

In the 1840s and 1850s, as with ether and chloroform, most medical studies examining opium as a cure for madness reported isolated cases or compared a few incidents. By the mid-1850s psychiatrists began to publish more comprehensive clinical studies on opium's therapeutic merits. In 1856, E. Binder, a medical student at the Faculty of Medicine in Strasbourg, wrote his thesis on opium's utility for the treatment of mental illness. Binder conducted clinical research as an intern at the Stephansfeld Asylum. For the treatment of mental illness, he claimed that "there is hardly an opium-based pharmaceutical preparation that has not been tested, and it would be difficult to say which is the most effective."[56] Despite this enthusiasm, Binder did express some concern over opium's potentially negative long-term effects. He warned against sustaining high doses of opium, necessary for the treatment of mania, for more than a few days, in order to prevent the "intellectual and physical torpor" caused by its immoderate use, as "everyone knows the story of the *thériakis*, who achieve a few happy dreams at this price." However, high doses of opium had a demonstrable effect on mania. Therefore, to justify this therapeutic intervention, doctors argued that mental patients had an unusual tolerance for medicines. Supposedly, mental patients experienced a diminished "impressionability" to drugs that made the absorption of medicines more difficult.[57] Doctors continued to use this argument about mental patients' abnormal tolerance to justify the administration of high doses of opiates into the early 1880s.

While early research suggested that opium was particularly effective for curing mania and agitation, eventually psychiatrists began to expand its therapeutic purview. In 1857, Dr Louis-Victor Marcé claimed opium had become such a classic treatment for melancholy that few experts had not vaunted opium's effectiveness.[58] One of Marcé's patients, Mme X…, was a forty-five-year-old woman suffering from melancholy. She had attempted suicide repeatedly. At first, she was placed under medical surveillance and treated with long tepid baths, purgatives, and cold showers. After a month of this treatment Marcé decided to try opium. In October 1856, he began to administer increasing doses of opium. In November, with a dose of 60 centigrams, Mme X… began to improve. She spoke of her children again and expressed a desire to see them. She also began to doubt her delirious ideas. The next month, she reached her highest maintenance dose of 80 centigrams and began to demonstrate signs of a return to reason. Gradually, "she felt her delirious convictions disappear one after another." In mid-December, Marcé began to decrease her opium dose gradually by 2 or 3 centigrams per day. By mid-January he had eliminated the opium entirely and noted that Mme X… was "completely returned to her normal intellectual state." Marcé concluded that the opium treatment was responsible for her remarkable recovery, as "improvement always coincided with the increase of the doses."[59]

Although French doctors did not recognize addiction as a pathological state of chemical dependence until the early 1880s, Marcé acknowledged that his patient became accustomed to the high doses of opium he administered. When he withdrew the opium, Mme X… experienced malaise, cerebral torpor, and an overwhelming drowsiness even as she became more sensitive than ever to the cold effusions administered.[60] Therefore, Marcé recommended weaning patients off of the opium gradually so as to avoid a nervous crisis that would waste all of the benefits of the treatment. Although doctors did not fully understand the physiological effects of addiction, they did recognize that their patients experienced symptoms of dependence.

Henri Legrand du Saulle also conducted extensive research on opium and mental illness. In 1851, as an intern under Professor Dumesnil at the public insane asylum in Dijon, he conducted research hoping to formulate a more precise methodology for administering opium to treat manic delirium and agitation. Legrand du Saulle viewed opium's ability to shock the patient's system as its greatest therapeutic advantage. He advocated administering opium in increasing doses. Then, instead of weaning the patient off the opium gradually, as other researchers did, he used opium to exacerbate his patients' manic symptoms and then abruptly suppressed their dose altogether. Legrand du Saulle claimed, "I have never seen a patient who displayed a noticeable exaggeration of all the pathological phenomena previously observed … remain incurable."[61] By this logic, Legrand du Saulle constructed opium as a litmus test for the "curability" of madness.

In the nineteenth century, to identify a mental patient as "incurable" was to condemn her to a sequestered life in one of France's asylums.[62] Catherine L… was one such patient. A sixty-six-year-old widow estranged from her children, she became destitute and lost her reason. When she entered the Dijon mental asylum in the mid-1840s, her doctors tried all the usual treatments. When these failed, she was deemed incurable, suffering from chronic mania. She remained in the *quartier des agitées* for years, fed, clothed, and washed but not subject to any active psychiatric treatment.

Incurable patients constituted a threat to the professional authority of the alienists responsible for the French asylum system. Despite alienists' widespread enthusiasm about the therapeutic benefits of isolating mental patients in asylums, their cure rates were relatively low – a fact that critics used to challenge their authority over the asylum system.[63] Asylum doctors thus had a vested interest in trying different remedies to see if they could elicit a cure. In 1851, five or six years after Catherine L… had entered the asylum, Legrand du Saulle gave her a potion containing 5 drops of Sydenham's Laudanum. He elevated her dose by one drop each day so that after two months, she was taking 65 drops of laudanum daily. During this time, she demonstrated extreme agitation: being "constantly straightjacketed," she did not eat, hardly slept, and "night and day let out screams intermixed with insults, cursing, blasphemy, [and] foul language."[64] It got so bad that she lost her voice. Then, all of a sudden, he suppressed the dose of laudanum altogether. Her agitation quickly diminished. She became calm and recovered her voice along with her reason. After her recovery, Legrand du Saulle contacted her estranged children and credited himself with their complete reconciliation. In this case, opium enabled Catherine L… to emerge from her alienation, transforming her from a hopeless, cloistered lunatic into a sane, functional woman returned to her family.

Legrand du Saulle boasted that forty patients had recovered from mental illness at the Dijon asylum during his internship with Dr Dumesnil in 1851 alone.[65] With the aid of opium, the psychiatrist could revisit a chronic case that might have seemed hopeless, for which all the habitual resources of therapeutic practice had failed, and in some cases provoke "an unexpected and completely undreamt of cure."[66] While acknowledging that treatments with progressive doses of opium often failed with patients who had been locked up in an asylum for four, five, or six years, Legrand du Saulle noted that in certain instances opium did offer hopeless cases a chance of recovery. Catherine L… was living proof.

Psychiatrists continued to experiment with opium as a cure for madness in the 1860s.[67] At times, when patients were agitated it was difficult to force them to take their dose. Often doctors had to resort to deception, administering opium without their patients' knowledge by slipping it into a *tisane* or a glass of wine.[68] Subcutaneous injections of morphine, opium's primary alkaloid, offered the same therapeutic benefits but were far more convenient to administer. One doctor argued that morphine injections "should be used for patients who are not conscious of their state of insanity and resist everything, to such an extent that it makes it impossible to take medicines orally."[69] In this light, morphine served as a technology of social order on the asylum wards, enabling doctors to subdue recalcitrant patients with greater ease and efficiency.

Although Professor Behier of the Hôtel-Dieu Hospital had introduced subcutaneous morphine injections in France in 1859, German psychiatrists appear to have led the first therapeutic efforts to use morphine injections to cure madness in the late 1860s. These experiments had mixed results. Between 1869 and 1871, the *Annales médico-psychologiques* published three different reviews of this research published in foreign psychological journals, including *Allgemeine Zeitschrift für Psychiatrie*.[70] Intrigued by the prospect of finding a medication to treat madness that could be injected rather than ingested, Dr Reissner of Hofheim experimented on his mental patients with six different alkaloids of opium. Although he found that morphine had an immediate effect, the calm it produced in his patients was only temporary. He concluded that morphine's utility in treating chronic mania was only palliative, useful for calming agitation and insomnia but without hope of producing a permanent cure.[71] Dr Tigges of Marbourg reached a similar conclusion. He claimed that "it is rare that the effect of an injection on the psychic state is [anything] other than temporary," and he observed that in some cases it even produced greater agitation.[72]

Despite these negative results, some psychiatrists still believed that morphine could serve as a curative treatment. In 1868, after working for several years as an assistant physician at the Illenau Asylum in Baden, Dr Richard von Krafft-Ebing published his research on the therapeutic use of morphine.[73] He found that morphine injections were particularly suited to cure madness complicated by neuralgia. This treatment became increasingly popular among German psychiatrists. Krafft-Ebing claimed that the Illenau asylum administered between 10,000 and 16,000 morphine injections per year.[74] Like Reissner, Krafft-Ebing also found morphine to be "the most effective means of combatting the insomnia so common among mental patients."[75] At Sainte-Anne Hospital in Paris, Drs Bouchereau and Ball achieved positive results using morphine injections to treat their patient's manic episodes.[76]

In France, the key proponent of morphine as a cure for madness was Auguste Voisin (1829–1898), an alienist of the Salpêtrière school.[77] He began his clinical research with mental patients at Salpêtrière in 1867 and published his initial results in 1874 in a paper titled "The Curative Treatment of Madness with Morphine Hydrochloride."[78] In 1876 he published additional observations, and in 1883 he republished all of his previous observations along with some new ones in a collection of clinical lessons.[79] In 1874, Voisin utilized both clinical observation and statistical analysis to determine the efficacy of this treatment. He documented each case he observed, even those in which morphine failed to produce a cure. Out of forty-three patients observed at Salpêtrière Hospital over the course of eighteen months, Voisin claimed that morphine cured twenty-five of their madness and produced notable improvement in eleven.[80] Although he treated his observations as a statistical whole under the umbrella rubric of "madness," he acknowledged that some mental pathologies were more susceptible to cure by morphine than others.

By administering gradually increasing doses of morphine, Voisin believed, a doctor could coax a mad patient slowly back to the path of reason. He observed that morphine had a "remarkably reliable effect" on his patients' agitation, delirium, and hallucinations, effectively calming them within two or three hours of a sufficient injection.[81] At first, morphine simply calmed patients' symptoms of agitation. Over time, however, "delirium disintegrates, delusional ideas, hallucinations ... they disappear one after another so that one day the patient finds himself having nothing but the memory [of them] ... as if the cerebral organ had suffered a shock from which it takes some time to recover." A patient experiencing this transition would begin take more interest in her surroundings, acknowledge the fact of her illness, and allow herself to be treated without resistance. "In a short time, the individual passes from the state of madness to the state of more or less total reason," Voisin noted, adding that it was difficult to express the satisfaction this brought him.[82] In morphine, Voisin believed he had found a cure for madness.

At a time when psychiatric medicine was still a relatively new specialty, morphine offered the alienist a rapid, concrete, and elegant therapeutic solution to psychiatric problems that were only just beginning to be classified and understood. Voisin found that morphine had the greatest therapeutic impact on melancholy, stupor, ecstasy, suicidal thoughts, religious and mystical ideas, neuralgia, melancholic anxiety, and manic agitation accompanied by hallucinations or delirium.[83] Like Legrand du Saulle, he acknowledged that morphine was much less effective for treating long-term maladies and mental illnesses with hereditary or anatomical origins.[84]

Voisin believed that morphine was particularly effective for treating lympemania, a condition similar to depression or melancholia. Many of the twenty-five patients Voisin cured had suffered from it. For example, one of his patients, Berg..., a forty-nine-year-old servant who had experienced intellectual troubles since the Paris Commune, suddenly experienced lympemania following the death of a friend and was admitted to Salpêtrière in 1873.[85] She also experienced mystical delirium and hallucinations. Just over a week after Berg... was admitted, Voisin began injecting her with increasing doses of morphine. Eventually, she reached a dose of 359 milligrams of morphine per day, after which point he decreased her dose, as she seemed to be improving. After seven months of treatment, she left his service cured – but he noted that she returned to see him every fifteen days to receive an injection of 15 to 18 milligrams of morphine, presumably as a preventive measure to ward off a relapse.[86]

While Voisin was enthusiastic about the patients he cured, he also published detailed accounts of eleven cases in which morphine produced only an improvement in the patient's state rather than a full cure. One of these patients was R***, a twenty-four-year-old woman who suffered from lympemania with alternating depression and agitation accompanied by terrifying auditory and visual hallucinations of animals and children in her clothes. Voisin administered morphine doses that eventually reached 390 milligrams. This maximum dose calmed her but did not completely prevent her hallucinations.[87] For other patients, morphine injections cured their hallucinations but not their melancholic states. These mixed results demonstrate not only the impossibility of using morphine as a universal cure for madness but also the remarkable variability of its therapeutic function depending on the individual case.

Voisin's procedure for curing madness with morphine was to administer progressively higher doses over time, just as earlier experimenters had done with opium. For the patients Voisin cured, the average duration of treatment was three to four months, with outlying hysterical cases cured after eleven months of morphine injections. For cases in which morphine improved but did not cure a patient's madness, the improvement usually occurred after eight to eighteen months of treatment. For cases in which morphine failed to produce any improvement, Voisin persisted in administering morphine for several months before giving up. In two cases he continued the treatments for over two years despite a complete lack of results.[88] His research demonstrates his firm belief in morphine's curative capacity.

In the 1870s, when conducting his initial clinical experiments, Voisin did not have the nosological vocabulary to discuss morphine addiction, as the earliest studies of morphine addiction were not published in France until 1876 and 1877.[89] However, his discussion of the physiological implications of prolonged exposure to morphine suggests that, although he did not understand addiction as such, he observed its symptoms. The duration of morphine's action varied according to the nature of the patient's mental illness, but Voisin noted that sometimes it was necessary to reinforce the morning injection with a second injection in the afternoon and sometimes even a third around eight o'clock. He also observed "rather curious phenomena" occurring around twenty hours after an injection, noting that

the patients have chills, a general malaise, aching, a feeling of obliteration, [they] are incapable of doing anything, and all of these problems cease as soon as the morning injection is done. This *need for the medication* is even more interesting to observe, as we are dealing with patients who, ordinarily, refuse any treatment and we see them await the time of their treatment with impatience and take the turn of those in front of them.[90]

Before doctors had researched the physiological impact of chemical dependence, Voisin interpreted his patients' eagerness for morphine as a bizarre reversal in the patients' previous unwillingness to be treated.

Voisin expressed concern over the potentially harmful long-term effects of his morphine treatments, not because he feared addiction but because he feared that it might make his patients anemic, given the effects of opium on blood circulation. He continued his research and in 1876 published a series of follow-up articles in the journal *Bulletin général de thérapeutique*. His concerns about anemia were unfounded. By studying the red blood cell count of patients who were taking high doses of morphine (between 44 and 88 centigrams) over the course of several months, he concluded that morphine had no ill effect on blood clotting.[91] This research suggests that it was ignorance of the nature of morphine addiction rather than indifference to his patients' long-term health that led Voisin to continue to administer such high doses of morphine.

According to the new observations he published in 1876, Voisin's enthusiasm for morphine only increased. He published several before and after lithographs of patients he had cured (Figure 3.2).[92] He also expanded his list of conditions for which morphine was an effective cure, including mental illnesses defined by memory loss, dementia, and even one case of amnesia.[93] For lympemaniacs suffering from hallucinations, he argued, "the treatment with morphine permits the doctor to make himself the master of the hallucinations."[94] Paradoxically, Voisin portrayed a cure as a question of the doctor's mastery over hallucinations rather than the patient's. Morphine made Voisin into an arbiter of sanity and authority. As long as the patient had not experienced hallucinations for too long, Voisin believed morphine could cure them. Even in cases of long-term hallucinations, he argued that morphine could moderate them by diminishing agitation, screaming, and insomnia with these patients.[95]

Voisin firmly believed in morphine's ability to cure madness. He administered injections with remarkable tenacity even when they seemed to have little effect. One of his patients, twenty-six-year-old Mme P, entered Salpêtrière in March 1875, suffering from lympemaniac madness with almost continuous visual and auditory hallucinations. She had visions of an army of soldiers shooting rifles, she saw fire, she smelled burning, and she heard voices telling her that her husband and

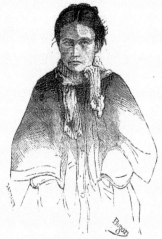

Fig. I. — Folle hypémaniaque accompagnée de démence et d'amnésie
(d'après une photographie prise par Noël).

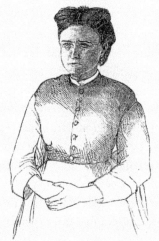

Fig. II.— La même malade est guérie (la photographie a été prise trois mois et demi
après la précédente ; la physionomie est tellement changée, que l'on a peine à croire
que c'est la même personne.

3.2 "Lithographs of B… before and after Treatment with Morphine."
This patient was a twenty-five-year-old woman suffering from
hallucinations, memory loss, and lympemania who entered
Voisin's service in August 1874. Voisin treated her with morphine
for over a year before releasing her, cured, in June 1875.

children were dead. She also engaged in "frantic onanism" and "indecent gestures." She refused to dress herself and struck anyone who vexed her. Voisin initially attempted to treat her with a morphine-wine mixture at a dose of 25 to 30 centigrams, but without success.[96] In August, he began treatment with 6-milligram morphine injections morning and night. Progressively her dose increased until it reached 75 centigrams of morphine per day by May of 1876. Despite this high dose, her symptoms did not improve. Voisin noted, "Same state, hallucinations. Sleeps little during the night; cries."[97]

Nevertheless, Voisin persisted. He increased Mme P's dose to over 1 gram of morphine per day in May and June. Although her hallucinations diminished at times, they did not fully disappear. Finally, her hallucinations began to subside in July, when she reached a dose of 1.5 grams of morphine per day. After she became calmer, Voisin began to decrease her dose again. By mid-October Mme P was able to recognize that she had been mad and speak about her hallucinations. Voisin finally declared her cured in November and ceased the injections by the end of December. She seemed fine when he saw her again in January, although he noted, "I recommended that her husband give his wife sub-cutaneous injections of morphine (of 1 centigram) if he observed her ill-humoured."[98] Voisin was surprised that it took a dose of 1.5 grams to dispel her hallucinations but postulated that this might be because Mme P was English and therefore might have a different constitution that enabled her to tolerate extremely high doses.

In 1883, when Voisin republished his morphine research in a collection of clinical lessons given at Salpêtrière, he added thirteen new observations collected since 1876, all of which had resulted in a cure.[99] His conclusions on the advantages of morphine in treating many varieties of mental illness had not changed much from his earlier work. However, by 1883 many French and German psychiatrists had published their research on morphine addiction, forcing Voisin to address the issue. He argued that there was no risk of addiction when doctors administered the injections themselves instead of relying on nuns, assistants on duty, or the patients themselves to administer them. Under his supervision, Voisin emphatically declared, he had never observed "a single case of *morphinisme*."[100] For Voisin, addiction could only be the result of ignorance or negligence on the part of nuns, assistants, and patients.

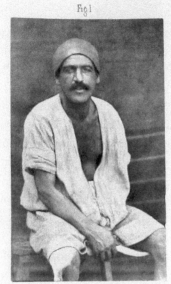

Fig I

Achmed 45 ans.

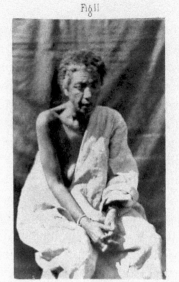

Fig II

X.Femme âgée de 55 ans.

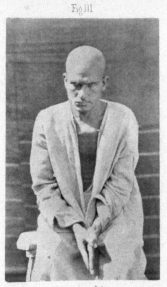

Fig III

Said Effendi. 20 ans.

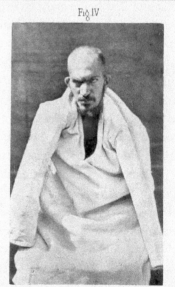

Fig IV

Mahambud Effendi. 25 ans.

3.3 Photographs of North African mental patients suffering from "hashish madness." Rather than depicting any kind of therapeutic intervention, these photographs reflect Voisin's classification of the condition of "hashish madness," which alienists at the time believed to be an intrinsic pathology of colonial subjects.

He refused to acknowledge the possibility that the therapeutic practices of exacting men of science could lead to such a disastrous side effect. Dismissing research that was "hostile to morphine," Voisin defended his prolonged use of the substance on mental patients, claiming that their "chronic constitutional states require treatments of long duration."[101] He insisted that morphine was a useful therapeutic treatment for madness. For Voisin, addiction was not something perpetuated by doctors.

Although Voisin adamantly denied that any of his patients had become addicted to morphine as a result of his treatments, he did acknowledge the possibility of drug addiction in other contexts. In fact, in the same collection of clinical lessons from 1883 he included a lesson titled "Madness by Intoxication," which included cases of mental alienation caused by opium abuse and *folie hachischique*, or "hashish madness."[102] Discussing toxic madness resulting from the abuse of opium and hashish, Voisin located the issue squarely within exotic spaces of psychotropic indulgence, referring to opium abuse in Persia or Malaysia and hashish abuse in the "Orient." To illustrate this exotic form of madness, he included several observations and photographs of individuals suffering from acute and chronic hashish madness that his former intern had collected from the Moristan Asylum in Cairo (Figure 3.3).[103] These mental patients were North Africans whose hashish abuse had led to a toxic madness, which took the form of extreme agitation and erratic behaviour combined with periods of depressed stupor. They are photographed seated slightly hunched, hands clasped between their knees, wearing vacant or hostile expressions. Voisin included the photographs of the North African patients simply to document a peculiar mental pathology, offering no suggestion for how to treat it. This reflected contemporary Orientalist assumptions about the inherently pathological nature of North African populations.[104]

These images of "hashish madness" contrast starkly with the photographs from Salpêtrière that Voisin included of the European women whom he cured using morphine injections (Figure 3.4).[105] To illustrate morphine's transformative effects, Voisin included before and after photographs. The photographs taken "before treatment" depict the women with their eyes downcast, one blurred with the motion of its subject. The "after cure" photographs depict the same women posing for a portrait, well groomed and coiffed after their rehabilitation through morphine administered by the capable hands of a medical professional. Voisin drew a line between the medical use and recreational abuse of psychotropic substances. For him, if hashish was a sign of colonial madness, morphine was a therapeutic tool of Western science that possessed the power to restore sanity.

THE PATIENT-ADDICT AND THE ADDICT-PATIENT

In the nineteenth-century asylum, psychotropic drugs operated as both regulators and instigators of mental pathology. By the time French doctors began to understand and write about addiction as a pathological condition in the 1880s, it had already become a considerable problem on the asylum wards. This was, in part, a result of alienists' attempts in previous decades to cure their patients' madness. The fact that psychotropic substances were also used as palliative treatments and agents of social control in the asylum wards to render mental patients temporarily calm further exacerbated the problem of the "patient-addict." By the 1880s, increased medical knowledge of the nature of addiction caused some doctors to re-evaluate their therapeutic practices. However, the ability of psychotropic drugs to produce results made the psychiatric profession reluctant to abandon them entirely.

Alienists found psychotropic drugs to be remarkably useful palliative tools for the regulation of the pathological symptoms of mental disorders, particularly that enigmatic condition of madness known as hysteria. In the fifth century BCE, Hippocratic physicians believed that hysteria was a female pathology caused by the uterus wandering around the body.[106] In the mid-nineteenth century, hysteria lacked a precise classification as a psychiatric pathology. Its complex series of symptoms included seizures, convulsions, fainting, paralysis of the limbs, loss of sensation in the skin, feelings of strangulation, and muteness. The symptoms were so diverse that Dr Charles Lasègue joked that hysteria was "the wastepaper basket of medicine where one throws otherwise unemployed symptoms."[107] While it was traditionally treated as an exclusively female problem, nineteenth-century doctors began to identify hysteria in men as well.[108] With few absolute indications, hysteria was difficult to diagnose and even more difficult to treat. In the 1870s, however, things began to change.

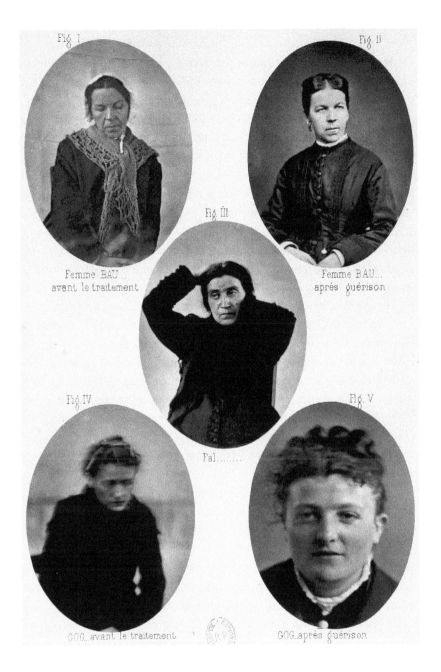

Fig. I

Fig. II

Fig. III

Femme BAU...
avant le traitement

Femme BAU...
après guérison

Fig. IV

Fig. V

Pal........

GOG..avant le traitement

GOG..après guérison

3.4 Before and after photographs of female mental patients
cured with morphine. Unlike the North African patients,
these images of European women reflect alienists' active
use of morphine in treatment.

Dr Jean Martin Charcot began researching hysteria at the Salpêtrière Hospital. By applying the principles of positivism, he transformed this collection of symptoms into an elegant nosological category.

Charcot, one of the founders of modern neurology, became famous in the 1870s and 1880s for his classification of "grand hysteria," which he defined through four successive stages: (1) the epileptoid period, defined by muscular spasms that mimicked an epileptic fit; (2) a phase of *grand movements* also known as "clownism" because of the acrobatic poses produced by the patient's contortions; (3) *attitudes passionnelles*, or "passion poses," in which the patient acts out vivid emotional states; and (4) delirium.[109] Like his colleagues at Salpêtrière and other French asylums, Charcot employed a variety of methods to try to control hysterical crises, including hydrotherapy, hypnotism, ovarian compression, and of course psychotropic drugs, particularly morphine, chloroform, and ether.

Foreign students, including a young Sigmund Freud, flocked to Salpêtrière to witness Charcot's famous clinical lessons, in which he used asylum patients to demonstrate the stages of "grand hysteria" for a captivated audience.[110] Salpêtrière's most famous resident hysterics were working-class women. The clinical lessons highlighted the power of the male physician, distinguished from his female patients by his masculinity, class, professional status, rationality, and self-control. In using drugs to suppress the symptoms of hysteria, Charcot and his colleagues sought to regulate the unruly minds of their patients.

Charcot's colleague, Désiré Magloire Bourneville, documented the frequent use of psychotropic substances to control hysterical attacks in the multi-volume *Iconographie photographique de la Salpêtrière*. For example, in 1877, after experiencing twenty attacks in a single day, V... C..., a twenty-four-year-old hysteric, was given chloroform. She was calm until morning but then experienced another seventy-two attacks. Thereafter, doctors administered chloroform each time her attacks became particularly volatile or frequent.[111] Although chloroform did not appear to influence the frequency of the attacks, it served as a palliative treatment to calm attacks as they arose.

Therapeutic practices at Salpêtrière were not standardized and doctors explored the palliative treatment of hysteria with various psychotropic substances through trial and error. The case notes of the patient Célina Marc demonstrate the frequency, variety, and longevity of these palliative psychotropic drug therapies. Marc, the only surviving child of a watchmaker and laundress, originally entered Salpêtrière in 1867 on Dr Delasiauve's service but then passed to Charcot's service in 1870.[112] She suffered from hysterical attacks and vaginismus, and, according to her doctors, she had extremely erotic tendencies. In the nineteenth century, doctors interpreted any overly explicit display of sexuality in women as a sign of mental pathology.[113] Among the "numerous medications" doctors had regularly administered over a decade at Salpêtrière were morphine injections, chloral, and thebaic extract (which includes opium), as well as amyl nitrite and ether, which were used to stop her attacks. Doctors used these substances, often administered all together, combined with ovarian compression, purgatives, hypnotism, and "metallotherapy" – the use of metals such as gold and copper to treat hysterical symptoms. With such a wide variety of treatments employed simultaneously, it was difficult for her doctors to distinguish which ones produced the positive results they observed.[114]

At the beginning of 1875, Marc constantly complained that she felt as though she was choking. In response, Charcot administered ether. Over a span of a few months she consumed progressively greater quantities: 125, 250, sometimes even 500 grams of ether per day. Bourneville noted, "Ether is now essential for her; she torments everyone until they give it to her. She has become much more difficult to restrain; she is very irritable, she screams, threatens, [and] sometimes breaks all the objects that she gets her hands on."[115] By May 1875, Marc was inhaling 125 grams of ether almost every day. When her doctors administered less than her habitual dose, she became violent, breaking windows and tearing the curtains when they refused to give her more ether.[116] Initially administered as a regulatory agent, ether acted upon Marc's mind and body to create a chemical dependence that provoked rebellious behaviour. Paradoxically, her increasing dependence upon ether's chemical action galvanized her to exercise a degree of individual agency within the limited boundaries of the asylum. Using her own intractability, violence, and capacity for destruction, she pressured the doctors and hospital staff to administer the ether to which she had become accustomed. Ether continued to regulate her behaviour, but not in the ways that her doctors had intended.

Ether also appeared to exacerbate Marc's eroticism. In March 1877, under the influence of ether inhalations, she sat on the floor in a cataleptic state, complaining, "He doesn't care enough!" Bourneville understood this to mean that they had not given her enough ether. When her doctors gave her more ether on a compress, she brought it to her nose and raised her skirt and apron over her head so the ether would evaporate more slowly. She experienced erotic delirium. Ten minutes later she clamoured for more ether, calling the doctors who refused it to her "savage beasts."[117] The next day, after more than two hours of hysterical attacks, she inhaled 250 grams of ether. Smiling after the inhalation, she experienced an erotic scene, exclaiming, "Oh! oh! … that feels good." Bourneville narrated: "(Kiss) … sends kisses, lies down again, presses her hand on her sexual organs, taps, is happy."[118] Bourneville reported this erotic, masturbatory scene as an illustration of Marc's pathological condition. He did not acknowledge his own disturbing voyeurism or the fact that he and his colleagues were the agents of her eroticism. Ironically, the ether treatments they gave her exaggerated the "erotic tendencies" they viewed as a symptom of her mental pathology.

Other patients experienced similar phenomena from ether inhalations. Blanche W… entered Salpêtrière in 1877 at the age of eighteen. She remained there for over a decade as one of the stars of Charcot's clinical lessons on hysteria.[119] In December 1878, Blanche's doctors administered ether to treat tremors she had experienced for a few days. This produced hilarity and delirium. Blanche cried out "Give me more ether" and then "she laughed, she wriggled, maintaining the compress against her nose and mouth," calling out to a lover in her delirious state to kiss her.[120] While ether had halted her tremors, it also exacerbated her erotic delirium. Under the influence of ether, vulnerable female hysterics exposed their bodies and erotic desires to the doctors who observed them, documenting their erotic displays without taking responsibility for their own role in producing them.

Although ovarian compression typically suspended Blanche's hystero-epileptic attacks, the attacks often returned when the compressor was removed. Doctors thus concluded that chemical agents were necessary to actually halt her attacks. Ether was highly effective, at first. However, "gradually, its effect diminished to such an extent that, to halt the attacks, an enormous dose was necessary."[121] Although Bourneville did not frame this case in terms of addiction, the fact that Blanche required larger doses of ether over time to produce the same results demonstrates that she had become chemically accustomed to the drug. Her doctors circumvented this problem by administering ether for ten to fifteen minutes and then administering chloroform as well. They used this "double anesthesia" a great number of times with Blanche and also administered chloroform alone.[122] In 1889, Blanche W… reappears in another set of clinical observations as an example of a nervous hysteric treated with morphine injections.[123] For over a decade, despite the administration of numerous psychotropic substances to treat her symptoms, Blanche continued to experience hysterical attacks. At Salpêtrière, psychotropic drugs were deployed to manage the unruly symptoms of hysteria rather than in pursuit of a definitive cure. Designed to treat the erratic symptoms of patients' hysteria, these drugs produced further erratic, and sometimes erotic, behaviour. They also produced a powerful chemical dependence.

When doctors began writing about chronic drug use in terms of addiction – a psycho-physiological dependence on a material substance – they often used the suffix -*manie*, or "mania." Toxicomania (*toxicomanie*), the general term for addiction, as well as the terminology used to describe specific addictions – morphinomania (*morphinomanie*), opiomania (*opiomanie*), etheromania (*étheromanie*), and later cocainomania (*cocaïnomanie*) – positioned psychotropic drugs as creators of pathological mental states.[124] This "artificial madness" that they produced took on two forms. First, doctors began to recognize symptoms of mental pathology in addicted individuals and argue that addiction led to hysterical symptoms, mania, excitability, and other abnormal mental states. Second, doctors began to construct the very condition of addiction as a mental pathology. Morphine had a regulatory impact over mental functions that placed the addict on the frontiers of madness and sanity.

In the mid-1870s, morphine addiction – which ten years later would represent a significant social problem – was just beginning to be studied by French, German, British, and American physicians.[125] In the late 1870s, two theses on the subject were published at the Paris Faculty of Medicine. Léopold Calvet's thesis, defended in December 1876, was the first monograph on morphine addiction in France. "There is certainly no [medication] whose use in therapeutics is more frequent," Calvet argued. However, he noted, "there is none that is less understood in terms of its physiological effects."[126] To remedy this lacuna of medical knowledge, Calvet focused on the physiological impact of morphine addiction on the body's vital functions, basing his conclusions on animal experimentation as well as clinical observation of acute morphine intoxication and chronic morphine addiction. While he focused on physiology rather than psychology, his clinical observations demonstrated that morphine addiction entailed a degree of intellectual trouble, if not full-fledged insanity at extremely high doses.[127] The second thesis on morphine addiction, published by N. Dalbanne in 1877, exposed the role of doctors in perpetuating morphine addiction among their patients.[128] Although these two early studies on morphine addiction exposed the devastating psychological and physiological consequences of its long-term use, widespread knowledge and understanding of morphine addiction did not permeate the French medical community until the early 1880s. In the meantime, asylum doctors continued to prescribe morphine to their patients as a sort of universal panacea for mental and nervous troubles.

Doctors unwittingly produced addiction in France's asylums. However, patients' morphine addiction did not only come from therapeutic treatments. It also occurred as a result of institutional pressures, negligence, and the use of psychotropic substances as agents of social control.[129] Writing in the early 1890s, Ernest Chambard denounced the all too frequent negligence of the hospital intern, "who by condescension or to guarantee a quiet shift, makes his rounds with his Pravaz syringe in hand."[130] Furthermore, perpetual overcrowding in hospital wards also led to systematic negligence, as doctors, interns, and nurses delegated the administration of injections down the line of command until eventually the patient was left to inject herself.[131] The hospital staff initially used morphine to regulate the disorderly behaviour of the mental patients on the wards, but this regulatory mechanism backfired and the pestering of addicted patients became a daily reality of hospital work. Chambard recalled that "in the year 1874, when I was an extern under [Dr] Behier at the Hôtel-Dieu, I had to struggle each evening against my patients in the female ward, clamouring for the injections to which they had become accustomed."[132] Here, addiction disrupted the authority that the medical man of science traditionally held over his female asylum patients.

Sometimes patients' addictions could be quite extreme. One patient-addict, initially injected by an intern on call, eventually reached the enormous daily dose of 1.5 to 2 grams of morphine.[133] One of Voisin's former interns told Dalbanne that at Salpêtrière, the mental patients "wait for the fixed hour of their hypodermic injections just as they wait for their meals." He explained, "if we wanted to eliminate injections overnight, *a veritable revolution* would break out."[134] Morphine injections imposed a regulatory time over patients' lives in the asylum. While the injections were designed to regulate their mental states, the chemical regulation of patients' bodies also contained the threat of disorder if their schedule for injection were disrupted. Dalbanne heartily agreed with the intern's assessment of Salpêtrière: "Woe to the nurses should they refuse the morphine flask! And this is hardly an exaggeration; to be convinced, just go check out M. Voisin's service."[135] Ironically, the drug that doctors used to exercise control over the erratic and enigmatic condition of madness caused patients to be even more intractable in their pursuit of additional injections.

Patient demand and fears of disorder on the wards shaped practices of morphine administration. Some addicted patients encouraged others to use morphine, causing addiction to spread rapidly through the wards. One hysteric at Hôtel-Dieu used morphine for the first time in January of 1886. One year later she was a seasoned addict. "An interesting fact to note in the story of this patient," her doctor wrote, "is that the example and the advice of many of her hospital companions who were *morphinomanes* played a large role in the birth and the development of her passion [for morphine]."[136] The extent and severity of morphine addiction in the asylum wards undermined the power dynamics between doctor and patient as doctors had to contend with patients constantly and forcefully clamouring for morphine even as they introduced other patients to the drug, further undermining medical authority.

To counteract this practice, Chambard proposed that hospitals should implement two regulations: that employees never provide any medication except by individual daily prescription; and that drugs or injecting instruments never be left in the hospital wards where patients could easily reach them.[137] The fact that Chambard had to propose these regulations in the early 1890s suggests that, despite the numerous articles and monographs published on the perils of morphine addiction in the 1880s, doctors continued to treat morphine as a miracle drug rather than a conduit for a potentially devastating addiction. This tendency was likely exacerbated by the persistent myth that mental patients had a much higher tolerance for opiates than the average patient.

Although morphine was perhaps the most widely discussed and documented "artificial madness" of the French asylums, mental patients also became addicted to ether and chloroform during their incarceration. One patient, who entered Salpêtrière in 1879, suffered from hystero-epilepsy and partial anesthesia. Likely as a result of overlapping psychiatric treatments, she had become addicted to morphine, ether, chloroform, and chloral simultaneously. Bourneville noted that she received daily morphine injections of 2, 4, or 6 centigrams and explained, "she gets excited as long as we do not give her subcutaneous injections or when we don't give her ether or chloroform." He lamented, "Unfortunately, we give in too often."[138] Addicted mental patients destabilized medical authority on the asylum wards. While ether, chloroform, and morphine acted directly upon the bodies of patients, over time they also influenced doctors' behaviour. When faced with an unruly patient in a state of withdrawal, the doctor responded by placating the patient with the drugs she demanded, allowing her addiction to influence his therapeutic regimen.

In the 1880s, the French medical community became increasingly aware not only of the fact of morphine addiction but also of doctors' own role in its rapid spread. In the popular imagination, *morphinomanie* became associated with pleasure-seeking women.[139] However, contemporary medical statistics on addiction actually cited more male addicts than female addicts. Furthermore, addiction researchers acknowledged that people became addicted most frequently as a result of encounters with medical men, either socially or as a result of therapeutic treatment.[140] While doctors were eager to try to deflect blame for the rapid spread of morphine addiction, they also began to consider how to reduce their own role in perpetuating this new pathology.

Asylum doctors began to re-evaluate their use of morphine in psychiatric treatment. In 1883, the *Bulletin de Société de thérapeutique* published a short debate about the effectiveness of morphine as a treatment for hysteria.[141] Some doctors continued to defend its therapeutic merit, but one doctor, M. Créquy, argued that it was ineffective. He claimed that he had a hysterical patient whose attacks had continued, even though he had administered up to one hundred morphine injections per day. Even considering Voisin's earlier argument that the doctor must persevere with morphine injections until they took effect, administering one hundred injections every day without any result seems excessive. Other criticism of the treatment was even more damning. Dr Blondeau argued that while morphine sometimes calmed hysterical attacks, on other occasions it actually provoked them.[142] Ironically, the once-lauded remedy appeared to cause the disorder it was supposed to cure. While these arguments illustrate the perspectives of only a few doctors, the lack of consensus suggests a shift in medical opinion. In light of a greater medical understanding of the principle of addiction, doctors began to express increased caution about the therapeutic utility of psychotropic substances.

After observing numerous cases of hysteria as an intern at Paris's Hôtel-Dieu Hospital, Jean-Joseph Terrail noticed that several of these women also presented symptoms of morphine addiction. He chose to write his 1889 doctoral thesis on the relationship between the two conditions. Terrail attributed the exaggerated abuse of opiates among certain hysterical patients to the fact that "doctors were less familiar with the psychological characteristics of hysteria and in opium they found a powerful sedative for pain, all while knowing almost nothing about its true physiological role." According to Terrail, medical ignorance bred addiction. Based on his clinical observations of morphine-addicted hysterics, Terrail argued that the hysteric was especially prone to morphine addiction because she was "more malleable, more irritable, [and] more sensitive" than other women. He cautioned that morphine should be used only as a last resort, because "the remedy can be worse than the illness." In addition to hysterical patients' particular propensity for addiction, the enigmatic nature of hysteria and its resistance to treatment perpetuated addiction, as it increased the psychiatrist's frustration. Terrail explained that "hysterical manifestations, [which are] often very persistent, can try the doctor's patience and cause him to leave his patients to use morphine in spite of himself."[143] However, relinquishing control over these powerful psychotropic substances had serious ramifications.

By perpetuating morphine addiction on the asylum wards, through therapeutic practice or otherwise, doctors created a new brand of mental patient: the addict. Like Dr Charcot's famous hysterics, these addict-patients were displayed and consumed as spectacles of madness.[144] In 1884, Dr Benjamin Ball presented a series of lessons at the Clinic of Mental

Maladies at Sainte-Anne Hospital on the subject of *morphinomanie*. To illustrate the incredible power of morphine over the addicted body with a touch of drama, Ball brought out a flesh-and-blood addict in a state of withdrawal – a woman who had become addicted to morphine while being treated for hysteria. Beginning his demonstration with a flourish, Ball announced, "I present to you one of the patients I told you about at the beginning of these lessons. She has been deprived of morphine since yesterday. The expression in her physiognomy is striking. Her gaze is lifeless, her vision is destroyed, the patient is blind and almost deaf: her face resembles a corpse, her intelligence is almost extinguished; finally she cannot support herself on her own legs."[145] The patient, blind, deaf, and weakened from morphine withdrawal, was entirely at the mercy of Dr Ball and of the morphine that her body craved.[146]

Although Ball described *morphinomanie* as a type of mental alienation, its pathological nature lay in its uprooting of the conditions of a "normal" state. In the absence of morphine – a normal condition for anyone who is not addicted – the *morphinomane* experienced intense psychosomatic suffering that left her in a state that seemed to be somewhat less than human. As with the manic patients treated by Voisin and Legrand du Saulle, Ball's patient could only function normally when she had morphine in her system. However, instead of treating a separate pathological condition, in this case morphine simply treated its own absence in a body that had become vitally dependent upon it. Wielding his syringe, Ball narrated: "I administer an injection of several centigrams [of morphine]. At this moment, her face expresses bliss: her faculties return, her mind awakens, she sees, she speaks, she hears. These are the general effects produced by an injection after a long abstinence."[147] By withholding morphine and then literally injecting the life back into his patient, Ball exerted incredible power over her. His declared goal was to demonstrate the effects of morphine on a patient experiencing withdrawal, but he also powerfully exhibits the medical profession's self-proclaimed control over morphine's curative and destructive properties. Through his demonstration, Ball dramatized the restoration of health and sanity through a visual spectacle enacted upon the body of a living patient. However, this spectacle of a cure obscured the fact that psychiatric treatment had caused her addiction in the first place.

Published around the time that medical knowledge of addiction was becoming more widely accepted, Daniel Jouet's 1883 thesis, *Étude sur le morphinisme chronique*, was one of the most frequently cited French studies that dealt exclusively with morphine addiction. Jouet argued that morphine addiction usually occurred after a period of injections lasting anywhere from a few weeks to two months.[148] However, patients in the Paris asylums often took morphine for much longer. One of these, Bonnaire, a thirty-nine-year-old ataxic patient, entered M. Berger's service in 1870. She suffered from serious cerebral troubles of unknown origin that caused delirium and comas. Bonnaire remained at Salpêtrière almost continuously over the next ten years. During this time, her daily morphine injections increased from seven to eight to ten and peaked at eighteen injections per day between 1878 and 1880. She had become entirely dependent upon the drug.[149] Her treatment reflected her doctors' ignorance or disregard for the potential consequences of prolonged exposure to morphine. Remarkably, Jouet's case report preserved Bonnaire's own testimony of how she experienced her addiction.

In her daily life at the asylum, Bonnaire experienced unpleasant mental and physiological side effects of morphine addiction. She lost weight from digestive and gastric problems. She was almost always constipated and experienced "excruciating pains" whenever she had to use the toilet. The morphine also made her feel as though she was living in a dreamlike stupor. It seemed to cloud her head and she found it difficult to follow conversations. She explained, "I only had dark thoughts, *I dreamed while awake.*" Bonnaire's addiction was so entrenched that she had difficulty functioning on a normal level intellectually, existing instead in a liminal space between waking and sleeping, unable to engage meaningfully with those around her. Physical discomfort and mental torpor made her frustrated. "I thought only of isolating myself," Bonnaire recalled, "waiting with impatience for the hour of my injection, I only feel good after having done it, but if by misfortune I happen to be unable to do it, I am beset by an atrocious crisis."[150] These injections punctuated Bonnaire's miserable life with brief moments of pleasure. However, these ephemeral pleasures also held the promise of continued addiction, reinforced by the fear of acute agony if she were to miss her required dose.

Morphine had a deleterious effect on Bonnaire's general health and mental state, but its absence was unbearable. She described her experience when, a few weeks prior, she had the misfortune to forget her morphine solution when she went out for the day:

> The hour [of injection] approaches and I begin to feel some chills, soon I start to retch and I vomit in the street, my ears are ringing, it seems like I am getting hit on the back of the neck. I'm all sweaty, my hands especially are drenched, they are swollen and covered with large painful veins, I have terrible colic, it seems like it's taking *my guts and tearing them from me*, then I feel a sort of large ball in the right side of my abdomen that is hard and horribly painful.
>
> Finally, no longer able to hold on, I have to sit down on the edge of the pavement and wait for a carriage.
>
> I find one, I can hardly give my address, when I arrive at Salpêtrière I demolish everything inside, window panes and cushions; finally going downstairs I grip the lantern so as not to fall, I break it and fall with it.
>
> I am transported to bed, given an injection, and twenty minutes later I sat down to dinner.[151]

Without her habitual dose of morphine, Bonnaire experienced the excruciating tortures of withdrawal from a substance that had reconfigured her body's state of equilibrium. Her body rebelled as she retched and shivered, helpless on the city streets. Then, once injected with morphine, she rapidly returned to normal. The therapeutic regimen that her doctors had followed for more than a decade had produced an addiction so entrenched that it made it impossible for her to forgo morphine and leave the asylum. To avoid the crisis of withdrawal, Bonnaire directed all of her energies toward morphine, "that harmful guest who slipped in so insidiously." For her, morphine "reigns as an absolute master and holds everything under its dependence."[152] Her story illustrates the devastating consequences of withdrawal and the incredible power that morphine, a material substance, holds over the addicted subject.

Addiction was a biochemical adaptation. *Morphinomanie* made the addict "revolt against a delay or suspension of the usual administration of the poison. It has already made a *second nature*, a *new interior environment*: to remove this new environment is to take the animal out of its element and it's no wonder that it struggles against this dispossession."[153] The addict was reduced to an animal, an organism stripped of culture and civilization, forced to adapt to a new internal equilibrium. Morphine fundamentally altered the individual's biological needs and instincts for survival.

Morphine produced significant physiological changes in the addicted body. Claudius Gaudry described *morphinomanie* as "a new physiological appetite created from the body's dependence on receiving a new food." Over time, appetite became necessity and then produced an irresistible "psycho-somatic *obsession*."[154] Addiction produced a fundamental shift in the balance of the bodily economy. For an addict, morphine became "a physical need for the cerebral cells, just like food and water are for the cells of the organism in general." It was so pressing that "the need makes itself felt at regular hours like the needs of hunger and thirst."[155] Georges Pichon understood that the psychoactive properties of morphine were connected to the brain. Although the agonies of withdrawal could be felt throughout the body, it was the brain, the seat of reason and intellect, that physically craved morphine. In this manner, morphine addiction became a mental pathology, an abnormal condition of a cerebral apparatus fuelled by a newfound chemical imperative.

Gaudry and Pichon both compared morphine to a food that the body craves and needs in order to function. However, far from providing nourishment, morphine actually inhibited the addicted body's capacity to nourish itself. As Bonnaire observed, morphine killed the appetite for food, disrupted the digestive system, and caused incredible constipation. Addicts were often painfully thin. At times realizing that morphine was poisoning his body, the addict would try to stop injecting. However, Gaudry argued, "his will is no longer whole; somatic problems appear with abstinence and he loses the free exercise of his intellectual faculties; he becomes delirious, or falls into a stupor, if not into *collapsus*; phenomena which a new injection will make disappear."[156] While morphine disrupted the body's physiological equilibrium, it also affected the addict's mental functions.

When a dose was delayed, the addict's most powerful impulse was the need to inject morphine as quickly as possible, whatever the cost. "Whether they find themselves at the theatre, at dinner, at a *soirée*, in lessons, there's no getting around it," explained Pichon. "At the usual time, as if they were obeying an internal order, they leave ... in such cases, they respond to an irresistible movement that it's impossible for them to restrain."[157] Pichon had a friend who was so addicted to morphine that within two or three minutes of an injection he felt the "ardent thirst" for morphine again.[158] German physician Friedrich Albrecht Erlenmeyer described *morphinomanes* "coming to prostrate themselves on their knees as veritable supplicants at the normal hours of injections."[159] Before injecting, addicts resembled automatons, powerfully led by the looming agonies of withdrawal to seek their required injection in the complete absence of free will. The liberal subject was turned on its head as the body led the actions of the organism, stringing the mind along behind.

As morphine's power over an individual's free will was so strong, attempting to cure morphine addiction proved to be incredibly difficult. There were three basic methods: (1) brisk suppression, in which the addict engaged in complete and immediate abstinence; (2) gradual suppression, diminishing an addict's dose of morphine over time; and (3) substitution, replacing morphine with a different substance designed to combat the symptoms of withdrawal, such as alcohol or cocaine.[160] With all three methods, success was rare and difficult and the likelihood of relapse was high.[161]

Brisk suppression was the most disruptive and painful method, as the patient's body experienced all of the agonies and miseries of detoxification at once. In theory, this method could cure addiction quickly, but the withdrawal was so agonizing that the addict required constant medical surveillance to prevent relapse.[162] From his clinical observations, Pichon noted that in eight out of fifty cases, patients in withdrawal had attempted suicide.[163] Nevertheless, several physicians, including Jules Voisin, continued to employ this technique.

The second method, gradual suppression, was designed to wean an addict off of morphine over time to avoid the harmful and agonizing shock to the system achieved through immediate and complete withdrawal. Many of the most prominent experts on *morphinomanie* were partisans of this gradual method, including Drs Zambaco, Ball, Notta, Pichon, Lancereau, and Grasset.[164] However, most addicts found it almost impossible to stop injecting altogether.

The third method, substitution, often caused more harm than good by producing overlapping addictions. Doctors experimented with a number of substances, including alcohol, pantopon, chloral, bromide, heroin, and cocaine.[165] In cocaine, doctors believed they had found the ideal substitute for morphine.[166] While substitution was more popular in England and America, it did find supporters in France.[167] As one would expect when treating addiction with another addictive substance, this method ended up replacing one addiction with another, or creating a new double-addiction: *morphino-cocaïnomanie.*

Given the tragic evidence of morphine's nefarious control over the addicted body, doctors wondered what impact these substances might have on the addicted mind. They debated the extent to which psychotropic drug addiction should be considered a mental pathology. Addicts certainly demonstrated extreme agitation in a state of withdrawal, but this was not the case when they were taking their habitual dose. One of the most widely discussed characteristics of morphine addiction was addicts' ability to conceal their addictions from the people around them. To the outside world, a morphine addict could function perfectly normally as a businessman or a state official, a doctor or a society woman, when injected with enough morphine. In this respect, *morphinomanie* could be considered a *névrose*, or "nervous disease," a kind of half-madness, like hysteria or neurasthenia, in which a patient with an underlying pathology could function more or less normally in society.[168]

Social thinkers found it disconcerting to think that concealed pathologies might lurk beneath the surface of seemingly normal individuals, undermining the social order. French sociologist Émile Durkheim conceptualized the individual in society as a *homo duplex*, whose inner life was driven by two forces in constant antagonism: the individual, defined by self-interested egoism derived from the "sensory appetites" of the profane material body; and the social, which constitutes "everything in us that expresses something other than ourselves."[169] This latter social consciousness was a higher faculty that encompassed civilization's collective ideals of reason and morality that "represent something within us that is superior to us."[170] The addict's "sensory appetite" for morphine undermined the social forces that would normally curtail self-interested egotism. However, under the influence of his habitual dose, the addict did not give the outward appearance of this *anomie*. At once normal and pathological, the addict's doubled self posed a danger to society.

Pichon argued that addicts demonstrated a "loss of moral temperament," which manifested in a complete indifference to everything around them: friends, misfortunes, family, appearances.[171] They exhibited a "surprising egoism" in that only "one single thing occupies them, interests them: *their injections of morphine.*"[172] This pathological egoism of the morphine addict, Gaudry argued, took on "the distinctive character of absolutism."[173] It produced an abnormal mental state in which the addict was no longer an engaged social being. Instead, the addict ignored everything external to the self other than the physical engagement with the syringe.

By the 1880s and 1890s, doctors began to see a correlation between morphine addiction and nervous disorders, particularly hysteria. While Terrail had argued that hysterics became *morphinomanes* because of the treatments they received in asylums, other doctors argued that morphine addiction actually produced hysteria.[174] In 1890, at the Société Médicale des Hôpitaux, Dr Jules Voisin (1844–1920) presented two cases in which morphine addicts demonstrated hysterical symptoms.[175] The first patient, a man addicted for five years, used 0.6 grams of morphine per day to treat abdominal pains related to tabes, a form of neural degeneration linked to advanced-stage syphilis. The second patient was a woman addicted for eighteen months who took roughly a gram of morphine per day to treat "violent head pains."[176] Voisin argued that morphine addiction often caused hysteria, especially among individuals with hereditary predispositions. Hysterical symptoms were most likely in the stage of withdrawal, when addicts experienced the "imperious need" to inject. Regular injections produced "well-being, a feeling of strength and vigor, of euphoria." With prolonged abstinence from morphine "agitation and obsession increase, the need becomes urgent, and at the same time the patients feel their reason leave them." Then, they would experience the symptoms of a hysterical attack: glottal spasms, suffocation, sensory issues, vertigo, and delirium.[177] Voisin believed that morphine withdrawal could actually provoke a hysterical attack. While most addicts could function quite normally while on morphine, in the absence of their habitual dose they experienced the physiological symptoms of withdrawal and nervous symptoms akin to those of hysteria. Ironically, morphine, deployed by psychiatrists to control hysterical crises, also had the power to cause them. Nor was morphine the only substance for which this was the case. In 1889, Émile Chambrin argued that ether, another common treatment for hysterical attacks, should be included among the substances that provoked hysteria.[178]

Shortly after Voisin published his findings on *morphinomanie* and hysteria, one of his students, Victor Neveu-Dérotrie, published a medical thesis on the subject. Neveu-Dérotrie argued that morphine addiction could reawaken hysterical symptoms or actually provoke hysteria among predisposed individuals.[179] In his thesis, he distinguished between two categories of addicts: those whose addictions had iatrogenic origins linked to pain management; and those who began to use morphine in the pursuit of pleasure. He claimed that the pleasure-seeking addicts were predisposed to nervous maladies like hysteria.[180] While all addicts in withdrawal experienced ghastly physiological symptoms – cold sweats, abdominal pain, extreme agitation, diarrhea, and "incoercible vomiting" – Neveu-Dérotrie argued that only pleasure-seeking addicts experienced "psycho-sensorial troubles."[181] This bizarre conclusion seemed to exonerate doctors from their role in the spread of mental pathology through the therapeutic use of morphine by suggesting that iatrogenic addicts only experienced the physiological symptoms of withdrawal, without psycho-sensorial problems.

This argument that *morphinomanes* were inherently pathological had traction with the French psychiatric community, for whom hereditary precedents played a large role in determining mental pathologies.[182] According to the statistics Dr Regnier published in his 1890 thesis on morphine, forty-five out of sixty-seven cases of morphine addiction had some kind of nervous pathology. Among these, fifteen were hysterics.[183] Although doctors often used morphine to treat the painful symptoms of hysteria, Regnier argued that hysterics had uniquely delicate constitutions that made them particularly vulnerable to *morphinomanie*. In his 1905 medical thesis, René Lefèvre came to the unequivocal conclusion that "every *morphinomane* is a hysteric."[184] By the early twentieth century, *morphinomanie* and hysteria had become associated pathologies.

Yet, because most addicts could function almost normally while taking morphine, *morphinomanie* could not be considered a complete state of mental alienation. In 1891, Charles Lefèvre, a medical intern of the Seine asylums, published a short article on the ethics of confining morphine addicts in asylums.[185] Germany, the United States, and England all had special facilities for treating addiction, with specially trained personnel, yet France had nothing comparable to these facilities, with the exception of a few incredibly expensive private institutions.[186] Addicts without the means to afford expensive treatment facilities could turn to hospitals, but Lefèvre argued that hospitals had insufficient surveillance and it was impossible to isolate patients there. Moreover, sending a morphine addict to a hospital could cause a "veritable epidemic of *morphinomanie*," as hospital wards could lead patients to engage in "reciprocal *morphinisation*."[187] Therefore, the only plausible refuge for a morphine addict was the asylum.

In the late nineteenth century, there were two paths to the asylum. The first, the *placement d'office*, involved the judicial system or the police, who had the power to commit individuals they considered to be a danger to society. The second method enabled families to have their relatives committed to an asylum under the *placement volontaire*. Of course, this "voluntary" process did not actually involve the consent of the patient, who was considered an *aliéné* under the 1838 law and thus denied citizenship rights and control over his finances while in the asylum.[188] Many families turned to *placement volontaire* as a last resort.[189] However, asylum critics viewed this as a form of arbitrary incarceration akin to the reviled *lettre de cachet* from the Old Regime, alleging that families exploited this system to rid themselves of relatives who were inconvenient, disobedient, or financially irresponsible.[190] During the Third Republic, such a blatant violation of individual liberty contradicted the government's emphasis on citizens' individual rights. Addiction only further complicated this issue.

Morphine addicts entering the asylum for treatment presented an ethical dilemma regarding consent. If an addict "in full possession of his intellectual faculties" expressed a firm wish to be cured of his addiction, then he could be admitted voluntarily. By the same token, internment in an asylum could be imposed on an addict "no longer in possession of his free will," whose intelligence had diminished through prolonged addiction. However, the law made no provision for the addict whose mental state was not yet compromised enough to commit involuntarily but who refused to enter an asylum and resisted all attempts at persuasion. Lefèvre posed the question: "Should we leave him to intoxicate himself until his reason is compromised, his memory weakened, his will annihilated?"[191] In so doing, he exposed one of the fundamental philosophical paradoxes underlying addiction. At what point in the process of addiction does the psychotropic action of the drug compromise the will of the individual? Or, to put it another way, when do the chemical imperatives of the addicted body subordinate the mind and seize control of its decision-making functions?

In asking whether one could circumvent an addict's consent in order to intern him in an asylum to receive treatment, Lefèvre acknowledged the delicacy of the issue and the serious potential violation of individual liberty that it entailed. Taking the interest of the patient as well as the interest of society into consideration, the asylum offered the best chances for the individual to be cured and to avoid contaminating the rest of society. Before lambasting against violations of individual liberty, Lefèvre argued,

> It would first be necessary to establish the rights of a *morphinomane* to enjoy freedom. In *morphinomanie*, is it clear that the notion of free will actually exists? – Are we really sure that a patient who is subjected to the fatal yoke of his morphine still possesses the moral qualities of a free man? – Take away his syringe and see your patient depleted, given over to irresistible impulses, to the most disturbing hallucinations, and fallen into a state nearest to bestiality.[192]

By Lefèvre's logic, to deny a morphine addict the choice to enter an asylum did not violate the principles of individual liberty, for by yoking himself to morphine, the addict lost his free will and, through it, his defining characteristic of humanity. To concretize the addict's "othered" status as distinct from free men, Lefèvre proposed adding a special piece of legislation on morphine addicts to the new law on *aliénés* that the public powers were in the process of reforming.[193]

Lefèvre's article revealed the addicted mind as a contested space in which a parasitical chemical substance had taken the reigns. It was morphine, rather than individual free will, that directed the addict's actions. This raised an interesting medical-legal dilemma for addicts who committed crimes. In a legal system founded upon the principle of free will, if an addict's captive body rather than his mind controlled his actions, could he still be held responsible for them?

ADDICTION ON TRIAL

In the late nineteenth century, morphine addicts began to appear in the docks of France's criminal courts.[194] However, at that time drug use was not a crime.[195] Instead, these addicted defendants faced other charges, ranging from petty theft to cold-blooded murder. From the mid-1870s onward, morphine addiction emerged in the courtrooms and the press as a subject of medical-legal debate. The issue at stake was the question of free will. As doctors investigated the physiological impact of addiction, medical-legal experts grappled with the thorny question of criminal responsibility: If morphine wielded such imperious power, should an addict be held responsible for criminal actions committed under its influence?

Within a broader framework of *fin-de-siècle* cultural anxieties over the excesses and decadence of modernity, critics argued that new "social pathologies" were diminishing both the quality and the quantity of the French population. Doctors and social reformers used the concept of "degeneration" to provide a common language for discussing seemingly unrelated social pathologies – alcoholism, hysteria, criminality, decadence, anarchism, morphine addiction – under a comprehensive scientific theory of national decline in which individual deviance threatened the collective fate of the social body.[196] Historians of *fin-de-siècle* criminology and degeneration have explored numerous tropes of courtroom defence, including kleptomania, hysteria, hypnotism, crimes of passion, and alcoholism, in which the testimony of medical experts played a significant role in determining the criminal responsibility of defendants.[197] However, the medical-legal history of drug addiction has been relatively neglected within this historiography.[198]

Morphine addiction became a subject of medical-legal fascination in the *fin de siècle*. However, the number of morphine addicts to appear before the courts was remarkably low, particularly compared with cases involving alcohol. Alcohol was involved to some degree in approximately 25 per cent of murder or attempted murder cases between 1880 and 1910.[199] In many ways, morphine and alcohol posed similar challenges to legal medicine.[200] Both were psychotropic substances that could produce states of delirium or mania, a form of artificial madness that defendants compared to a state of temporary insanity. However, while social reformers associated alcoholism with working-class irrationality and moral failure, morphine addiction seemed to represent a new and uniquely modern pathology that emerged as an unanticipated side effect of medical treatment.[201] Morphine, a material object, exercised a disconcertingly powerful effect over the behaviour of the addicted subject. Medical-legal experts focused on a handful of cases of morphine addiction, which they used as case studies to investigate the limitations of free will.

Morphine addiction forced experts to interrogate criminal defendants as embodied subjects. Drawing on the methodologies of positivist science, including clinical observation, diagnostic experimentation, and chemical urinalysis, medical-legal experts explored the complex ways in which addicts' altered physiology contributed to their criminal behaviour. Addicted defendants claimed that morphine produced in them a state of temporary insanity. In contrast, medical-legal experts emphasized the more complex regulatory influence of morphine over the addicted body – specifically, morphine's capacity to relieve pain, soothe anxiety, and stave off withdrawal symptoms of its own making. In so doing, they attempted to reconcile new deterministic arguments about the role of physiology in criminal justice with traditional juridical arguments about the primacy of free will and moral responsibility.

The French Penal Code of 1810 was founded upon an "uncompromising moral arithmetic."[202] It prescribed standardized, irrevocable sentences for specific crimes in order to eliminate arbitrary sentencing and to deter others from crime. Guilt or innocence under this system depended upon the individual's capacity for reason and possession of free will. As the alienist Jean-Pierre Falret (1794–1870) explained, "Man is free to choose between good and evil, free by his will to decide between the different motives that draw him in different directions … Consequently, he is morally responsible and legally punishable when he willfully commits an action rejected by morality and condemned by law."[203] If legal responsibility hinged upon free will, then, by the same logic, individuals who did not "willfully" flout law and morality could not be held responsible for their crimes.[204] Article 64 of the Penal Code explicitly recognized this distinction and served as the statutory foundation of the insanity defence. It states, "there is neither crime nor misdemeanour when the defendant was in a state of insanity at the time of the act, or when he was constrained by a force which he could not resist."[205] Furthermore, judges and, after 1832, juries had the power to grant extenuating circumstances for defendants whose free will had been compromised at the time of the crime. The law compelled the courts to issue a milder sentence than the one prescribed by the Penal Code if a jury found extenuating circumstances.[206] Therefore, while the Penal Code prescribed a rigid system of punishments, in practice the courts could exercise a certain degree of flexibility in sentencing.

Although the insanity defence dated back to the Roman period, the methods that French courts used to establish insanity shifted at the turn of the nineteenth century.[207] Previously, judges had treated insanity as an absolute state, defined by the absence of reason. They believed that anyone with common sense could easily identify the disordered intellect and impaired judgment of the insane. Consequently, they relied primarily on witnesses who knew the defendant well rather than medical experts to establish the credibility of an insanity plea.[208] In the early decades of the nineteenth century, however, French alienists introduced new categories of "partial insanity," including *manie sans délire* (mania without delirium), homicidal monomania, and lesions of the will.[209] These conditions affected volition rather than reason. Afflicted individuals experienced uncontrollable impulses and emotions but demonstrated no impairment of intellectual function or judgment. As a result, they appeared perfectly normal and sane to the untrained eye, undermining straightforward divisions between sanity and insanity. As Jan Goldstein has demonstrated, French alienists, and particularly Esquirol's student Étienne-Jean Georget (1795–1828), used the complex symptomology of homicidal monomania to expand the alienist's role as a medical-legal expert and, in so doing, "enhance[d] the standing of the *médecin des aliénés* by integrating his functions into those of the state."[210] Therefore, by the mid-1820s, distinctions between "madness and badness" in the courtroom had become contingent upon specialist knowledge.[211]

French courts had called upon medical-legal experts to testify on issues of the body since the medieval period. Over the course of the nineteenth century, these experts played an increasingly important role in assessing issues of the mind to determine the extent of defendants' criminal responsibility.[212] Ruth Harris has argued that under the influence of these medical-legal experts, French jurisprudence experienced a shift during the *fin de siècle* from moralistic to deterministic under-standings of crime.[213] Medical-legal experts advanced new theories of criminology that emphasized the role of hereditary degeneration, the "unconscious," morbid impulses, and other social, environmental, and physiological factors, undermining the emphasis on free will that had defined classical jurisprudence.[214] Despite the increasing popularity of these new deterministic theories within the medical community, the principle of individual moral responsibility continued to dominate the French justice system. Morphine addiction offered medical-legal experts a unique case study for exploring how physiology influenced criminal behaviour. By challenging straightforward conceptions of individual free will, it exposed the often ambiguous boundaries between responsibility and irresponsibility in criminal cases.

The earliest cases that shaped medical-legal opinion on morphine addiction emerged in the late 1870s and 1880s alongside debates over another medical-legal defence: kleptomania, the "distinctive, irresistible tendency to steal."[215] As department stores faced a rise in retail thefts in the 1880s, medical experts increasingly used the kleptomania diagnosis to explain the bizarre behaviour of bourgeois women who impulsively stole useless items that they could easily afford.[216] The kleptomania de-fence rested upon bourgeois social privilege and assumptions about the inherently pathological nature of female physiology.[217] Experts focused on the apparent uselessness of the items stolen. They considered poor and working-class women, who stole from a real need, to be rational, if immoral, thieves. In contrast, respectable bourgeois women were kleptomaniacs. As such, they were not held legally responsible for their actions because experts believed that such irrational behaviour necessarily entailed a loss of reason, connected to perceptions about the inherent instabilities and weaknesses of the female body.

At first glance, the earliest cases of criminal *morphinomanie* resembled cases of kleptomania. In both instances, female defendants committed petty theft of items from novelty shops. Furthermore, both cases involved an overpowering urge for an object that compromised the defendant's free will. For the kleptomaniac, it was the obsessive desire to possess a trinket. For the *morphinomane*, it was the overwhelming physiological need for morphine to stave off withdrawal, as stolen items could be sold to buy morphine. Like kleptomaniacs, addicted defendants pleaded that they were not responsible for their actions because, in a state of morphine intoxication, an overpowering force had propelled them to steal. However, in spite of these similarities, experts contended that the particular pathological action of morphine over the human organism distinguished these thefts from cases of kleptomania.[218]

To establish criminal responsibility, medical-legal experts first needed to assess the severity of the defendant's addiction. Then they had to determine how and to what extent that addiction might have inhibited the defendant's free will at the time of the crime. In June 1878, Paul Brouardel (1837–1906), who lectured on legal medicine at the Paris Faculty of Medicine, conducted a medical-legal examination of C…, a thirty-eight-year-old morphine addict accused of stealing items from the stalls at the *magasins du Louvre*. Brouardel sought to determine whether kleptomania or morphine addiction might have motivated her actions.[219] As the medical community was just beginning to recognize morphine addiction as a new pathology, there were few legal precedents.[220] Nevertheless, cases of *morphinomanie* provided opportunities for multiple strategies of medical-legal investigation, including observation, interrogation, and chemical analysis.

Brouardel began his examination by observing C…'s physical appearance, expressions, and manner as he interviewed her about her medical history. Throughout the interview, C… displayed a calm indifference, giving only partial responses when prompted. Although her movements and responses were slow, Brouardel noted that her answers to his questions were correct and that "[her] judgment is perfectly healthy."[221] C… reported that she had injected herself with morphine for years to treat chronic neuralgic abdominal pains. She secured a steady supply of morphine from her husband's dental practice and claimed to consume a gram of morphine daily, approximately one hundred times a typical dose. Despite contemporary arguments that morphine addiction was both a cause and a symptom of the degeneration of modern society, C…'s addiction – like those of most morphine addicts of the time – had therapeutic origins. Whether it began from self-medicating or from a physician's prescription, the morphine she had used to regulate her abdominal pains had gradually produced an insidious physiological dependence.

Unlike most social pathologies associated with diminished criminal responsibility, morphine addiction left measurable physical evidence.

Brouardel used chemical urine analysis. He treated a 10-cc urine sample with iodized potassium iodide to detect the presence of alkaloids. A large amount of precipitate formed, indicating that C… had consumed a much higher than average dose. He then applied Fröhde's reagent to determine what the alkaloid was. It revealed the "distinctly purple" colour characteristic of morphine.[222] Brouardel's chemical investigations bolstered the authority of his empirical observations of C…'s behaviour and demeanour. The laboratory tests gave him both qualitative and quantitative scientific means of corroborating her story. C… was definitely a morphine addict. Nevertheless, as there was nothing in the nascent medical literature on morphine addiction to suggest that it could cause morbid impulses like kleptomania, Brouardel concluded that C… was responsible for her actions. However, he equivocated that "the state of intellectual stupor into which she was plunged, by the fact of her intoxication, can be taken into consideration and should be considered as partially attenuating this responsibility."[223] Brouardel's report demonstrates the challenges of reconciling moralistic legal arguments about free will with emerging medical knowledge about the physiology of morphine addiction.

The medical community, and French society as a whole, had become more familiar with morphine addiction by the mid-1880s. In 1886, Dr Paul Garnier (1848–1909), a medical-legal expert attached to the Infirmerie Spéciale of the Paris Prefecture of Police, observed that the abuse of morphine was being invoked more and more frequently in trials as an excuse for criminal behaviour.[224] The Infirmerie Spéciale was an important centre for medical-legal research. It served as clearing house for a wide variety of individuals, including criminals, vagrants, prostitutes, and the mentally ill. Doctors had to work quickly to diagnose individual cases because the facility had only a limited number of holding cells.[225] A greater number of cases of criminal *morphinomanie* enabled medical-legal experts to develop more specific rules for determining the extent of an addict's criminal responsibility in such cases. Garnier's own 1885 report on H… became one of the foundational case studies of criminal *morphinomanie*.

In June of 1885, the police arrested H…, a thirty-seven-year-old seamstress, for stealing various items from stalls at the Place Clichy and outside the Printemps department store. A search of her person uncovered a Pravaz syringe, a small bottle of morphine, and several stolen items worth approximately 55 francs. When the police commissioner interrogated her, H… explained that she had recently lost her job owing to a workshop closure and that her desperate state of destitution had driven her to steal something she could resell. She later changed her story for the magistrate, arguing that she remembered taking items from the stores without paying but had no idea why she had acted in that manner. "It's a sort of madness which took possession of me," she explained. "I would have taken the whole store! … I wasn't hiding, everyone could see me." She attributed this inexplicable, temporary madness to the morphine she injected five or six times a day to sooth her painful hepatic colic.[226] While at first she described a premeditated theft driven by her desperation after the loss of her job, her altered version of the events drew on tropes of the kleptomania defence.[227] However, H…'s state of poverty distinguished her from the bourgeois women typically acquitted as kleptomaniacs. Furthermore, like Brouardel before him, Garnier contended that there was nothing in the medical research to suggest that morphine addiction would lead to "irresistible impulses" or "kleptomaniac tendencies." Both experts distinguished *morphinomanie*, driven by physiological need, from kleptomania driven by impulsive desire.

Garnier used the medical-legal examination he conducted at Saint-Lazare Prison to test the strength of H…'s addiction. He watched her experience several violent hysterical crises accompanied by desperate screams, insensibility, and terrifying hallucinations. Fortunately for him, the physiology of withdrawal provided a straightforward diagnostic test. If a doctor administered a morphine injection to an addict during a crisis of withdrawal, Gautier argued, it should immediately "calm the storm unleashed by the reflex excitability of the nervous centres suddenly deprived of [their] usual moderating agent; the [bodily] economy resumes its more or less artificial equilibrium."[228] Each time he applied this test to H…, a 2-centigram injection of morphine returned her to normal almost instantly, suggesting that morphine withdrawal rather than hysteria was provoking her attacks.[229] Garnier also conducted a physical examination, which revealed numerous grey and purplish indentations on her right side that were consistent with frequent and prolonged morphine injection.

In the intervals between crises, H… was completely lucid. She asserted that she had felt strange on the day she was arrested. Seized by a violent dizziness, she went into the public toilets to administer four injections of morphine. "Leaving the water-closets," she explained, "I was dazed, I felt seized by vertigo and, I don't know how, passing in front of the stalls of the Magasins de la place Clichy, I was driven to take a cape. Yet I recall that I did. What could make me act in such a manner, I cannot say, but I am not a thief."[230] H… described her actions on the date of her arrest as automatic, divorced from free will or intention. However, Garnier found this inconsistent with his observations of her behaviour at Saint-Lazare. The absence of morphine produced crises; its presence returned her to a state of reason and lucidity. Therefore, he determined that H… should be held responsible for the theft as, by her own admission, she had injected morphine in the public toilets immediately before committing the crime.[231]

Withdrawal, rather than morphine, compromised an addict's mental state. Garnier's report suggested that H… could be considered in her right mind only when morphine was present in her system, making it a fundamental part of her status as a moral subject. Based on his medical-legal observations and an examination of twelve years of French medical research on chronic morphine addiction, Garnier concluded, "it is much less by regular continuation than by the sudden cessation of habits of intoxication that disorders of the mind break out … delusional disorders directly caused by morphine injections are relatively rare." Nevertheless, he qualified that H…'s "neuropathic temperament" exacerbated by her morphine addiction should attenuate her responsibility to a certain extent because it weakened her resistance to impulses.[232] On the basis of Garnier's report, the court found H… responsible for her actions but granted extenuating circumstances and condemned her to only a few days in prison. For H…, morphine functioned more as a moderating force than a catalyst of instability. Ultimately, Garnier attributed any extenuating circumstances she might have deserved not to her morphine addiction but to an underlying nervous temperament connected to contemporary assumptions about the constitutional weaknesses of the female body.

Garnier's conclusions about morphine as a regulatory agent shaped fin-de-siècle medical-legal debates on addiction. In 1886, Claudius Gaudry wrote a medical thesis on the penal responsibility of morphine addicts, in which he codified a series of medical-legal tenets for experts to follow to determine criminal responsibility in cases involving addiction. He argued, unequivocally, that an addict in a state of withdrawal should be considered irresponsible, particularly in cases in which the crime was committed in order to procure more morphine. Withdrawal produced agonizing physiological symptoms, including vomiting, diarrhea, chills, profuse sweating, respiratory anxiety, and sensitivity to touch.[233] The intense desire to avoid the torments of withdrawal drove a distinguished lawyer to steal morphine from a ship's pharmacy after having lost his entire provision of morphine during a bad storm on the journey from Genoa to Marseille.[234] The accentuated physical and psychosomatic disturbances of withdrawal could produce sudden violent delirium and intense, furious mania. In addition to its unpleasant physiological effects, Pichon argued that there were three main psychological symptoms of withdrawal: a manic state, which could vary in intensity from simple manic excitement to violent acute mania; hallucinations; and impulses ranging from stealing to suicide to murder.[235] In a state of withdrawal, "the human being has lost command of himself, his will and his reason no longer direct his actions." Gaudry held that it would be unreasonable to reproach a morphine addict or to hold him responsible for actions driven by impulse and physiological withdrawal rather than free will and reason.[236]

For crimes committed by addicts in a state of withdrawal, doctors turned to metaphors of hunger to describe the intensity of the body's physiological need for morphine. Chambard and Pichon both compared the addict in withdrawal who steals to buy morphine to the "individual who, needy and starving, steals a piece of bread from a baker's stall."[237] The poor starving man steals bread, in spite of the principles of law or morality, because his biological existence depends upon the bread's material sustenance. It was the same for the addict, if not worse, for, as Pichon asserted, addiction made the need for morphine "one hundred times more tenacious than the needs of hunger or thirst."[238] One addict even claimed, "I do not believe that lacking food I would ever have stolen a penny to procure myself some bread ... I would have preferred ... to die of hunger ... but being deprived of morphine when one is addicted is a completely different thing. Then I would do *everything* to have it."[239]

Considering the addict's complete subordination to the chemical imperatives of addiction and the extreme agonies and mental disturbances of withdrawal, French medical-legal experts concluded that morphine

addicts who committed crimes in a state of withdrawal should be granted full criminal irresponsibility. This became the fundamental tenet of
medical-legal rulings. Morphine undermined criminal responsibility,
not by its presence but by its absence.

Nevertheless, French medical-legal experts generally recognized
a certain diminution of responsibility even before an addict reached
a state of withdrawal, particularly when his supply of morphine was
dwindling.[240] "When one who commits [a crime] is absolutely pressed
by need; when the privation of morphine will throw [him] into a state
threatening his vital functioning and plunge him into a horrible torment,"
Gaudry explained, "then the will is no longer whole, the moral sense is
most often affected and the unfortunate [addict] obeys a pathological
impulse."[241] Withdrawal, or even the anticipation of withdrawal, crippled
the addict's free will.

The physiological need for morphine compelled the addict to take
whatever action necessary to satisfy the needs of her addicted body.
For example, in 1883 the police arrested Mme J... for stealing 120 francs
worth of novelty shop items, which she planned to sell for morphine. She
had resorted to petty theft only after she had exhausted her credit with
the pharmacist, borrowed money from friends, and pawned clothing
and furniture for morphine.[242] After observing the intense mental and
physiological disturbances that Mme J... experienced during withdrawal,
her medical-legal examiner Auguste Motet (1832–1909) concluded that
"her will is overpowered, the discomforts she feels when she is deprived
of the narcotic to which she has become accustomed no longer permit
her to suspend injections of morphine hydrochloride."[243] The court
accepted his conclusions and acquitted her of all charges.

The question of whether the addict was under the influence of morphine at the time of the crime became the primary measure of criminal
responsibility. As addicts appeared to function normally under the
influence of their regular dose of morphine, most French medical-legal
experts argued that they should be held fully responsible for their actions.
Dr Évariste Marandon de Montyel, the director of the public asylum
in Dijon, argued that in the initial state of "euphoria" that followed an
injection, "responsibility is complete, because then morphine, far from
lowering or disturbing the economy, gives it increased life; moral energy,
like intellectual energy, asserts itself more."[244] German medical-legal

experts even argued that addicts were *more* responsible for crimes while under morphine's influence, because of the stimulating action morphine had on the intellect, though French experts rarely went so far.[245]

While medical-legal convention linked irresponsibility to a state of withdrawal for most addicts, in certain cases the excessive, prolonged use of morphine could lead to a general deterioration of an addict's mental state akin to more traditional understandings of insanity. Pichon posited that the salient feature of this degree of addiction was "that state of dejection, of obnubilation [the clouding of consciousness] that renders [the addict] incapable of resisting the bad advice of the imagination."[246] German psychiatrists referred to this mental state as *psychische-Schwäche*, literally "psychic weakness."[247] In this state, the addict's mind displayed a certain passivity, or "inertia," in which he "lets himself be dominated by his bad instincts, failing to resist his mind's incitement to bad actions, whereas in a healthy state, his normal good sense would be immediately appalled."[248] In these cases, morphine inhibited the individual's will and ability to resist the dangerous influences of his own mind and imagination, transforming him into a passive automaton. This level of mental incapacity invited a more straightforward application of the insanity defence. Therefore, doctors believed that in these exceptional cases, criminal responsibility should be somewhat attenuated even when defendants were on morphine.[249]

In the 1870s and 1880s, the relationship between morphine and mental illness was ambiguous. Some doctors, like Pichon, were beginning to recognize the dangers of addiction as a potential cause of mental illness, particularly in cases of excessive, prolonged use. Others, like Auguste Voisin, continued to explore morphine's therapeutic potential as a treatment for mental illness. Therefore, medical-legal experts occasionally had to assess cases in which nervous conditions and morphine addiction offered competing visions of criminal irresponsibility.

On 9 November 1885, the police arrested twenty-six-year-old Annette G… for stealing and selling a blanket that belonged to her landlord. The court sentenced her to three months in prison for the crime.[250] However, at Saint-Lazare Prison she was sent straight to the infirmary, where doctors diagnosed her as a *morphinomane hystérique* of the highest degree. The appeals court called upon Charcot, Motet, and Brouardel, three of the leading medical-legal experts in Paris, to examine her mental state.

The medical-legal experts attributed Annette G...'s nervous troubles to childhood trauma. At age eleven, she had witnessed soldiers execute a group of insurgents by firing squad during the Paris Commune. This left a strong impression on her "predominantly nervous temperament."[251] With the onset of puberty, she regularly began to experience intense throat pain during menstruation. In September 1875, she began to experience more intense nervous crises, which included frightening visions and hallucinations, delirium, rigidity, and throat pain so intense it kept her from eating. She soon began to use morphine injections to relieve her throat pain and manage her hysterical crises. Although Annette G... continued to experience crises even under the influence of morphine, they took on a different, less disruptive form. Morphine revitalized her and enabled her to perform small tasks at home. She regained more control over her life. However, it was not long before "the appetite, the need for injection became more and more imperious, more and more tyrannical." She gradually increased her dose to as much as 1 gram of morphine per day spread out over twenty injections.[252] While morphine regulated her hysterical crises, it also produced a new physiological need.

Annette G...'s addiction was so entrenched that when she arrived at Saint-Lazare, she experienced an acute crisis of withdrawal, which manifested in vertigo, spasms, fainting, and a state of depression and weakness. In the prison infirmary, doctors administered morphine injections to halt the crisis. They sustained her in this manner for several days, managing her crises with morphine before replacing the injections with lower doses of opium. The normalizing effect of morphine over this addicted defendant illustrated the extent of her addiction. However, Annette G...'s hysteria complicated matters. Ultimately, Charcot, Motet, and Brouardel attributed her crime to this underlying nervous condition rather than to the influence of morphine per se. They acknowledged that the dual influence of nervous troubles and morphine addiction had produced in her a state of "moral and intellectual disarray." The medical experts determined that she had stolen the blanket out of desperation, misery, and hunger. She committed the crime "as one of those instinctive solicitations that do not find sufficient counterweight of deliberation and resistance in a mind debilitated by the malady."[253] They recommended that she be exonerated. The court accepted the doctors' conclusions and Annette G... was immediately released. The medical-legal report portrayed morphine as a normalizing force used to combat, however imperfectly, an underlying hysterical issue as well as the agonies of withdrawal.

Medical-legal experts reached a comfortable consensus on the criminal irresponsibility of a morphine addict in withdrawal who stole for the express purpose of acquiring more morphine. Such a theft could be considered the desperate act of an organism whose very survival depended upon securing another dose. In the case of violent crimes, however, the issue became more complex. What was an addict's responsibility when the crime was against a person rather than property?

The first major incident of murder involving morphine abuse was the "Affaire Fiquet." In 1882, in the city of Dijon, a morphine addict known as Mme Fiquet lured a five-year-old girl to her home after school. Later that evening, she and her husband carried the girl's lifeless body to the Bourgogne Canal, where the police found it the next morning. What happened during the intervening twelve hours remained shrouded in mystery, as Mme Fiquet kept changing her story.[254] First she denied all knowledge of the incident; then she claimed that her husband had murdered the girl and she was merely an accessory; and finally she argued that she must have kidnapped the girl because of an impulse caused by her morphine addiction.[255] She claimed she could not remember the specific events of the day of the murder. In turn, the medical experts wryly noted that the holes in her memory seemed to coincide perfectly with the important facts of the case that could incriminate her. Such a "mental condition" was "scientifically inadmissible."[256]

Mme Fiquet's medical-legal examiners observed the physical symptoms of withdrawal. However, they believed that she was fabricating the psychological symptoms she claimed to experience, modelling them on a description of morphine-induced psychotic disturbance provided by a naïve hospital attendant and on the famous cases of hysteria popularized by Charcot at Salpêtrière Hospital.[257] Dr Marandon de Montyel argued that Mme Fiquet's calculated deception and simulations of madness were in fact signs of her intellectual capacity. The medical-legal experts determined that Mme Fiquet was responsible for her actions, as she had been under the influence of morphine on the day of the girl's disappearance. Nevertheless, they did allow for some extenuating circumstances, possibly owing to the bizarre and inexplicable nature of the crime. The court sentenced Mme Fiquet to twenty years of hard labour.

In other cases, experts found addicts not responsible for acts of violence. In November 1891, *Le Figaro* published a series of articles on a case in which M. Gennevraye, a composer of music and a morphine addict, was accused of abusing his children and encouraging his wife to become addicted to morphine.[258] After hearing rumours about the extent of the Gennevrayes' addiction and that M. Gennevraye had shoved his infant son so forcefully that the child's leg was broken, the Union Française pour le Sauvetage de l'Enfance called upon the justice system to intervene. One witness testified that she had seen a box containing over two hundred broken needles at the family's home and that every evening M. Gennevraye's valet brought him four 30-gram flasks of morphine, which were emptied by the morning.[259] After conducting an official inquiry, the magistrate issued a warrant for Gennevraye's arrest, because "it is imperative before all else to examine the mental state of the *morphinomane* and to prevent M. Gennevraye from becoming dangerous." *Le Figaro* noted that Gennevraye's state of overexcitement was such that the director of admissions deemed it prudent to place him in a padded cell.[260]

Unlike earlier cases that highlighted the regulatory influence of a habitual dose, this case depended upon an examination of the responsibility of an addicted defendant in a state of acute morphine intoxication. Consequently, it more closely resembled cases of alcoholism, in which crimes were committed in a state of excess rather than deprivation.[261] The court assigned Garnier and Motet to determine Gennevraye's mental state, in order to decide whether to prosecute him or take protective measures so he could not harm himself or others.[262] These medical-legal experts concluded that morphine intoxication made him dangerously impulsive and "partly obscured the consciousness of his actions."[263] As Gennevraye had become calm and was no longer delirious, they argued that incarceration in an insane asylum was unnecessary. The judge granted him provisional liberty to be treated in a convalescent home. Nine days later, based on the medical report, the magistrate issued the official order of dismissal declaring that Gennevraye was not responsible for his actions.[264]

In cases of alcoholic intoxication, the courts displayed considerable class bias against working-class defendants who brutalized their families but they rarely held bourgeois alcoholics accountable for their actions.[265] Furthermore, as France's Civil Code granted fathers considerable latitude in punishing their children, it is perhaps unsurprising that the court did not see fit to sanction the bourgeois M. Gennevraye for the violence he had committed against his son.[266] The justice system recognized the danger Gennevraye posed, yet it treated him as a mental patient rather than a criminal, placing him in a padded cell and prescribing convalescent treatment. The court ruled that Gennevraye, by consuming excessive amounts of morphine, had compromised his sanity and thus his moral responsibility.

Three months later the French press bristled over another sensational incident of morphine-induced violence. In March 1892, Léon Porteret, a morphine-addicted doctor from Lyon, murdered his young wife, shooting her three times in the chest before shooting himself in the head.[267] He died of his wound in hospital a few days later, pleading for morphine.[268] Purportedly, the day before the murder Porteret had performed eighteen morphine injections on himself and had taken cocaine. His state was aggravated and overexcited and he appeared to be hallucinating. Two hours before the murder, Porteret wrote a long letter to the newspaper *Gil Blas* to explain his crime of passion. He denounced his wife for having committed adultery with his own brother and one of his colleagues, denied paternity of their infant son, and claimed that most of the women in his wife's family were widows whose husbands had died under suspicious circumstances.[269] Given the scandalous nature of the accusations, the newspaper posed this question: Was this the letter of "a madman, a *morphinomane*, or a man truly suffering from the misconduct of his wife?"[270]

Social ideas about gender shaped the legal defence for crimes of passion.[271] Male defendants often asserted that a violation of honour, typically infidelity, had produced an overpowering passion that caused a state of temporary insanity.[272] To demonstrate the purity of their motives, they acknowledged premeditation and attempted to publicize their actions as retribution designed to restore their honour.[273] Male defendants frequently attempted suicide in the aftermath of a crime of passion. The credibility of this attempt was one of the methods that courts used to establish the legitimacy of the crime-of-passion defence. However, courts also measured a male defendant's responsibility "based on how much the female victim was considered to have lived up to her social and familial obligations."[274]

Aside from his morphine addiction, Porteret's case possesses all the main features of a crime of passion: he announced his intentions to murder as an act of justice to restore his tarnished honour; he publicized his motives, outlining his wife's infidelities; finally, he attempted suicide, with eventual success. However, Porteret knew that people would assume that his addiction had motivated his actions, so he deliberately attempted to establish his own sanity and credibility through his letter to the editor of *Gil Blas*. He claimed that he had considered the idea that his jealousy and suspicions might be a result of mental disturbances caused by his addiction but then had dismissed this thought and reasserted that he was in his right mind. He declared, "I am not crazy, I assure you, and whatever the medical-legal experts who conduct my autopsy might say, I am very certain that I have all my good sense and reason with the most perfect logic."[275] Porteret deliberately attempted to circumvent the medical experts' line of argument by asserting his own mental stability and articulating specific grievances against his wife.

Despite these efforts, discussion of the extent of Porteret's morphine addiction overshadowed all other concerns in both the press and the autopsy report. Antonin Poncet and Alexandre Lacassagne, who conducted the autopsy, concluded that although the bullet passed straight through Porteret's head from one temple to the other, "these lesions do not appear to have been the true cause of death. This was mainly caused by the inveterate habits of morphinism," which produced a state of delirium and paranoia that ultimately led to his outburst of violence.[276] Therefore, according to medical experts, the morphine that had poisoned Porteret's brain beyond reason was more responsible for his death than the bullet that had passed through it.

For the most part, medical experts measured a defendant's addiction and criminal responsibility through clinical observation in a prison or an asylum. In these spaces, they could question the defendant and observe any symptoms of withdrawal that might indicate the severity of his or her addiction. On occasion, however, the powerful grip that morphine held over the addict revealed itself in the courtroom. In 1896, Guillaume-Louis-Joseph Aubert, a thirty-year-old wine seller, appeared before the Assizes Court of the Seine. Aubert was accused of luring his victim, Emile Delahaef, to his apartment in order to steal his valuable stamp collection and then brutally murdering Delahaef with an axe and stuffing his corpse into a large trunk. Aided by his mistress, Aubert moved the trunk between the baggage checks of various train stations around Paris before sending it to Courville. There, the stationmaster, disturbed by the noxious odour emanating from the trunk, opened it to discover the body.[277] When Aubert and his mistress returned to collect the trunk, the police arrested them on the spot.

Whatever Aubert's mental state might have been at the time of the murder, during the trial his morphine addiction manifested dramatically, at times interrupting the proceedings of the court. Aubert had been addicted to morphine for several years. His addiction was so entrenched that before the trial he wrote to the judge requesting permission to buy morphine. The judge denied his request. When Aubert entered the courtroom he appeared to be suffering from withdrawal. The *Gazette des tribunaux* noted that his entrance provoked curiosity from the audience, as he "moves and shakes his head from a nervous tic that makes his two bright little eyes blink."[278] The defence lawyer asked the court to grant a mental examination of Aubert, claiming that two doctors had already proclaimed him to be an unstable degenerate.[279]

When the prosecution asked the court to reject this request, Aubert stood up and began to "gesticulate like a madman." The guards had to intervene to calm him down. At first glance this might appear to be a carefully timed theatrical display meant to gain the sympathy of the court. However, Aubert's subsequent behaviour in the trial suggests that his state of morphine withdrawal, rather than any rational calculation, was dictating his actions. The presiding judge rejected the defence's request for a medical examination.[280] In so doing, he transformed the courtroom into a space where the audience, and particularly the jury, had the opportunity to assess the defendant's addiction for themselves.

Aubert exposed the severity of his addiction through erratic behaviour and explicit oral testimony. During questioning, Aubert was excitable. He gesticulated frequently. At one point, he exclaimed, "I cannot, I cannot; allow me to go and inject myself and I will be calm. I must defend myself; I was not able to do it at the *instruction* [before the trial], I must do it before public opinion." Morphine withdrawal compromised Aubert's ability to mount an adequate defence in court. After a few more questions, the judge ordered a recess so that Aubert could compose himself. When they reconvened, however, Aubert was just as agitated as before, suggesting that he had been unable to get his fix. When cross-examined about inconsistencies in his testimony, he became irate, "hit the bar with anger," and accused the magistrate of unfair treatment during his pretrial investigation.

Aubert's outbursts during the trial demonstrated his mental and physiological imbalance when separated from the psychotropic drug that had become a vital component of his daily life and an integral part of his subjectivity. When the judge asked Aubert to calm down, he responded, "I cannot, M. le président; I am suffering from a nervous malady; inject me with morphine and I am calm; without it, it's stronger than me, I cannot control myself."[281] Aubert recognized his own inability to function in a reasonable manner without the drug. Morphine addiction had permanently altered his consciousness and his body's vital needs, fundamentally changing the parameters of his "normal" state. For Aubert, normality required morphine.

Aubert's agitation heightened on the second day of the trial. After a violent outburst during a witness's testimony, guards had to forcibly remove the defendant from the court. The trial was suspended for twenty minutes, after which Aubert returned pale, groggy, and notably subdued after having been injected with morphine. When he returned, "he leaned on the balustrade, his face shaking with nervous spasms; the guards made him drink a potion and Dr Floquet [sat] next to him." The shift in Aubert's behaviour was so dramatic that on two separate occasions the judge asked the doctor to confirm whether Aubert was in a fit state to follow the debates. Before the morphine injection, Aubert had protested vehemently against particular points of the case and persisted in his claims that he had acted in self-defence. After the injection, he appeared disengaged and drowsy. On the third day of the trial, "during the entire time that the civil party's lawyer pleaded [his case], Aubert slumbered, his head resting on the balustrade, indifferent to the plea pronounced against him." On the fourth and final day of the trial a huge crowd gathered to hear the verdict. However, rather than demonstrating concern or even interest in his fate, Aubert "appear[ed] to sleep, his head nodding slightly as it rested constantly on the palm of his right hand."[282] The court used morphine to discipline the unruly behaviour of this defendant. After Aubert received a morphine injection in the middle of the trial, everyone in attendance could witness his dramatic transformation from impassioned, erratic, and agitated to groggy, disinterested, and unaware.

In light of Aubert's volatile behaviour during the trial, it is surprising that the court denied his lawyer's request for a mental examination.[283] The defence lawyer did call several witnesses who all testified that Aubert had had a nervous tic for years and that they had long considered him to be unstable. In his closing statement, Aubert's lawyer argued that his unusual behaviour in court should indicate that something was not quite right with the defendant's mental state:

> I did not say that Aubert was insane, because I have no idea, but he is an unfortunate person who has committed follies in his life that should have granted that mental examination that I requested in vain. Do you not regret [the refusal of a mental examination], when you see this man who today is no more than a cadaver [now] that we have witnessed this singular and unusual spectacle of a defendant obliged to be taken outside the courtroom to receive an injection of morphine and then brought back to his bench insensible to all that is happening around him[?][284]

Regardless of whether Aubert had been of sound mind during the murder itself, during the trial for murder he appeared unstable at the very least. Wrapping up his closing remarks, the defence lawyer implored the jury not to send Aubert to the scaffold, "because you do not know what mystery is hidden in his sick brain, if, in a word, he is really responsible for his actions. This man is unhinged, a sick man, the kind of man we treat but do not guillotine."[285] The jury found Aubert guilty and responsible for his actions but granted him extenuating circumstances. Instead of the death penalty prescribed by Articles 302 and 304 of the Penal Code, the court sentenced Aubert to a lifetime of hard labour.[286]

Aubert's case exposed the court's resistance to the deterministic arguments of medical-legal experts regarding the origins of criminal behaviour. In his closing statements, the prosecutor, M. Bonnet, explicitly condemned the deterministic theories of criminology then in vogue, insisting, "we must rise up ... against this current trend of seeing madmen everywhere."[287] Asserting that Aubert was clearly and entirely responsible for his actions, Bonnet implored the jury not to grant Aubert extenuating circumstances. The court's refusal to grant Aubert a mental examination suggests that the presiding judges sympathized with the prosecution's condemnation of the growing popularity of deterministic theories, particularly as the court had allowed other expert witnesses during the trial, including a handwriting expert, the doctor who conducted the autopsy, and an expert chemist who tested for bloodstains. The law of 1832, which granted juries the right to find extenuating circumstances, compelled the court to reduce the sentence in such cases by one degree from the punishment prescribed in the Penal Code. However, for crimes punishable by death or hard labour, judges also had the authority to reduce the penalty by an additional degree.[288] They declined to do so in Aubert's case.

The peculiar conditions of Aubert's trial make it difficult to determine the extent to which his addiction might have served as the mitigating factor in the jury's verdict. Typically, French juries were least lenient in cases of premeditated murder. They found defendants guilty in approximately three-fourths of trials for premeditated murder in the 1890s.[289] At the same time, juries also frequently ruled in favour of extenuating circumstances for individuals accused of capital crimes. Between 1891 and 1900, juries granted extenuating circumstances to 88.2 per cent of the 1,951 defendants convicted of capital crimes, sentencing only 231 (11.8 per cent) to death.[290] There was no question that Aubert had killed Delahaef and the prosecution provided ample evidence demonstrating that Aubert had plotted Delahaef's murder.[291] Furthermore, the death blow – an axe wound to the back of the victim's head – undermined Aubert's claim that he had simply acted in self-defence. The case for the defence rested entirely on the argument that morphine had made Aubert mentally unstable. However, without a mental examination conducted by experts, the jury was left to assess the extent of Aubert's guilt based on the oral testimonies of witnesses and Aubert's own performance in court.

The French judicial system did not require juries to list the reasons for granting extenuating circumstances.[292] Therefore, one can only speculate as to whether the jury believed that Aubert's morphine addiction had compromised his reason or free will sufficiently to attenuate his responsibility or whether, in granting extenuating circumstances, they were following the established tradition of French juries using their discretionary power to mitigate the legally prescribed punishment.[293] If the logic of the jury's verdict remains subject to conjecture, Aubert's performance of his addiction and the court's response to it are far more revealing. Aubert's addiction revealed itself dramatically in the courtroom through his agitated and erratic behaviour, his violent outbursts, and his pleas for relief in the face of withdrawal. In response, the judge called for a recess, during which a doctor injected Aubert with morphine, rendering him calm and docile. In so doing, the court actively acknowledged the regulatory influence that morphine had over this defendant. Despite an unwillingness to grant him a mental examination, by using morphine to control Aubert's behaviour the court conceded that he was unstable, dependent on morphine for any semblance of a normal state.

Morphine occupied a privileged and paradoxical position in legal medicine. Whether seen as an essential therapeutic tool or a dangerous catalyst of addiction and mental disturbance, medical-legal experts acknowledged its powerful influence over the individual. They recognized that this alkaloid, injected directly under the skin, produced a far more tenacious form of addiction than other forms of drug consumption, such as opium smoking.[294] Furthermore, as morphine addiction was frequently a side effect of medical treatment, medical-legal experts tended to view morphine addicts as less blameworthy than opium smokers, whose habits were associated with deviance and decadence in the popular imagination.[295]

The verdict in the infamous Ullmo spy case highlighted this distinction and morphine's privileged status in medical-legal defence. In 1908, Benjamin Ullmo, a young naval officer, faced charges of treason. He had photographed important naval documents, attempted to sell them to foreign agents, and then blackmailed the French navy for over 100,000 francs to pay off gambling debts, finance his opium smoking, and support his opium-addicted mistress.[296]

For over six years, Ullmo had smoked opium regularly while serving in both France and Saigon. He usually smoked about 30 grams of opium per day divided among 30 to 40 pipes. He rarely went for three days without it, so he used opium pills to stave off the shivering, sweating, and diarrhea he experienced when he was separated from his pipe. While incarcerated awaiting trial, he had no access to opium. However, the medical-legal experts who examined him noted that they were surprised at the "relative ease" with which Ullmo withstood the withdrawal.[297]

This did not bode well for his defence. Ullmo claimed that he had committed treason under the unique mental state produced by opium addiction but told the medical experts that "now that he is weaned from the poison, he would be absolutely incapable of a such a crime."[298] He explained that he had concocted the plan to steal military secrets under the influence of the cloudy torpor of opium addiction, which caused him to act "quasi-automatically."[299] The experts disagreed. They argued that Ullmo was not sufficiently addicted to opium to be considered irresponsible. Clinical observations of other opium smokers revealed that they only experienced effects like the ones Ullmo described when taking doses of 100 to 120 pipes per day. Ullmo took a far more modest daily dose of 30 to 40 pipes.

Ullmo's ability to maintain a stable daily dose and the relative ease with which he endured withdrawal and recovered his health following his arrest suggested that his opium addiction was relatively mild. The experts noted that injecting high doses of morphine had much more disastrous effects on an organism than smoking opium, because a lot of the opium's potent alkaloids were lost through combustion and in the residue left in the bowl of the pipe.[300] Furthermore, Ullmo's crime was not impulsive. He executed a detailed plan over the course of six months that required careful planning, perseverance, and calculated risk. As Dupré wryly noted, "he did not commit treason in order to procure opium."[301]

The court found Ullmo guilty. Rather than declaring him a victim of the nefarious influence of an imperious drug, the experts labelled Ullmo a weak-willed man, whose dominant psychological trait was "the incapacity to resist the solicitation of his appetites": opium, gambling, and women. He was stripped of his military rank in a large public spectacle and deported for a life sentence on Devil's Island, where he occupied the same cell that Alfred Dreyfus had during his own incarceration there. The French legal system punished Ullmo for an act of willful treason, in which he placed his own selfish desires for sensual pleasure above the welfare of society. Unlike the innocent Dreyfus, whose incarceration was a miscarriage of justice that tarnished France's republican ideals, Ullmo's imprisonment was justified punishment for a crime that exposed the social danger of *anomie*.[302] Despite the court having found Ullmo guilty, the medical-legal report reaffirmed the status of opiates in legal medicine, noting that "opium, the poison *par excellence* of moral strength, is an agent of destruction for the will, for initiative, and for action ... Then it affects ethics and affective sentiments, and finally it alters the intelligence."[303] Unfortunately for Ullmo, the court ruled that opium had not altered his intelligence enough. Insufficiently addicted, Ullmo had to pay for his crime.

In the early twentieth century, new legislation transformed encounters between drug addicts and the judiciary. The government passed a new poisonous substances law in 1916, which criminalized the *use* of psychotropic drugs for the first time under certain conditions. However, the legislation was designed to target social drug use and did not criminalize individual private consumption.[304] As French society increasingly stigmatized other pleasure-seeking forms of drug consumption as dangerous vices in the years leading up to the 1916 law, morphine retained its status as an important staple of therapeutic medicine. Even within this more hostile climate, medical-legal experts continued to emphasize the overpowering influence of morphine over the addict's free will.[305]

Debates over the criminal responsibility of morphine addicts in the *fin de siècle* should be understood as part of a larger shift in the history of criminology toward a consideration of physiological, social, hereditary, and environmental factors. Medical-legal experts who specialized in mental maladies contributed to the formation of numerous new tropes of legal medicine – including hysteria, alcoholism, kleptomania, hypnotism, and crimes of passion – that increasingly challenged the moralistic logic of classical jurisprudence. Morphine addiction introduced into criminal cases a new variable, which fit uneasily into these established categories of legal medicine. For addicts, morphine served as a regulatory technology to correct a physiological imbalance of its own making. Doctors used medical-legal examinations to determine the extent of a defendant's addiction by analyzing physiological evidence and observing morphine's power over a defendant's actions. In so doing, they deployed the strategies of positivist science, typically associated with deterministic ideas about crime, to emphasize the continued importance of moral responsibility and free will.

From the asylum to the courtroom, doctors interrogated how drugs regulated the mind. Psychiatrists believed that psychotropic drugs could produce dramatic and, in some cases, permanent changes in their patients' mental states. These drugs served as crucial legitimizing mechanisms for the emergent psychiatric profession in France by enabling doctors to return previously "incurable" patients to a state of sanity. However, these treatments also had unexpected consequences. In a quest to cure madness, doctors ended up creating addiction. Psychotropic drugs served both as therapeutic tools and as corrupting agents of mental pathology. By creating a new form of "artificial madness," doctors destabilized their own role as healers and raised new questions about individual free will.

Morphine addicts who committed crimes resisted clear distinctions between legal responsibility and criminal insanity. In some cases of acute morphine intoxication, excessive amounts of the drug could compromise an addict's sanity through a loss of reason reminiscent of traditional judicial understandings of total insanity. More frequently, however, addiction did not serve as a straightforward legal defence because doctors recognized the regulatory power of morphine over the addicted body. Without a normal dose of morphine, the addict suffered agonizing withdrawal. In such cases an addict's status as a legal and moral subject was contingent upon morphine's normalizing influence. Therefore, morphine became a fundamental component of the addicted self, required for the individual to be considered legally sane and morally responsible. Through medical-legal debates over *morphinomanie*, experts forced the courts to consider the role of the addicted body as well as the mind. Such cases effectively shifted the seat of moral responsibility from the addict's brain to the drug that controlled it.

{ 4 }

SEX AND DRUGS

The spasm of love: when ether hallucinates
The young woman in the grip of Lucina's torments
O from a double mystery of ineffable power!
At the moment she gives birth, she believes
she is conceiving.

This excerpt from Auguste-Marie Barthélemy's *Zodiaque poétique* (1847) suggested that ether could act as both anesthetic and aphrodisiac. In the poem, ether not only eliminated the painful sensations of parturition but actually turned birth into an erotic experience. Paradoxically, ether, an anesthetic agent, transformed agony into orgasm.

Psychotropic drugs became ubiquitous in nineteenth-century society because of their capacity to relieve pain. However, these drugs also offered users access to a world of chemical delights. Over time, psychotropic drugs gained a reputation as sources of indulgent pleasure, associated with illicit sex and sexuality. Paintings depicted drug use as erotic.[1] Novels described the seductive powers of psychotropic substances, portraying them as "vengeful mistresses" who ensnared their victims in a tantalizing web of pleasure and desire.[2] Newspapers printed titillating descriptions of *demimondaines* in Toulon and Brest who ran private opium dens and Montmartre prostitutes who supplied cocaine to their clients, fusing sex and drugs together into a single erotic economy.[3] Through this entanglement of erotic and narcotic indulgence, psychotropic drugs became inextricably bound to anxieties over sex and sexuality.

Doctors had to tread carefully to distance themselves from the aphrodisiac reputation of these substances while simultaneously appropriating them as legitimizing mechanisms of medical authority. During the *fin-de-siècle* degeneration debates, doctors and moral reformers expressed concerns over the impact of psychotropic drugs on sexual desire and virility for both the individual sexual body and the social body of the French nation. Social critics condemned the individual's selfish pursuit of chemically enhanced pleasure.[4] Paradoxically, they depicted psychotropic drugs both as dangerous aphrodisiacs that would corrupt public morality and as debilitating impotence-inducers that would cripple the reproductive capacity of the French nation. These were powerful arguments amid anxieties about France's demographic future.[5] However, in the case of certain pathological conditions like vaginismus, a vaginal condition that made sexual penetration impossible or prohibitively painful, drugs like cocaine offered some couples their only hope of conceiving a child. If drugs threatened the French nation when misused, they also held the potential to restore its vitality.

ANESTHESIA AND APHRODISIA

When the Academy of Sciences and the Academy of Medicine first discussed the anesthetic potential of ether and chloroform in 1847, doctors had mixed feelings: their elation at the prospect of painless surgery was coupled with anxiety over the vulnerability of the unconscious, insensible body of the patient. More skeptical than many of his colleagues, the physiologist François Magendie expressed concern that anesthesia placed a patient completely under the control of another human being. "In acting upon the patient in this manner," Magendie asserted, "you take away the awareness of his being; you surrender him entirely to the people surrounding him. To plunge a woman into a state of *ivresse*, making her insensible, making her lose consciousness, is this a moral thing? Have you reflected upon all that could result from it?"[6] Magendie's questions highlighted the absolute power of the doctor over his unconscious female patient and the ease with which he could take advantage of her in such a state.

Over fifty years later, Magendie's fears were realized. In 1901, the courts condemned Auguste Pillot, a pharmacist in a small village in Burgundy, for running an illegal dental practice out of his pharmacy in order to perform "lecherous acts" on his female patients under the influence of chloroform anesthesia.[7] He faced sixty-eight counts of assault or indecent behaviour against married women, single women, and young girls over a seven-year period.[8] In 1893, Mme Louise Desbois had visited Pillot complaining of an extremely painful molar and he administered chloroform. Though it dulled her consciousness, Mme Desbois testified that she felt him engaging in "reprehensible acts" on her person. Another patient, Mme Gauliard, accused him of attempted rape, which was prevented only because another client interrupted him before he could finish. Two patients accused Pillot of raping and impregnating them under the influence of chloroform anesthesia. The first was Eugénie Potonnier, a young woman whom Pillot submitted to chloroform anesthesia during a tooth extraction in January 1900. She began to feel the first signs of pregnancy in April and gave birth to a daughter on 2 October. In the second case, Pillot submitted a young woman named Jeanne Baudron to chloroform for complaints of stomach pain on 21 February. Mlle Baudron remembered Pillot raping her. She became pregnant, and she gave birth on 22 November.[9]

Yet despite these two cases of impregnation and numerous other charges brought against Pillot by a wide range of women who were well regarded by their communities, some medical professionals still wondered whether the pharmacist had really abused his power. Pillot's defenders questioned whether these two unmarried women were taking advantage of cultural biases about anesthesia in order to absolve themselves of the stigma of single motherhood. Dr Auguste Lutaud, a gynecologist from Burgundy, summarized Pillot's case in the *Revue de psychiatrie* in an article shockingly titled "Can women be raped during anesthesia?" Chloroform anesthesia produced a grey area of consciousness for Pillot's accusers, which undermined both the women's status as victims and their credibility as witnesses.

At the beginning of the nineteenth century, rape convictions rested upon the victim's ability to prove that her assailant had used physical violence to force himself on her. However, judicial understandings of what constituted rape gradually began to shift. After 1850, jurists began to acknowledge that victims' free will could also be compromised by non-violent forms of coercion, like threats or blackmail; a loss of consciousness from fainting, a coma, or anesthesia; or an altered consciousness from intoxication caused by alcohol, opiates, or anesthetic gases. Yet they continued to approach victims with suspicion.[10] In the Pillot case, Lutaud argued that if the women were aware enough to remember his assaults, they would have been able to struggle against him. As evidence, he cited Dr Paul Brouardel's descriptions of the initial period of excitation in which surgical patients attempt to push the anesthesia mask away.[11] Nineteenth-century legal experts consistently argued that a woman would be capable of defending herself against a sexual assault from one man acting alone, a claim that seems particularly illogical given contemporary arguments about women as the "weaker sex."[12] Although Lutaud admitted that Pillot had engaged in inappropriate touching and lecherous acts with his female patients, he would not label it rape. He explained, "it is more or less impossible that he consummated the sexual act with a large number of women without their consent."[13]

Female victims, presumed to be duplicitous and irrational, struggled to be taken seriously by bourgeois men of science. Lutaud recounted another case in which a woman claimed that she had been forcibly impregnated under anesthesia. Six months previously, she had visited a hypnotist who claimed he could cure her unspecified ailment by hypnosis. However, one *louis* and twelve failed attempts later, he proposed to put her to sleep using chloroform. "I agreed [to the chloroform]," she explained to Lutaud, and "when I woke up I was all confused, and I had dreamed that a man introduced something into my genital organs. It's since that day [six months ago], Monsieur, that I have been pregnant."[14] Lutaud dismissed her claims and informed her that it was impossible to rape a woman under anesthesia. However, the woman insisted that the hypnotist had used chloroform to rape and impregnate her against her will. Despite the irrefutable evidence of her pregnancy, Lutaud refused to entertain the possibility that she might have been telling the truth.

By the end of the nineteenth century, the use of psychotropic drugs to commit rape had become a subject of medical-legal debate. While the number of reported cases of rape using chloroform or ether was relatively low, the issue provoked much debate in medical circles, probably because doctors and dentists were most likely to be implicated in cases of anesthetic rape.[15] Lutaud aside, most doctors acknowledged that anesthetic drugs could be used to facilitate sexual assault. Some even acknowledged that a rape could be committed without a woman's knowledge if her rapist administered ether or chloroform while she was sleeping.[16] The courts agreed. Just over ten years prior to Pillot's case, a dentist from Marseille had been condemned to forced labour for an "indecent assault" on a woman whom he had anesthetized for a tooth extraction.[17]

The use of psychotropic drugs as tools of dastardly seduction was also a popular plot device in drug literature and theatre.[18] Xavier de Montepin's 1874 novel, *Drames de l'adultère*, illustrates the role of anesthetic drugs as tools of rape.[19] The premise of Louis Bechét's three-act comedy, *Doctor Morphine*, first produced in 1906 bears a striking resemblance to Pillot's case.[20] In the play, Monsieur Baumelon, a pharmacist nicknamed "Dr Morphine," used morphine to weaken the resolve of attractive women so that he could rape them. The central focus of the drama surrounds the two children born of his exploits who unknowingly develop an incestuous romance. The trope of the doctor or dentist using psychotropic substances to commit rape was well established, both in the medical community and in society at large. So, the question remains: Why was Lutaud so adamant that Pillot's accusers could not have been raped under the influence of anesthesia?

Popular associations of psychotropic drugs with eroticism and assumptions about their aphrodisiac qualities informed Lutaud's skepticism. It is not that he denied the possibility of a sexual encounter under the influence of anesthesia; rather, he believed that such an experience could not be considered rape because of chloroform's aphrodisiac effect on the body. Defendants used this argument as well. One Parisian dentist who had been accused of rape in 1869 claimed by way of defence that "under the sway of chloroform, these young women had erotic hallucinations."[21] Chloroform divorced the body from the restraining influences of free will, modesty, and morality. Unrestrained by rational consciousness, Lutaud suggested, the sexual body embraced its natural carnal desires. Contemporary gender ideology also shaped his perspective on anesthetic rape. While men supposedly had superior reason, free will, and self-control, which they used to justify their exclusive rights as full political citizens, women were considered particularly vulnerable to emotions, desires, and the physiological caprices of their reproductive bodies.[22] In a society that defined women by their physical bodies above all else, Lutaud dismissed women's claims of anesthetic rape by substituting unconscious physiological arousal for conscious consent.

Cast in this light, the female body erotically charged under the influence of chloroform threatened the dispassionate professionalism of the male doctor. Lutaud thus recommended that doctors and dentists should never submit a woman to chloroform anesthesia without the presence of a third party in order to protect themselves from accusations of inappropriate behaviour. A third party could corroborate a doctor's story if a patient mounted an accusation. Additionally, Lutaud implied, a third party might serve not only as a witness to the doctor's unfailing propriety and professionalism but also as a restraining force to prevent a doctor from giving in to his baser desires when faced with the vulnerable body of a patient. Lutaud emphasized, though, that the third party present during surgery *should never be the husband.*[23] He used an anecdote to illustrate this point. Dr Z… owned a small sanatorium outside of London, which his wife administered on a day-to-day basis. When Mrs Z… needed a small surgical procedure, Dr Jules K…, a young, active, and intelligent medical resident, acted as anesthetist in her husband's presence. After the first inhalations, "Madame Z… lost consciousness, seized the chloroformist by the neck, kissed him sensually and cried 'Come into my arms, Jules, the old man has left.'" Lutaud sardonically remarked, "one can judge the effect this had on the husband … who wasn't called Jules, but Ernest."[24] The chloroform revealed Mrs Z's hidden passion for her husband's medical resident – passion that had not necessarily been acted upon but that chloroform had brought out into the open. It was imprudent to allow a husband to be present while his wife is anesthetized, Lutaud argued, because "chloroform *ivresse* often awakens in women the idea of voluptuous sensations, especially in the case of genital operations. *In chloroformo veritas.*"[25]

Ether and chloroform reputedly provoked erotic dreams in anesthesia patients, particularly women.[26] Yet doctors disagreed over whether these anesthetic gases produced the erotic dreams or simply revealed an underlying erotic desire. At stake was the very nature of women's sexuality. Dr Alexandre Lacassagne viewed the erotic dreams that some women reported experiencing under general anesthesia as an indication of pre-existing erotic desires.[27] "In the absence of any regulatory brake," explained Lacassagne, "the passions appear and flaunt themselves shamelessly."[28] Ether incapacitated the rational will, the regulator of social propriety and sexual morality.

The anesthetized body revealed repressed desires, passions, and habits that would mortify a conscious individual. Yet, despite doctors' presumptions about women's latent eroticism, anesthesia also revealed men's erotic desires. One of Lacassagne's colleagues, Dr Bouisson, administered ether to a young man for the extraction of an ingrown toenail. Under its influence, the patient "revealed with lascivious gestures a harmful habit that he was no longer able to restrain."[29] In this instance, the patient's impaired will caused him to masturbate unselfconsciously on the operating table, transforming Bouisson into a voyeur in the process. Lacassagne's interpretation of the perceived aphrodisiac effects of psychotropic drugs suggests that they revealed an individual's authentic sexual "habits."

Surgeons who made contact with a patient's genitals during the normal course of surgery could provoke the physical manifestation of erotic desire. When Dr Courty inserted a catheter into an anesthetized military sergeant, that patient achieved an erection and "demonstrated with gestures, the expression of his physiognomy and a few unequivocal words, that he believed he was with a *femme publique* whose hands were engaged in impure caresses; when he awoke all was forgotten."[30] With his senses compromised by the chloroform, the sergeant mistook his male physician for a female prostitute. The doctor unintentionally became the object of the sergeant's erotic desires. Chloroform transformed a routine medical procedure into a scene of same-sex eroticism – at least for the doctor. The sergeant, who perceived his genital sensations as the erotic caresses of a female prostitute and retained no memory of the experience afterward, remained entrenched within a heterosexual matrix of desire, despite his arousal at another man's touch. Dr Courty recognized his awkward position as the potential agent of another man's arousal – an agency he tried to displace onto the chloroform.

Observations about the arousal of patients under anesthesia were part of the medical research agenda in the nineteenth century. Doctors sought to understand the physiological progression of insensitivity on different parts of the body, including the genitals. Dr Bouisson observed

that the genital mucus membranes seemed to conserve their impressionability long after sensitivity had been extinguished in the rest of the
body. Therefore, he claimed, a woman under ether anesthesia who did
not react to her skin being pinched might experience a "very evident
sensation" when a catheter made contact with her vulva.[31] Doctors also
observed that male patients' penises frequently became erect during hip
operations. While manipulating the dislocated hip of a fourteen-year-old
boy under a mild chloroform anesthesia, Dr Lacassagne observed that
bending the boy's thigh over his pelvis caused a strong erection almost
immediately.[32] Although touch could stimulate the erectile tissues,
Lacassagne noted that he had never witnessed a patient ejaculate during
surgical anesthesia, nor did he know of any other surgeons who had.
Still, the fact that the erectile tissues could be stimulated even after the
loss of cutaneous sensitivity sparked experimental curiosity. Lacassagne
conducted some informal experiments to demonstrate that erectile tissues
still functioned when patients were anesthetized. He claimed that he was
able "to provoke the erection of the nipple with repeated titillations"
among several unconscious – and unconsenting – female patients.[33]

The vulnerability and unrestrained physical arousal of unconscious
anesthetized bodies structured medical debates over sex and drugs in
the context of anesthesia. In popular culture, however, people associated
sex and drugs with the production and enhancement of pleasure. In
turn, the pursuit of pleasure fuelled morphine addiction.[34] Dr Georges
Pouchet explained that "the search for the aphrodisiac action of opium
was very often the point of departure for *morphinomanie*." Such addicts
consumed opium and morphine to "exaggerate the sensations that one
experiences during the sexual act."[35] Cocaine gained popularity in France
in the *fin de siècle* on the heels of morphine, and for similar reasons.
Users subscribed to the aphrodisiac "legend" of cocaine, which claimed
that cocaine "increases virile power tenfold, augments the pleasure of
venereal orgasm, and momentarily restores the use of a lost function
to genital impotents."[36] These purported elixirs of love offered users a
shortcut to uninhibited passion and pleasure.

Opium had a long-standing reputation as an aphrodisiac, dating
back as early as the seventeenth century.[37] Orientalism enhanced the
drug's erotic reputation. In his 1813 study on aphrodisiacs, Julien-Joseph
Virey described opium as "the most powerful aphrodisiac in all of the

East Indies."[38] Images of opium smoking often linked Orientalism and eroticism. Henry Émile Vollet's 1909 painting *Le Vice d'Asie: Fumerie d'Opium* depicts an opium den, possibly in Marseille or one of the other port cities (Figure 4.1). A naval officer lies smoking opium out of a long pipe with his head in the lap of a beautiful Asian woman. Various other smokers, male and female, lie sprawled near them, their clothing dishevelled, lost in their own internal sensations and opium dreams. The Asian woman sits, her arm extended holding out another pipe as though bestowing the gift of opium onto her clientele. She might be the proprietor of the opium den. Or, she might serve as an allegorical representation of an imagined Orient, conjured up out of the naval officer's opium dreams. Whether she is real or imagined, the painting portrays the experience of smoking opium as both exotic and erotic.

The construction of psychotropic drugs as aphrodisiacs and their association with eroticism in art, literature, and popular culture contributed to the widespread integration of psychotropic substances into France's sexual economy. During the Third Republic, the associated pleasures of drugs and illicit sex troubled social reformers concerned with France's flagging population. They believed that, through prostitution, men were engaging in the egotistical pursuit of pleasure for its own sake, which threatened the demographic future of the nation by delaying marriage and diverting men's sexual energies away from the conjugal bedroom.[39] Between 1900 and 1920, a large number of the individuals arrested for selling opium, morphine, or cocaine illegally were women who had sexual connections to the drug trade. Some were the mistresses of drug traffickers or crooked pharmacists who had drawn them into the business. Others were prostitutes who offered opium or cocaine to clients as a part of a larger menu of services for sale. Still others were themselves addicts who had turned to prostitution and drug trafficking to ensure a steady supply of these increasingly regulated substances.[40] These women capitalized on the aphrodisiac reputation of opium and cocaine to increase their clientele and secure future profits from the sale of these highly lucrative and addictive substances.

French port cities became hotbeds of opium consumption at the turn of the twentieth century. Located along long-distance trade routes that connected France to North Africa, India, and the Far East, port cities had large garrisons of sailors and naval officers – ideal conditions

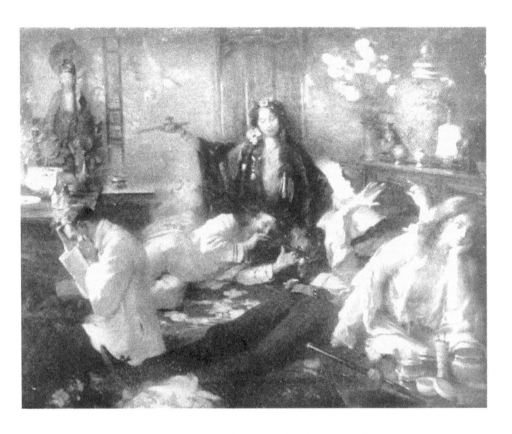

4.1 Henry Vollet's painting of an opium den depicts popular associations
of opium with Orientalism and eroticism.

for the propagation of opium smoking, which connected supply with
demand. In 1906, the police chief of Brest estimated that approximately
40 per cent of the officers in the city "abandoned themselves to this
unfortunate passion."[41] Many colonial functionaries and naval officers
acquired a taste for opium abroad and continued their habit when
they returned to France. Opium consumption was particularly high
in Brest, Marseille, and Toulon but also a significant problem in Nice
and Lorient. As with any city containing a concentrated population of
mobile single men, port cities also attracted a considerable population
of prostitutes and *demimondaines*. To cater to the dual demand for sex
and opium, *demimondaines* and *filles galantes* in these port cities ran
private opium dens, known as *fumeries*, out of their lodgings. By offering

opium as one of many services available to their clients or lovers, these women threaded opium into the commerce of sex.

The French government was concerned about rampant opium abuse in the French military, particularly in light of broader anxieties over the degeneration of the French population at the turn of the twentieth century. The existing poisonous substances legislation restricted the sale of opium and other drugs to individuals with a medical prescription but did not regulate consumption, frustrating police efforts to regulate the illegal trade.[42] To combat the alarming spread of opium smoking, the Ministry of Justice issued a decree in 1908 that made it illegal for individuals to "encourage the possession or illegal use of opium." While this measure was designed to facilitate the prosecution of opium den proprietors and smugglers, the fines and prison sentences for violating this decree remained low and opium smoking remained a widespread problem in France's port cities.[43]

Correspondence from Ministry of Justice investigations of opium consumption and trafficking reveals that sex and drugs were fused into a lucrative network of illicit pleasure. The police and officials at the Justice Ministry worried about the corruptive influence of these pleasure dens on impressionable young military officers. Doctors and moral reformers echoed this sentiment. "The *demimonde* adopted [*fumeries*] with enthusiasm," explained Félix Brunet, a doctor in the French navy. "Almost all the *demimondaines* in Toulon keep an opium *fumerie*, which thus becomes a double centre of contamination," spreading the twin vices of sex and opium smoking.[44] Although police had some limited success in pursuing the proprietors of public opium dens, most opium smoking occurred in private residences converted into exclusive *fumeries*, which easily evaded detection.

In March of 1912, the Sûreté Générale, a centralized national police force that supplied detectives to help local law enforcement, sent an inspector to Brest to research the extent to which opium dens had spread throughout the city.[45] The inspector discovered numerous *fumeries* in Brest, "the majority [of which] were operated by women who had naval officers for lovers." Female opium den proprietors used pseudonyms such as "Loulou," "La Taïtienne," "Zette," or "Mimi le Bazar," which evoked the diminutive pseudonyms commonly used by prostitutes in the *maisons de tolérance*, France's system of officially regulated yet technically illegal brothels.[46] However, most of these *fumeries* were closed to the public. Potential users were admitted only if they knew a naval officer who could vouch for them. The report noted that "the rare 'civilians' who had access there were the young *Brestois*, almost always the 'romantic lovers' of the proprietresses."[47] The report also acknowledged the apparent existence of several "very closed private opium dens" but admitted that the official enquiry had been unable to uncover any of them.[48] These exclusive spaces of drug consumption tempted patrons with discreet, unrestrained, chemically enhanced pleasure.

One of the largest *fumeries* in Brest walked the line between prostitution and the *demimonde*. A woman known as "Loulou" ran this popular opium den on the rue du Comédie. Her lover, M. Montgolfier, a naval ensign and inveterate opium smoker, had provided her with a furnished apartment. The Sûreté inspector's report noted that "every evening [her lover] sees her leave the 'Grande Brasserie de la Marine' in the company of several naval officers who accompany her to her place to 'smoke' while he played cards with other friends."[49] The inspector used quotation marks to suggest that the naval officers who followed Loulou home to "smoke" might have satisfied other desires there as well. He suggested that she spent more time with these other "smokers" than with her lover. When the police tracked down Montgolfier in July of 1912 to get his testimony, he said that he and Loulou had lived together in Brest, but that their *fumerie* had been for their own private use. However, according to the woman who denounced them to the police, Montgolfier and Loulou ran an open *fumerie* where naval officers and *demimondaines* had illicit rendezvous.[50]

Most of the women mentioned in the Sûreté report ran opium dens financed by their lovers and frequented by other naval officers. However, the report made a point to note the peculiar fact that one *fumerie* proprietor, Marguerite Thomas, had no proclaimed lover. Whether she was an independent businesswoman or had a lover particularly adept at eluding police investigations, the fact that the report noted the oddity of her single status indicates how firmly entrenched the commerce of opium in Brest was within the amorous couples of the *demimonde*. Despite her single status, Marguerite Thomas ran a very popular opium den. When the police searched her apartments, they uncovered some opium, a lamp, nine pipes, and a naval ensign, who had presumably showed up to avail himself of her services.[51]

It is unclear whether the exchange of sex and drugs in the *demi-mondaine* establishments included a monetary transaction or if these *fumeries* operated as informal economies of exchange that simply bound sex and opium together as associated pleasures. However, for women who engaged in formal prostitution, opium was a lucrative venture. In 1912, the police commissioner of Toulon claimed that high-quality opium could be sold for 1,200 francs per kilogram and average-quality opium for 500 to 600 francs per kilogram.[52] One woman from Brest was denounced to the police for running a furnished house where she lodged *filles galantes*, the majority of whom were opium or morphine addicts.[53] A 1913 report from the Procurer General of Rennes explained that although Brest and Lorient did not have public *fumeries* per se, *filles galantes* ran private dens attached to their lodgings where "to double their funds, they charge their clientele for love or for opium without distinction."[54] The fact that these prostitutes offered opium as part of a variety of sexual services suggests that they viewed opium and sex as compatible pleasures. Officials worried about the malign influence of these clandestine *fumeries* on young and naïve officers. Curious about the possibility of enhanced pleasure, these young officers were "lured to the homes of women of loose morals and trained to smoke."[55] The women would sell opium at a high price to their *amis de rencontre* in order to double their profits.

One official from the Cour d'Appel de Rennes suggested that if the government wanted to know the full extent of the consumption of opium in Brest, it should send "an agent from the Sûreté capable of mingling with the society of young men who could frequent opium dens. Frequenting the places of pleasure, the *brasseries des femmes*, this agent would attach himself to the idlers who form their company." The official predicted that such an undercover agent would discover the addresses of all the opium smokers in Brest, their suppliers, and their meeting places within a month or two.[56] While this plan would surely yield valuable information about the underground economy of sex and drugs in Brest, it would also implicate the Sûreté agent as a collaborator in that economy, as it would be impossible for the agent to gain the trust of other young smokers or the *filles galantes* without participating in their excesses.[57]

On occasion, police investigations uncovered far more than anticipated. In May 1913, the Brest police opened an inquiry against two singers who worked at the Eden Concert, a popular *café-concert* that had previously been associated with illicit opium smoking.[58] Marguerite-Louise Volger, called "Meg-Love," and Marie-Louise Girod, called "Yanna," lived and worked together and were reputed to be avid opium smokers who provided opium to others. When the police commissioner of Brest made a visit to their residence, he noted, "'A Monsieur' was found in Girod's room lying with that girl; the girl Volger was sitting in proximity of the bed. An opium pipe was posed on the night table."[59] One can imagine not only the surprise of the police commissioner on walking in on this intimate scene but also what he might have walked in on had he arrived a bit earlier. When the commissioner burst in on them, Girod was actively under the influence of opium.[60] While this brief scene captured in reports to the Ministry of Justice does not provide much information, it demonstrates the intimate nature of opium consumption.

Despite police efforts to unearth the opium brothels and the harsher penalties of the 1916 drug legislation, sex and opium remained firmly linked in the port cities after World War I. In 1923, the minister of the Navy remarked that in Brest and Toulon it was increasingly urgent for the authorities "to find the opium dens and hinder the business of *demi-mondaines* notorious for corrupting our young officers in their homes."[61] Such was the strength of the connection between illicit sex and psychotropic drugs that one reformer tried to argue that the police should be able to use the stricter regulations that applied to houses of debauchery to prosecute individuals who consumed drugs collectively, because the consumption of narcotics "is most often followed [by] scandalous scenes."[62] While consumers treated opium and sex as kindred pleasures, social reformers bound them together as mutually reinforcing vices.

While opium was the aphrodisiac of choice among *demimondaines* in the port cities, Parisian prostitutes turned first to morphine, then to ether and cocaine. By the first decade of the twentieth century, cocaine had infiltrated networks of prostitution in Montmartre.[63] Prostitutes gained a reputation for cocaine use, and they propagated the legend of cocaine's aphrodisiac effects in order to increase their clientele.[64] Like opium in the port cities, cocaine and sex in Montmartre were pleasures consumed simultaneously. Social reformers blamed the women who sold them for the spread of a double vice. Although a lot of men were also involved in the "lamentable career" of cocaine trafficking, Dr Courtois-Suffit observed that "often, they were initiated to the pleasures that the drug brings through contact with a mistress."[65] Little packets of cocaine marked with "enticing labels" such as "Captivating Coco" and "Universal Idol" circulated through the bars, cabarets, and nightclubs of Montmartre.[66] Offering an enhanced sexual experience with the aid of cocaine, prostitutes created new cocaine users to increase business. The association of cocaine with prostitution was so strong that the drug became known as the "white whore."[67]

In her study of drug users in interwar France, Emmanuelle Retaillaud-Bajac demonstrates the links between drug use and prostitution through a statistical analysis of the addresses of arrests for infractions of the Poisonous Substances Law of 1916 during the period from 1917 to 1937.[68] Individuals prosecuted for drug consumption and possession were particularly common in the greater Montmartre area, particularly around Grande Carrières and Saint-Georges, the neighbourhood containing the infamous Place Pigaille, the "heart of 'hot' Paris," where the surrounding streets housed a large number of clubs, cabarets, places of solicitation, and hotels that rented rooms for brief encounters.[69] Places where prostitution operated on a more modest scale, including the Latin Quarter and the Place Maubert, also appear in her statistics as significant spaces of drug consumption, though to a lesser extent than the area around Montmartre.[70] In light of this geographical data, Retaillaud-Bajac determined that the social diffusion of drugs occurred along the "vector of prostitution."[71]

The consumption of drugs and sex had a complex, symbiotic relationship. Far from acting as simple drug pushers to clients and lovers, many prostitutes and *demimondaines* who offered these substances to their clients and lovers as extra services were themselves addicts. Some women even turned to informal prostitution in the first place as a result of drug addiction, to make the money needed to secure their required dose. "Dominated by the *idée fixe* of procuring the poison [that is] indispensable to their existence," Dr Chambard argued, when morphine addicts belong to the "seductive sex, they pay for morphine with their person when they can no longer pay with their purse."[72] Chambard also chastised the immorality of "gallant apothecaries" who offer morphine to "pretty clients, richer in willingness than money, who pay them with the currency of women."[73] Dr Guimbail concurred, explaining that women, who had no other assets at their disposal, would "surrender themselves entirely to the first to come along (against the price of several grams of morphine)."[74] Unfortunately, since doctors often prescribed cocaine to treat *morphinomanie*, these women often ended up trading one addiction for another. In his 1912 medical thesis, André Chevallier argued that *femmes galantes* were particularly afflicted with cocaine addiction.[75]

Louise Van…, called "Symiane," was a well-educated actress from a good family. She had no children and was separated from her husband. At the age of twenty-five, she began using morphine on the advice of a friend who wanted to share her "deadly passion." Symiane soon became addicted, but the soporific action of the morphine interfered with her career, so "she had to resort to cocaine, a stimulant of the nervous system that gave her some energy when she had to appear on stage."[76] At one point she was injecting between 1 and 1.5 grams of morphine and snorting 7 to 8 grams of cocaine per day – an enormous expense given that cocaine was priced anywhere between 20 and 80 francs per gram between 1918 and 1922.[77]

Addicts often became dealers to guarantee a steady supply of a drug they could not do without. In order to augment the allowance she received from her father, Symiane began to engage in "reprehensible acts" and to sell cocaine for a man known as "Grand Charles." He provided her with twelve packets of cocaine for the price of ten. She kept two packets for herself and sold the rest. As Symiane herself explained, "the anticipation of withdrawal is even more difficult that the withdrawal itself."[78] Young actresses, cabaret performers, prostitutes, and other women enmeshed in the nightlife of Montmartre became the intermediaries in the dual economy of sex and drugs.[79]

The role of prostitutes and nightclub performers in the black-market cocaine trade at the turn of the century further fuelled cocaine's associations with sexual pleasure in the popular imagination. Although opium's reputation as an aphrodisiac had long preceded its incorporation into France's formal and informal sexual economies, the simultaneous consumption of sex and drugs in brothels and *demimondaine* opium dens reinforced opium's associations with erotic pleasure. This simultaneous consumption of illicit sex and psychotropic drugs provided a backdrop to debates over drugs, depopulation, and degeneration in the late nineteenth and early twentieth centuries.

THE INDIVIDUAL SEXUAL BODY

Despite their growing reputation as aphrodisiacs in the popular imagination, opium, morphine, and cocaine were portrayed in *fin-de-siècle* medical literature as agents of impotence that were contributing to the rapid demographic decline of the French nation. While the French birth rate had begun to decline in relation to those in other European countries by the beginning of the nineteenth century, anxieties over this plummeting rate heightened after France's crushing defeat in the Franco-Prussian War. Between 1872 and 1911 the French population grew by an average of 89,700 per year, for a total increase in size of 10 per cent, while the German population grew by an average of 600,000 per year, for a total increase of 58 per cent.[80] The French birth rate was so low that in 1890, 1892, 1895, 1900, and 1907 deaths actually exceeded births.[81] As France's marriage rate remained one of the highest in Europe, doctors, moral reformers, and social hygienists had to consider the ways in which fertility and changing sexual practices and values might have altered the dynamics of marital sex during the nineteenth century.[82] The depopulation crisis shaped debates over national decline and became the "master pathology" with which doctors and reformers measured other social contagions.[83] It was in this context that doctors paradoxically condemned psychotropic "aphrodisiacs" as destroyers of sexual desire.

Beginning in the 1880s, psychotropic drugs – particularly morphine, opium, and, later, cocaine – were constructed as forces of physical and moral degeneration, which jeopardized the individual sexual body and, by extension, the French nation. Doctors worried that chronic use of these substances would damage the individual's reproductive capacity, reducing the French birth rate even further. They also feared that widespread indulgence in psychotropic drugs would distort public morality and lead to massive social alienation. By providing alternative experiences of pleasure, psychotropic substances diverted the carnal pleasures that drove the act of sexual reproduction toward unproductive ends. Emblematic of other so-called pathologies of modernity – cerebralism, asociability, decadence, libertinism – psychotropic drug abuse contributed to anxieties over the deterioration of the modern self and the degeneration of the French nation.

Medical opposition to the abuse of psychotropic substances during the depopulation debates followed several lines of argument. First, doctors claimed that although opiates and cocaine provoked sexual excitement in the early stages of their use, with prolonged use these drugs transformed users into impotent individuals, sapping both desire and physical prowess. Second, in cases in which drug addicts did manage to conceive, doctors argued, their offspring would be degenerate, according to the contemporary neo-Lamarckian theory of species evolution by which environmental factors and deviant behaviours could lead to hereditary degeneration.[84] Third, social reformers believed that opiates and cocaine uncovered and strengthened latent pathological sexual desires, including homosexuality, sadism, masochism, masturbation, and exhibitionism. Simultaneously portrayed as agents of both impotence and sexual perversion, psychotropic drugs threatened both the quality and the quantity of France's population.

Medical debates over the sexual impact of psychotropic drugs vacillated between two contradictory poles: aphrodisia and impotence. Ironically, the very substances that prostitutes claimed would enflame their clients' venereal desire were the same substances that doctors blamed for diminished virility. "Anaphrodisia and Aphrodisiacs," an article published in Dechambre's 1870 medical encyclopedia, attributed these two contradictory actions of opium to differences in dosage and tolerance.[85] In small doses opium acted as an aphrodisiac, in more elevated doses it was an anti-aphrodisiac, and with chronic use it could produce a state of permanent anaphrodisia.[86] Like alcohol, which the author argued had similar action over the sexual apparatus, opium's aphrodisiac properties were contingent upon moderation. However, as morphine caused physiological addiction, the ideal of moderation would have been difficult to sustain in practice.

In the context of the depopulation crisis, social hygienists considered diminished virility to be a major obstacle to the propagation of the French nation. Doctors understood human sexuality to function through a combination of psychological desire and physiological arousal. Thus, sexual pathology could have either mental or physical origins. In a 1903 book, popular medical writer Jean Fauconney attributed male impotence to four possible factors: a lack of sexual desire, an inability to produce an erection, an inability to ejaculate, or a lack of venereal pleasure.[87] The pathological disturbance of these elements, alone or in combination, would impede the completion of the sexual act. Doctors sought to counteract the popular aphrodisiac reputation of psychotropic drugs by highlighting the potential long-term dangers they posed to the individual as a sexual being.

During the last three decades of the nineteenth century, the French medical community reached a level of consensus about the action of opiates on sexual physiology. Most doctors agreed that in the early stages of use opium and its alkaloid morphine had an aphrodisiac effect but concluded that with prolonged use these substances produced a state of impotence.[88] In the early twentieth century, Drs Courtois-Suffit and Giroux reached a similar conclusion about cocaine.[89] However, some doctors challenged the idea that these substances could ever be considered aphrodisiacs. Chambard, an expert on morphine addiction, emphasized the limitations of its aphrodisiac effects even in the initial stages of use. He argued that genital arousal from opiates "is as misleading as it is ephemeral." With the male genitalia, he explained, "the erection is perhaps more prompt, the desires are perhaps more vivid, but this arousal loses in duration and effectiveness what it gains in intensity." Still, he advised, "[Be] happy if it doesn't suddenly droop at the moment when it ought to prove its worth!"[90] Successful insemination depended on a man being able to sustain an erection long enough to ejaculate. Therefore, men who traded erectile strength and longevity for chemically enhanced pleasure impeded the proliferation and regeneration of the French nation.

Even more troubling for reformers hoping to increase the French population was the idea that the quality of men's sperm deteriorated with prolonged opiate use. In his 1893 analysis of the evolution of sex, Alfred Fouillée characterized the sexual differences between men and women in terms of their reproductive cells, explaining that "the egg, voluminous, well-nourished, and passive, is the cellular expression of the characteristic temperament of the mother; the lesser volume, less-nourished aspect and preponderance of activity of the father sum up the masculine element."[91] Fouillée highlighted the sperm's activity as its distinctive feature. Among male morphine addicts, Dr Noirot observed that spermatic secretions were altered; specifically, the semen became "more liquid, without spermatozoa or with short, skinny spermatozoa that are restricted in movement" such that it was "unfit for fertilization."[92] Its movement crippled by prolonged opiate use, the sperm of the male addict lost the energetic activity that distinguished the masculine reproductive cell and began to resemble the "passive" female egg.[93] Over time, opium diminished seminal virility, emasculating the male opiate user by making him "unfit" for procreation.

Historians have discussed in great detail the perceived gender crises that reformers believed were destabilizing the social order in the early decades of the Third Republic. While many have focused on the role of the "new woman," others have focused on the ways in which the anxieties of modernity contributed to a "crisis" of masculinity.[94] A product of increasing social mobility, the proliferation of sedentary "white collar" professions, and the feminizing impact of excessive individualism and intellectualism, the figure of the bourgeois intellectual embodied this late nineteenth-century "crisis of masculinity."[95] Cerebral, sedentary, physically weak, and sexually insufficient, the bourgeois intellectual undermined the demographic future of France by privileging intellectual pleasures over physical ones. Drug use exacerbated this image of degenerate masculinity. While prolonged opiate use led to physical impotence, the intellectual pleasures of opiates lasted longer. Some doctors, like Pouchet, argued that certain individuals, especially poets, who sought psychological exaltation through the use of opiates would experience an extended aphrodisiac action that was more mental than material.[96] This psychological pleasure threatened to supplant reproductive sex by offering the user an alternate experience of cerebral aphrodisia, which simultaneously inhibited both his desire and capacity for physical relations.

The intimacy and subjectivity of the sexual experience made it difficult for medical researchers to study the impact of psychotropic drugs on the sexual mechanics of the human body. However, unwilling to rely on observation alone, one medical student from Montpellier enthusiastically volunteered his own body in the pursuit of medical knowledge. Honoré Nicolas collected the evidence for his 1884 doctoral thesis, *Some Investigations on the Physiological Effects of Chandoo (The Opium of Smokers)*, by questioning opium smokers about their experiences and by experimenting on himself. Nicolas used his own body to explore the physiological effects of opium smoking on the circulatory, respiratory, nervous, and digestive systems as well as opium's impact on the genital organs.[97] To research the exact nature of opium's reputed aphrodisiac powers, he smoked opium and tested his own body's sexual responsiveness under its influence.

Nicolas found that many of the supposed effects of opium were myths. Neither he nor any of the opium smokers he questioned had experienced spontaneous ejaculation. "As for the aphrodisiac action," he explained, "I have never seen it produced if it was not provoked."[98] In Nicolas's experience, opium dens were asocial spaces of self-pleasure, in which "the smoker is almost always alone facing his lamp, he dreams, happy to forget his troubles." Therefore, to research opium's impact on sexual physiology, Nicolas would have had to stimulate himself to "provoke" the experience he wished to observe.[99]

Opium prolonged and enhanced the mental experience of sexual pleasure. "When one smokes pushing the dose just until the beginning of *ivresse*," Nicolas claimed, "erection occurs easily, voluptuous sensations exist, just as strong as in the normal state, but ejaculation is delayed."[100] One doctor, writing forty years later, observed that some opium smokers retained erections for sixty or even ninety minutes before being able to ejaculate.[101] The degree of the intoxication determined opium's impact on genital function and arousal. At the highest doses, erection became impossible. Nicolas found he could not provoke an erection above a certain dose of opium. In this research, Nicolas demonstrated a remarkable willingness to expose the most intimate details of his own body and its erotic relationship with the opium he consumed. Throwing social and professional conventions to the wind, he exposed his sexual body in an extreme state of ecstasy as well as in a debilitated state of impotence. He placed himself in a compromising position, as an object of both experimentation and emasculation.

While opium could enhance sexual pleasure and prolong orgasm in the short term, the long-term abuse of opium could cripple sexual function to such an extent that "an inveterate smoker is an impotent man." Nicolas saw opium-induced impotence as a problem of the nervous system. He defined ejaculation as "the final stage of a reflex action whose starting point is the extremities of the pudendal nerve and termination is the contraction of the spermatic vault."[102] With occasional opium use, everything returned to its normal functionality within twenty-four hours. However, with prolonged exposure to opium, Nicolas cautioned, "the testicles, no longer receiving nervous excitement ... become permanently unfit for providing sperm, as with any gland that no longer secretes."[103] A man who overindulged in opium's immaterial pleasures could irreparably harm his ability to have reproductive sex.

Gender played a significant role in determining how drugs impacted sexual function. In the context of the depopulation debate, doctors' primary concern was drug-induced impotence in men, the "active" party in reproduction. Successful generation depended upon male erection and ejaculation. Many doctors overlooked the sexual impact of psychotropic drugs on women because they viewed women's sexual role to be essentially "passive." However, at least one doctor challenged medicine's silence on this subject. Observing a patient whose menstruation had ceased completely during her morphine intoxication inspired André Noirot to write his 1902 doctoral thesis on the genital troubles caused by morphine addiction.[104] One of the most remarkable aspects of this thesis is that it explicitly focuses on the female reproductive system, rather than treating women as an afterthought. Noirot included men only in his first chapter on the genital sense, devoting his second chapter to menstruation and his third to pregnancy and childbirth.

In the seventeenth and eighteenth centuries, doctors believed that the female orgasm played a vital role in fertilization. By the late nineteenth century, however, doctors no longer viewed female sexual pleasure as a necessary component of reproduction.[105] One doctor explained that because ovulation is not linked to exterior sensation, "fertilization happens in spite of resistance, frigidity, aversion, or disgust."[106] Noirot attributed morphine's purported aphrodisiac action to imagination and the cerebral excitation during the early stages of use, which heightened all functions of the bodily economy, including genital function.[107] However, Noirot argued that in women as well as men, prolonged use led to "complete indifference [to sex] and the absence of all voluptuous sensation."[108]

Doctors worried that this might be an obstacle to reproduction in that women who did not experience sexual pleasure would "refuse their conjugal duties."[109]

For one addict, morphine heightened arousal but stifled sexual pleasure. Mme B explained that "she experiences a great sexual arousal after an injection," Noirot reported, but she "finds no pleasure in sexual relations. Without an injection, on the contrary, the reverse occurs. She does not experience any arousal, but she feels the pleasure that accompanies venereal orgasm."[110] Morphine divorced Mme B...'s sexual arousal from the act of sexual intercourse and transposed it onto the act of injection. Morphine prevented her from experiencing pleasure during intercourse. Furthermore, it monopolized her state of arousal so that she could not experience sexual arousal independent of injection. As she took high doses, from 30 centigrams to 1 gram per day, it is unlikely that she would or could choose sobriety and pleasurable sexual relations over the stimulation of a morphine injection, which had the added force of chemical dependence to incentivize continued use. While morphine's impact on sexual pleasure and desire varied from patient to patient, in some cases it seemed to appropriate the function of sexual arousal entirely.

Even if female *morphinomanes* ignored their lack of pleasure and managed to have sexual relations, they might have had difficulty becoming pregnant because of morphine's impact on menstruation. Amenorrhea, or the abnormal absence of a menstrual period in women of reproductive age, was one of the "most constant symptoms of chronic morphine abuse."[111] Noirot cited observations of women who had not menstruated during months or even years of morphine addiction. One patient, Mme D..., stopped menstruating after a year of morphine use once she reached a dose of 60 centigrams per day. After five years of addiction, she managed to stop injecting and her period returned. She became pregnant and gave birth to a healthy child. Three months after her delivery, she began injecting morphine again and, once again, her menstruation ceased.[112] Noirot concluded that as long as addicts were under the influence of morphine, "the uterine life is momentarily extinguished."[113] Therefore, for women as well as men, morphine undermined the body's normal reproductive physiology. It diverted pleasure and desire from the physical act of reproductive sex to the cerebral experience of narcotic bliss.

While drug abuse seemed to weaken an individual's reproductive physiology, doctors also asserted that psychotropic drug use was linked to deviant sexual behaviour. In the late nineteenth century, French sexologists believed that a weakened sexual drive could "deflect the [reproductive] instinct in abnormal directions."[114] As the extensive use of psychotropic drugs led to a loss of virility, doctors feared that drug addiction would pervert normal sexual instincts and lead to sexual fetishes, perversions, and abnormalities.[115] The implications for the demographic future of the French nation were troubling. According to Charles Féré, chief physician at Bicêtre Hospital, "the sexual preoccupations [of individuals] are often in inverse ratio to their sexual powers. Nations that perish through sterility are remarkable for their licentiousness."[116] In this light, individual drug abuse threatened the sexual health of the nation as a whole. Instead of neutralizing drug addicts by removing them from the sexual landscape altogether, psychotropic impotence produced a population of pleasure-seeking "degenerates" whose peculiar tastes and vices threatened to contaminate others.

Degeneration theory bound individual vice to the nation's current and future strength. In 1857, Bénédict Augustin Morel published his famous *Treatise on Degenerations*.[117] Morel built on neo-Lamarckian heredity theory, which held that the pathological environmental factors to which one generation adapted would weaken the hereditary makeup of the following generation. Therefore, the drug use and deviant sexual behaviours of the current generation would have a lasting impact on future generations, should these "degenerate" individuals be able to reproduce. Given the severity of the depopulation crisis in France, French sexologists pathologized any form of sex that deviated from the heterosexual reproductive framework of the married couple. Thus, they tended to be less sympathetic to sexualities that departed from the norm than their English or German counterparts.[118]

Researchers believed that psychotropic drugs unearthed a variety of underlying sexual "perversions," including exhibitionism, fetishism, sadism, masochism, and homosexuality. In his 1919 study on cocaine, Hippolyte Piouffle argued that cocaine unleashed an individual's inherent perverse desires by freeing the impulsive elements of the brain from the restraints of the will. "We cannot say that cocaine is the creator of sexual impulses," Piouffle clarified, "but in all degenerates where they exist in a latent state, barely restrained by education and the will, the poison makes them appear, strengthens them and makes them chronic."[119] Therefore, while a typical exhibitionist might experience the irresistible need to expose himself in public, a *cocaïnomane* would take a more active approach, practising "exhibitionism accompanied by the act of masturbation with provocation of debauchery to those present."[120] Reformers and social hygienists wanted to encourage reproductive sexual relations in order to expand the national population. However, they feared the hypersexuality that cocaine produced might divert the user's reproductive potential toward unproductive pleasure.

Literary works also depicted the role drugs played in exposing hidden perversions. Jean Lorrain's 1901 novel, *Monsieur de Phocas*, portrays psychotropic drugs as substances that unlocked morbid eroticism and cruel fantasies. A noted ether addict, Lorrain was no stranger to decadent vices himself. In the novel, his wealthy protagonist, the Duc de Fréneuse, is plagued by a fetishized obsession with the search for a "gaze." He seeks this gaze in jewels, dreams, and portraits, and in the eyes of men and women alike. Fréneuse becomes dependent upon Claudius Ethal, a depraved artist who takes pleasure in images of suffering and death. Ethal offers to cure Fréneuse of his obsessions but instead fuels his baser desires, perhaps reflecting the role that ether played in Lorraine's own life.[121] In this light, *Monsieur de Phocas* could be interpreted as an account of an ether addict's descent into depraved fantasy and illicit desire.[122]

In the novel, psychotropic drugs call forth violent images of salacious eroticism. At Ethal's suggestion, Fréneuse consumes a drug that he initially believes to be opium but turns out to be hashish.[123] Under the influence of this mysterious substance, Fréneuse has visions of an enchanting nude dancer whose face had "the ghastly charm of a death's-head." Then, the dancer's morbid eroticism transforms into a grisly scene of street violence. Fréneuse watches as "two horrid louts" drag a "blonde and delectable" woman wearing a ballgown into a deserted Paris street, knock her down, and saw her head off with a cutlass, as blood spurts out to stain her white silk dress. The horror Fréneuse experiences at the nightmare of the woman's brutal murder is mingled with sadistic fascination and excitement.[124]

Later in his hashish state, Fréneuse's erotic fantasies move beyond mere sadistic voyeurism. Finding himself in a crypt, he feels "frightful kisses from little pointed mouths." He explains, "I was a captive of hopeful caresses, my entire being tortured with cunning little bites until I lost my strength. From top to toe I was prey to innumerable blood-suckers: fetid beasts shared my body between them, insidiously violating the entirety of my naked form." Horror and pain mix with excitement and pleasure again as an "army of enormous bats" titillate and consume his naked flesh, sucking his blood and kissing his body. He explains, "The caress persisted, sometimes so precisely that I was forced to quiver with atrocious pleasure."[125] The intermingled pain and pleasure he experiences as the vampiric bats conquer his flesh and violate his naked body highlights the masochistic inclinations of his particular brand of eroticism. At the beginning of the novel, Fréneuse is a bored dilettante, disenchanted with modern society and unsatisfying sexual liaisons, but smoking hashish uncovers the subconscious violent and obscene desires that plague him through the rest of the novel.

French moral reformers included drug use on a long list of degenerative vices, including fetishes, sexual excesses, and "perversions." They were particularly concerned about the associations of drug use with homosexuality. As "sodomy" was not explicitly prohibited by law under the Napoleonic Code of 1810, France had a more liberal attitude toward homosexuality than most other European legal systems. However, police still prosecuted individuals suspected of homosexual acts under Article 330 of the Penal Code, which prohibited "public offences against decency."[126] In the first half of the nineteenth century, amid the upheavals of industrialization and urbanization, writers and novelists had treated sexuality and gender as more fluid categories and used them to explore the permeability of social and economic boundaries in France's rapidly changing society. In contrast, after the violent working-class uprising of the Revolution of 1848, bourgeois elites sought to re-establish and maintain order increasingly by rigidly categorizing sexuality and demarcating distinct gender roles in the 1850s and 1860s. Male homosexual relationships frequently transcended class boundaries, and as a result, doctors like Ambroise Tardieu viewed these relationships as a threat to the French social order.[127] In the 1880s during the degeneration debates, French sexologists began to classify homosexuals as "sexual inverts," a term that conflated same-sex desire with gender inversion. By associating "sexual inverts" with a host of other deviant behaviours, including effeminacy, immorality, masturbation, and fetishism, fin-de-siècle medical practitioners pathologized homosexuality as both a symptom of and a catalyst for widespread national decline.[128]

Social reformers considered homosexuality and drug use to be dangerous, mutually reinforcing vices. A 1921 report from the Mental Hygiene League claimed that both of these vices spread rapidly through society because they sought company. "If, in a community, there are two inverts who do not know one another," the report explained, "they will certainly become acquainted very quickly. It is the same for drug addicts."[129] The Mental Hygiene League emphasized that the police must not hesitate to pursue addicts because, like homosexuals, they will find one another and spread their vice throughout society. Moreover, reformers also feared that through the common pursuit of illicit erotic pleasure, these two vices could merge. Dr Paul Michaut, who researched opium addiction in the Far East, claimed that "one of the first effects of opium is the perversion of the reproductive instinct, the loss of the moral sense, and the weakening of the will." Michaut associated homosexuality with the abuse of opium, arguing that "pederasty follows opiomania very exactly ... and the morphinism of smokers has no companion more faithful than pederasty."[130]

One high-profile case from 1916 demonstrated the police's belief in opium's close association with transgressive sexuality. A naval administrator in Nice, M. Borie, faced the accusation of "smoking opium and spreading these unfortunate habits to his entourage." After receiving several anonymous tips about Borie, the Naval Ministry conducted an inquiry. The investigators found that Borie had installed an opium den in the home of his mistress in the Pavillon Victoria, where friends frequently accompanied him to smoke. When confronted, Borie promised to stop smoking opium and close the *fumerie*. However, despite his promises, "gradually, the irresistible passion for opium took hold of him once more and he began smoking again, doing his utmost to share his vice and to inculcate people too weak to resist him."[131] He recruited more smokers at the Hôtel de la Marine. Eventually he installed another *fumerie*, "furnished in the oriental style," on the rue Cotta in the home of a different mistress, Madame Raymonde Banes. By locating his *fumeries* in his mistresses' residences, Borie's opium smoking reflected the conventions of the *demimondaine* opium networks in the port cities. However, Borie's opium smoking was somewhat unique in the port cities, in that it bridged the conjugal world and the *demimonde*. Not only was Borie's wife aware of his opium smoking, but she was actively involved in the opium business. The police claimed that both Monsieur and Madame Borie offered gifts to their entourage to fortify their opium habits and secure future profits.

Police worried about how quickly a man of Borie's influence could spread his vice throughout the city. However, his *fumeries* were exclusive spaces. Only Borie and his intimate friends – including a princess, two Persian princes, a doctor's wife, and a pharmacy technician, who was also his opium supplier – were admitted. After Borie and his second mistress broke up, he closed the *fumerie* on the rue Cotta. Then, he and his entourage transferred their activities to a villa known as "La Cabane." It had a discrete entrance blocked by doors and gates, shielding it from prying eyes. Its clientele included "people who came from foreign colonies and had habits of peculiar [sexual] mores."[132] As Frank Proschan has demonstrated, French writers in colonial Indochina constructed pederasty, opiomania, and syphilis as interrelated colonial social vices that threatened to corrupt the French population in Indochina.[133] Clearly these stereotypes about colonial sexuality held sway in the French hexagon as well. Yet, notably it was Borie, the French naval administrator, who ran the opium den, not a colonial subject.

The police commissioner of Nice noted in his report that smokers congregated at "La Cabane" in the evenings after nine o'clock for "scenes of pederasty, which extended into orgies [of] everything imaginable."[134] The secretive, exclusive nature of the private opium den raised questions as to what might take place behind its closed doors. The report implied that among a large group of smokers, indulgence in one vice could easily devolve into indulgence in another, making opium smoking and transgressive sexual practices mutually reinforcing pleasures. As a result, the Justice Ministry and the navy treated Borie's activities as a social and moral contagion. They feared what might result if Borie and his wife continued actively persuading others to partake in their opium debaucheries, particularly given Borie's high rank. Ultimately, the Naval Ministry removed Borie from active service and forced him to step down.

Eroticism and metaphors of seduction permeated discourses of drug addiction in the late nineteenth and early twentieth centuries.[135] Addicted bodies and drugs constituted a particular kind of intimate relationship. They replaced interpersonal sexuality with subject-object intimacy. Like the legendary "green fairy" of absinthe, medical and popular writers alike constructed the "white whore" of cocaine, the "grey fairy" of morphine, and the "black idol" or "brown fairy" of opium as dangerous female seductresses who used their feminine wiles to ensnare unsuspecting users.[136] Richard Millant described opium as an "exclusive mistress who forbids her lovers any delights except those that she dispenses herself."[137] Here, the "monogamy" of the addict and the drug was not one of choice. Opium portrayed as a jealous mistress denied the addict all other sensual pleasures, forcing him to renounce material sexuality for the pursuit of immaterial pleasure. A 1913 debate in the Chamber of Deputies described medical students' use of morphine in similar terms. The report claimed that during stressful exam periods, medical students turned to morphine and "without suspecting it, morphine takes her place as mistress of their bodies; thereafter they meekly accepted her tyrannical grip."[138] As a mistress who ruled with a "tyrannical grip," morphine rendered the addict weak and dependent, overturning the expected power dynamics between subject and object.

An abstract view of psychotropic drug use – the penetration of the body and mind by an external object – mimicked the sexual act. In this context, by ingesting, injecting, or inhaling psychotropic substances, the drug user adopted a passive, "penetrated" role in which the psychotropic substance dominated the mind and body, provoking voluptuous sensations. In the case of morphine addiction, this penetration took on a literal form as the phallic hypodermic syringe penetrated the user's flesh to deposit the liquid morphine. Morphine's addictive properties subjected the addict to a life of regulated doses to avoid the agonies of withdrawal. If an addict missed an injection or delayed it, "the mistress regains her authority," wreaking havoc on his body until he takes another dose.[139] Morphine, constructed as the archetypal femme fatale, penetrated and dominated the addict. By submitting his free will to the impulses of addiction, the addict subordinated himself as a tributary of a material object. In this relationship between a male addict and the material substance that has become his "mistress," woman dominates man as object dominates subject.

Yet addicts were by no means exclusively male. In fact, some authors contended that women's "impressionable" or nervous character made them particularly susceptible to seduction by psychotropic substances.[140] In light of the drug-as-mistress metaphor, the image of a drug gendered female seducing a female addict transgressed purported ideals of heterosexual desire. At the turn of the twentieth century, images and descriptions of eroticized female morphine use captivated the popular imagination. At the same time, constructions of female sexuality vacillated between a belief in the inherently excessive sexual desire of women and the "myth of female sexual passivity." French sexologists worried that the denial of women's sexual desire might lead to nymphomania, lesbianism, or other sexual pathologies. Similar to perceptions of the corruptive influence of impotence on male sexuality, specialists treated female frigidity as "less a question of absent desire than one of potential perversion."[141] Despite the popularity of morphine among members of both sexes, in the 1880s *morphinomanie* joined kleptomania and hysteria among the modern pathologies that society imagined to be specifically feminine ills.[142]

Contemporary iconography portrayed intimate moments in interior spaces in which women injected themselves with morphine in the company of other women, baring skin to one another and to the viewer. Albert Matignon's painting *La Morphine* (1904) portrays three women in evening finery in various states of undress and morphine intoxication (Figure 4.2). One woman is sprawled face down, her hair cascading down the side of the bed. A second sits on the bed, hair down, back arched and eyes closed in a state of ecstasy, one breast protruding above the plunged neckline of her gown. A third woman sits at a small table, elaborately coiffed and fully clad in evening gown, jewels, and long white gloves. Her gloved fingers grip the back of a chair as she leans forward, staring intently at the ecstatic woman seated on the bed. A syringe rests inside a clear bottle of morphine on the table, next to a china tea set and a lamp that illuminates the contours of the dark room and the women within it.

Matignon's painting exhibits male imaginings and anxieties over the potential transgressions women might commit in domestic interior spaces. Rather than enacting a new femininity in public on the fashionable boulevards of Paris, these women brought the threat of moral degeneration inside the bourgeois home, the quintessential space of motherhood and domesticity.[143] The abandoned tea set on the table next to the open bottle of morphine suggests an inversion of traditionally acceptable forms of

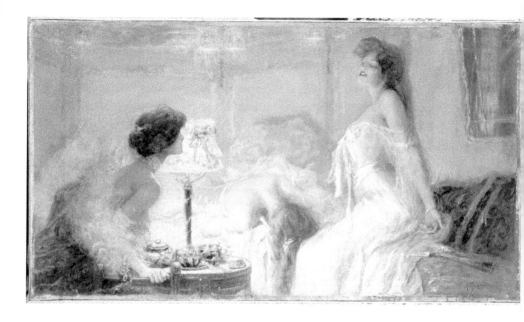

4.2 Albert Matignon's 1905 painting, *La Morphine*, depicts three
women in various states of morphine intoxication, highlighting
the eroticism of self-induced pleasure.

female sociability. The women's evening finery and the darkness of the
room suggest that the women had returned from a night at the theatre.
While in the middle of the afternoon the tea set might have facilitated
conversation during a social call, after dark it is abandoned on the table
while the women experience more sensuous amusements.

The women's body language reflects pleasure experienced individually. Rather than depicting the women engaged in polite conversation
around the table, Matignon illustrates the physical effects of morphine
injections that preclude verbal communication. The two women on the
bed focus on internal sensations. The woman lying face down on the
bed is the very image of closed-off physical sensation.[144] Her arms are
folded underneath her body, not visible, suggesting that she might have
been combining one sensuous pleasure with another. The viewer of the
painting joins the seated woman in her voyeurism of the half-clad ecstatic
woman arching her back on the bed. Whether she is enraptured by a
desire for the woman on the bed or a desire to achieve a similar sensual

experience from morphine, the eroticism of the image is apparent. The painting reflects anxieties over the dangers of self-pleasure and the possibility of homosociability slipping into homosexuality.

An earlier image of female morphine use, published in *Le Petit Journal* in 1891, is less explicitly erotic but also privileges physical sensation over discursive interaction (Figure 4.3).[145] One woman stands, staring empty-eyed out of the image as she injects herself with morphine. Another woman lies sprawled on a chaise longue with her eyes closed, a novel open beside her. Since the Enlightenment, moralists had condemned the reading of novels because they overstimulated the erotic imagination.[146] The two women do not interact with each other in a social manner; instead, each woman focuses on her own individual sensation. These images of collective female *morphinomanie* demonstrate *fin-de-siècle* anxieties over a form of female sociability defined through physical sensation rather than discursive communication.

Anxieties over the physical sociability of collective female morphine use also permeated medical and popular writing on addiction. In the 1890s, doctors expressed concerns over the rise of female morphine clubs. These spaces, popular among upper-class women, supposedly played a large role in recruiting new morphine addicts.[147] In 1893, Chambard remarked, "it is not rare … to see society women disillusioned and tried with sorrows, real or imagined, form veritable *morphinomanes* clubs where, after having properly slandered the untrustworthy sex, they obtain, together, a sweeter intoxication than that of love."[148] Chambard suggested that *morphinomanes* sought the company of other women to overcome the dissatisfactions of disappointing heterosexual relationships.

In a memoir from his time at the Sûreté, former Paris police chief Marie-François Goron claimed that different morphine clubs catered to women from all walks of society. "La Morgue" was one of the most famous upper-class morphine clubs, run by an illustrious princess. It got its sinister nickname because "on her salon's large divans, women in visiting clothes under the influence of the poison, lie like cadavers without moving."[149] Less affluent women also had spaces where they could "intoxicate themselves in unison." In a brasserie in the environs of the Place Pigaille, the notorious red-light district at the base of Montmartre, prostitutes and "*demoiselles* of the *demi* or even *quart du monde*" congregated to inject themselves with morphine.[150] "Many were dressed

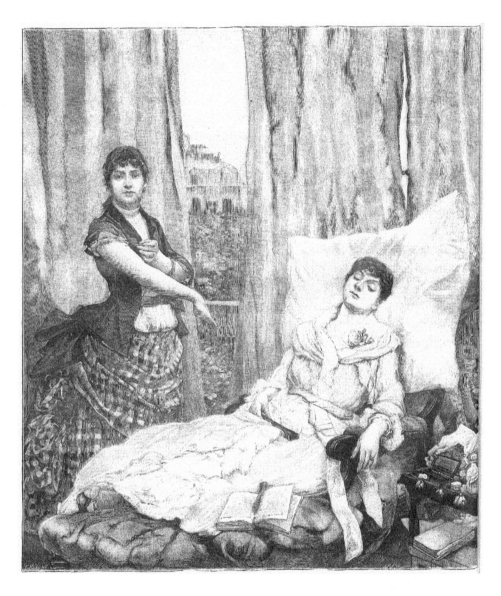

4.3 Georges Moreau de Tours's 1891 illustration of female morphine users, from *Le Petit Journal*, reflects anxieties over the consumption of drugs by bourgeois women in domestic spaces.

in negligee, without a corset, in a peignoir," Goron remarked, "having thrown an overcoat or the traditional waterproof over their shoulders." They sat at the brasserie tables staring in silence, "with the bored apathy particular to *morphinomanes*." The brasserie was known as the Cabaret des Spectres, or the "Ghosts' Cabaret," because its patrons resembled ghosts and shadows more than living beings. The women sat immobile, except when, "from time to time, one perceives a cloud of fabric under a table; it's one of the regulars hitching up [her skirts] and pushing the needle of her Pravaz syringe into her thigh."[151]

Both the poor women of the Cabaret des Spectres and the affluent women at La Morgue mimicked death, or something close to it, resting motionless, without speaking, lost in their own mental and physical sensations. Rather than engaging in conversation, their social experience was defined solely through physical proximity and the common enterprise of self-injection. Prostitutes and *demimondaines* depended on their physical attractiveness and sexual vigour for their livelihoods. At the Cabaret des Spectres, however, their role as sexual beings existed in tension with the degenerative and immobilizing effect of morphine on their bodies. While many of the women were still young, Goron lamented, "their beauty is no more than a memory ... their skin is flabby ... their eyes are ringed with brown ... it is complete decay; these sad brasserie patrons hardly have the strength to bring a glass to their lips."[152] For the ex–police chief, these women's bodies served as painful illustrations of the decay and physical degeneration of modern society. Death at La Morgue and the Cabaret des Spectres was gradual and incomplete.

As closed-off feminine spaces of collective drug use, the morphine clubs provoked male insecurities. In the female morphine clubs of Paris, "men are received but not sought out; one can do without them." Professor Ball claimed, "it is in the secret of these feminine orgies that we find the explanation for almost all morphine addicts' passion for proselytism." Ball and other writers like him worried that collective morphine injection could lead to sapphic pleasures that would render heterosexual relations superfluous. While the spectre of lesbianism loomed large in male descriptions of the morphine clubs, these venues may or may not have actually included orgies or even explicitly sexual interactions between women. Ball explained that for women "morphine causes a voluptuous semi-anesthesia that makes them dream of scenes even more delicious than reality."[153] Morphine facilitated autonomous pleasure. Injecting morphine as an act of self-pleasure resembled masturbation. Both acts rendered men redundant.[154] Female morphine clubs exacerbated male fears over the degeneration of the French population. They fuelled anxieties over physical degeneration, same-sex desire, and self-pleasure that might threaten women's willingness or capacity to engage in interpersonal reproductive sex.

In late nineteenth-century debates over depopulation and degeneration, doctors attempted to debunk the aphrodisiac myth of psychotropic drugs. They emphasized the ways in which these drugs hindered the body's reproductive mechanisms and corrupted sexual desires. However, depicting these purportedly aphrodisiac substances as agents of physical and moral degeneration forced doctors to contend with sexual practices defined by, and in some cases subordinated to, the pursuit of self-pleasure.

THE REPRODUCTIVE FAMILY

In the *fin de siècle*, the conjugal family was the bastion of France's demographic future. As Judith Surkis has demonstrated, republican reformers viewed the monogamous, reproductive family as "at once a motor and measure of 'civilization.'"[155] In the context of the depopulation crisis, this "motor" was more crucial than ever if France hoped to recover from its demographic decline. In 1896, Jacques Bertillon, the famous demographer and repopulationist, emphasized the need to increase the number of legitimate children born within conjugal families to improve the quality of the population and not just the quantity.[156] Doctors and social reformers demonized psychotropic substances as a threat to this conjugal bastion that could derail and distort sexual desires away from reproductive ends. Although reformers tended to construct drug addicts as degenerates, they also acknowledged that psychotropic substances could corrupt and pervert "normal" citizens. Yet their condemnation of psychotropic drugs was not as straightforward as it might appear at first glance. In certain instances, doctors actually prescribed these substances to overcome physical or mental barriers to reproductive sexuality.

Social reformers blamed the expansion of drug addiction in French society on drug addicts who enthusiastically proselytized the pleasures of morphine, opium, and cocaine to their friends. To help publicize the disastrous consequences of morphine addiction, Marcel Mallat wrote a novel designed to frighten and deter individuals who were curious about the artificial pleasures of morphine.[157] *La Comtesse Morphine* was published in 1885, at the height of France's demographic crisis. This morality tale exposes the tragic life of the beautiful Countess Iva de Volnay as morphine addiction transforms her from a devoted wife and mother to an addicted adulteress engaged in the relentless pursuit of pleasure.

The Count and Countess de Volnay begin their marriage with six months of conjugal bliss and sexual passion. Doctors order them to refrain from all sexual activity following the birth of each of their two children and then again after Iva's husband fell ill. Iva's mother-in-law, who disapproves of their marriage, schemes to further delay the couple's sexual rapprochement following his illness.[158] Iva is bored in the provincial setting prescribed for her husband's convalescence. Her sexual frustration manifests in painful headaches, which she treats with morphine. Craving sexual gratification, she indulges in sexual fantasies about a former admirer. When the married couple finally give in to their sexual desires, against medical advice, Iva's headaches disappear without recourse to morphine. However, her husband's health deteriorates and he begins to cough up blood.[159] Although Mallat reaffirms the authority of medical expertise, he also strongly suggests that sexual intimacy within marriage is both natural and necessary. Significantly, Iva's headaches, the psychosomatic manifestation of her sexual frustration, can be cured either by renewed sexual intimacy or by morphine injections, suggesting that sexual and narcotic pleasure are interchangeable.

To give Iva's husband the time to recover his health, Iva's mother-in-law persuades her to enter a convent and renounce worldly pleasures.[160] In the celibate isolation of the cloistered environment, Iva's headaches return. Miserable with loneliness and on the edge of despair, she discovers a syringe and a small supply of morphine in her bag. From that point forward, "she was no longer alone; morphine adorned her cell with its golden dreams, its voluptuous oblivion from life's miseries, the celestial ecstasy that prayer denied [her]."[161] She quickly increases her doses, passing the days in a morphine-induced stupor.

In the convent, morphine reasserts itself as an agent of self-pleasure. One day, after sleeping through a visit from her children, Iva awakens to inject herself with morphine and begins her *toilette*. She lets her chemise fall to the floor and takes pleasure in examining herself, smiling as she admires and caresses her breasts. At her own touch, "a voluptuous trembling shook her whole being; then she continued her examination, infatuated with herself! Forgetting all modesty, she studied her secret beauties with indulgence, moving slowly over her luscious flesh."[162] Morphine replaces the physical intimacy of a lover and inspires Iva to indulge in self-pleasure. With her syringe in hand, Iva can penetrate herself, experiencing the ecstatic pleasures of self-love. Significantly, Iva's indulgences in erotic, psychotropic pleasure cause her to neglect her maternal duty. She misses most of her children's visits while lost in an unconscious state. When she finally returns to her husband only to be barred from physical intimacy once again by her mother-in-law, she turns to morphine to gratify her erotic desires.

Morphine lowers Iva's inhibitions as it gradually consumes her. She begins a passionate love affair with a former admirer, neglecting her children and her husband when she sneaks out to be ravished by her lover in a nearby villa. Iva's life rapidly spirals out of control. In the early months, morphine heightens her energy and sexual passion to a frenzy. Over time, however, she increases her dose to such an extent that she becomes an invalid trapped in a drug-induced haze, deaf to worldly pleasures and incapable of acknowledging the outside world except to beg for another injection. In such a state, "even maternity was unable to make an impression on her softened brain."[163] When doctors attempt to cure her addiction, Iva returns to life, screaming for morphine like a wild beast as she suffers the agonies of withdrawal. Without morphine, her sexual appetite returns; "in the grip of erotic delirium, she rolled violently in the bed, calling in a pleading voice for … all those that she had loved. She begged for their kisses with the expressions of a passionate tenderness, swooning under the caresses of these invisible lovers."[164] Morphine has satisfied her bodily need for pleasure but at the cost of her husband, her family, and her reputation. Unable to overcome her addiction, Iva finds a servant willing to administer morphine injections. Tragically, "the Morphine Fairy had reconquered her victim and was leading her to the land of eternal sleep."[165]

La Comtesse Morphine demonstrates how easily morphine could destroy a family. Before her addiction, Iva and her husband are an ideal couple: young, attractive, fertile, and completely besotted with each other. Mallat highlights their ideal conjugal family through the foil of the Marquise Léonie de Saint-Ys, the woman who introduces Iva to morphine. The Marquise de Saint-Ys marries a man twenty-five years her senior who indulges her whims, "taking pleasure in making her recount her escapades and count her lovers."[166] Both their age difference and her husband's cuckold fetish inhibit reproductive sex. Thus, the marquise and her husband divert their sexual energies to more lascivious ends. Unlike this anti-conjugal couple that is doomed to sterility and perversity from the outset, Iva and her husband have been happily married. Unfortunate circumstances and scheming antagonists lead Iva away from her marital responsibilities toward the deviant pleasures of morphine and adultery. Morphine destroys Iva's sense of maternal duty and conjugal fidelity as it gradually takes possession of her mind and body, directing all her thoughts and actions. Without morphine, Iva could have grieved her husband's early death from a wasting illness and then moved on with her life, possibly to remarry and have more children. Instead, morphine destroys her at the age of twenty-five, leaving her two children orphaned and destitute.

While most families would not encounter the scheming antagonists and unfortunate circumstances depicted in *La Comtesse Morphine*, doctors contended that one of the most nefarious threats to the reproduction of the bourgeois family came from within. The medical community lamented the all too common practice of morphine addicts encouraging addiction in their spouses, extinguishing their sexual desires in order to shirk conjugal responsibilities.[167] Dr Pichon found that among married *morphinomanes* the frequency of sexual encounters "falls well below the usual figure."[168] Despite widespread assumptions that women were the most dangerous proselytizers of drug addiction, within the conjugal couple husbands who had become impotent through their own excessive morphine use shouldered the majority of the blame for conjugal *morphinomanie*.

In 1891, Dr Guimbail published a remarkable medical-legal study of conjugal *morphinomanie*. M. Dida, a violent and jealous man rendered impotent though his morphine addiction, became wild with suspicions that his beautiful young wife would commit adultery because he was unable to "fulfill his husbandly duties." As Dida lacked a medieval chastity belt, Guimbail quipped, he turned to morphine "to extinguish all stirring of sensuality in his unfortunate companion."[169] He used morphine "with the secret intention of killing the temptations of the flesh" in his wife. Guimbail viewed this wilful destruction of his wife's sexual desire as indicative of the degeneration of "our ultra-civilized era."[170] To compensate for his own impotence, M. Dida converted his wife's physical desire into psychotropic pleasure.

Doctors had particular contempt for husbands who used drugs to stifle their wives' sexual desire so that they would not have to perform sexually.[171] In 1884, France had reinstated divorce so that individuals could extricate themselves from sterile marriages in order to find partners with whom they could engage in reproductive relations. Populationists like Jacques Bertillon supported this legislation as a way to stimulate population growth in the midst of a demographic crisis.[172] However, if a woman's first husband got her addicted to morphine or cocaine to stifle her sexual appetite, he not only doubled the obstacles to reproduction within their marriage but also threatened his wife's future reproductive capacity. Mme Dida had two children with her husband before morphine rendered him impotent. By encouraging her morphine addiction, he ensured that she would be unable to have any more.

A singular feature of Guimbail's account of this case of conjugal *morphinomanie* is that it came to light in the wake of Mme Dida's brutal murder at the hands of another man. Pierre Wladimiroff was an impoverished man, twelve years younger than the recently widowed Mme Dida. He became infatuated with her wealth and beauty and contrived to marry her. She accepted his proposal, but after it became apparent that he was a violent spendthrift she broke off their engagement. Wladimiroff pawned a gold and diamond pin she had given him as a gift and bought a revolver. He threatened to kill himself unless she married him and when she stood firm in her refusal, he shot her multiple times in the head. He claimed the murder had been a crime of passion.[173] Despite the dramatic violence of the "Wladimiroff Affair," the main focus of Guimbail's article was Mme Dida's victimization by her dead husband, the morphine addict. Guimbail explained that Mme Dida's morphine addiction weakened her will and sense of propriety such that "she gave in and abandoned herself to Wladimiroff's first advances. She lost all control of herself: she compromised herself to pleasure, forgetting that she has custody of her family's honour."[174] Guimbail did not trivialize the gravity of Wladimiroff's crimes. However, he held her dead husband to account for encouraging the morphine addiction that had compromised her moral compass, allowing her to get involved with Wladimiroff in the first place. Guimbail portrayed the individualism of a woman abandoning herself to pleasure as fundamentally incompatible with her social responsibility as custodian of the family's honour.

Conjugal *morphinomanie* could have a lasting impact on a woman's sexual economy. In a lecture on *morphinomanie*, Dr Ball explained that addiction typically produced an anesthetic effect on the sexual organs. However, abstaining from morphine could cause an addict's sexual organs to become overexcited. These "manifestations of exaggerated eroticism" were, according to Ball, especially common among women.[175] One of Lutaud's patients, Mme E…, was a thirty-nine-year-old mother of two who had become addicted to morphine "by her husband's bad example." By July 1883, her daily dose of morphine had reached 75 centigrams and she had stopped menstruating. After numerous failed attempts to cure her addiction, in 1886 she was interned in an asylum in Paris. At the asylum, Drs Legrand de Saulle and Motet, who were experts on morphine addiction, cured her addiction through rigid surveillance and a progressive diminution of her daily dose. A few months later, her menstruation resumed and she returned to live with her family. However, she remained excitable. Every time she menstruated, she experienced "the most disturbing symptoms of nymphomania." Menstruation provided material evidence of her body's fertility and capacity for reproduction. However, Lutaud noted that her excessive sexual desire had made her family long for the period when addiction had stifled her reproductive instinct and made her menstruation disappear.[176] That her family would prefer her addicted and sterile suggests the extent to which her former morphine addiction had disrupted and then amplified her sexual desire. For this former addict, unbridled lust seemed to supplant reproductive sexuality.

In a society plagued by depopulation, which extolled the ideals of "republican motherhood" and championed feminine virtue as a moralizing force, women's hedonistic pursuit of artificial pleasures was considered particularly reprehensible.[177] The excessive individualism of morphine addiction threatened to undermine the individual's duty to her family and society. At the moment of withdrawal, when the body is "hungry for the poison," one medical-legal article explained, "the appetite [for morphine] dominates and smothers ... reason."[178] The fear of agonizing withdrawal made addicts' search for a reliable supply of morphine an obsession that eclipsed all other thoughts and responsibilities. Reformers were particularly concerned that women would neglect their maternal obligations if they became addicted to a drug that vaunted self-interest and sensual pleasure.

Dr Guimbail argued that the addict's imperious need for morphine was stronger than a mother's love for her children. In January of 1891, the police arrested Louise K..., a twenty-nine-year-old mother of two, for attempted theft in a novelty shop on the Faubourg du Temple. When they searched her residence, a "revolting hovel" on the boulevard Belleville, the police found her two children, ages five and eight, suffering from pulmonary consumption. A search of the property revealed a drawer filled with "a considerable quantity of new cloth, which came from thefts." The police reproached Louis K... because she was a *morphinomane*, who "steals to get morphine and not to provide any well-being for her unfortunate children."[179] The squalid conditions of her home and her contemptible neglect of the consumptive children shocked the police commissioner far more than the fact of her theft. He even implied that her crime could have been understandable or justified had she stolen the cloth in order to provide comfort for her sick children. However, in this case, the addict's sense of self-preservation overpowered her maternal compassion.

Addiction wreaked demographic havoc in the short term by producing impotent, pleasure-seeking individuals who shirked their reproductive responsibilities and spread immorality and vice to others. However, reformers were also highly concerned that addiction would damage the quality of France's future citizens by causing birth defects. Although doctors frequently argued that drug abuse caused impotence, they acknowledged that some addicts still managed to reproduce, but in a way that perpetuated national degeneration. "Cocaine strikes more than the individual," asserted Dr Courtois-Suffit; "it compromises descendants and, consequently, the future of the race."[180] He gave the example of a cocaine addict who snorted 4 grams per day. The patient had four children, born at different stages of his addiction. His oldest child was a healthy, intelligent thirteen-year-old girl who had been born before he began using cocaine. His second child, a frail, sickly eight-year-old girl, had been conceived after he had started using cocaine. His last two children were both conceived at the height of his cocaine addiction. Both boys were born with mental problems and his youngest, only six months old, was born with microcephaly, an abnormally small skull.[181] The progression of the patient's cocaine addiction was dramatically inscribed on the minds and bodies of his children.

Listing the progressively degenerate progeny of psychotropic drug addicts became a trope of medical literature on addiction.[182] Dr Brouardel gave the example of the children of a diplomat who took 30 centigrams of morphine per day: "the first died at three days old; the second, [who was] simple, died of a wasting disease at age 16 or 17; the third was an imbecile, depraved, then insane."[183] Doctors concluded that in cases when addicts were still able to conceive children, their offspring would be of an inferior quality – evidence that future generations would suffer both physically and mentally from the irresponsible decadence of their parents.

Since the 1880s, when the medical community had begun to re-search and classify morphine as a new pathology, doctors recognized the dangers that addiction posed to French society. This early research had acknowledged the role that the medical profession itself had played in spreading addiction by overprescribing morphine to treat pain and other symptoms. Nevertheless, when doctors discussed the degeneration crisis, they condemned pleasure-seeking degenerates for spreading this vice throughout society and continued to believe that, with appropriate professional caution, medical practitioners could still deploy psychotropic drugs to treat their patients' ills. Therefore, while opium, morphine, and cocaine became associated with deviant sexuality and degeneration in both medical discourse and the popular imagination, in certain cases doctors actually prescribed cocaine to facilitate reproductive sex be-tween married couples who would otherwise have been incapable of reproduction. For example, Dr Piouffle believed that cocaine lowered inhibitions and revealed hidden sexual desires. While it might reveal underlying sexual perversions in degenerates, Piouffle argued that co-caine could be productively administered to "phobics, obsessives, and timid individuals [who], under the influence of cocaine intoxication of the first degree, can forget their fears, see their anxiety reduced, and complete the coitus that normally would be denied to them because of their pathologically troubled psyches."[184] Piouffle sanctioned the use of cocaine to overcome medically diagnosed psychological obstacles to reproductive sex. In this case, cocaine acted to reduce anxiety rather than to increase desire or pleasure.

When doctors prescribed cocaine to facilitate reproductive sex, they deliberately removed it from its context as an agent of pleasure or desire and reclaimed it as a medical tool designed to treat a specifically diagnosed pathological issue. Nowhere was this distancing of cocaine from the pleasure complex more apparent than in the case of vaginismus. Vaginismus is a painful vaginal condition in which the pathological contraction of the vagina makes it difficult or impossible to engage in penetrative sex. Although doctors had recognized the condition in France since 1834, vaginismus did not become part of medical nosology until 1861. According to Auguste Lutaud, an expert on vaginismus, the delay in classifying the disease was a result of doctors' discomfort with the condition and its implications for normative sexual relations.[185] Lutaud believed that vaginismus was a relatively common condition, citing studies by colleagues that included dozens of observations (and in one case, over a hundred).[186] Doctors did not really understand what caused vaginismus, but they proposed a wide range of theories. These included the reading of erotic books, masturbation, an erotic disposition, hysteria, or a highly resistant hymen.[187] Many doctors blamed the husband for the condition; however, they disagreed over why this was the case. Some argued that if the husband was overly weak and timid in the bedroom, he could not copulate with sufficient force to break through his wife's membranes. Others argued that it was the husband's excessive brutality and lack of sympathy during sexual penetration that caused both physical and psychological trauma.[188]

The extreme pain of penetration made it very difficult for gynecologists to examine and treat vaginismus patients. Before the advent of local anesthesia, doctors had a very limited number of treatments for vaginismus.[189] Most of these treatments were drastic and excruciatingly painful. Doctors could perform incisions to widen the vaginal sphincter, rapid forced dilation of the vagina, or cauterization of vaginal lesions. These agonizing procedures required surgical anesthesia and did not guarantee success.[190] Instead of suffering through such procedures, or even the embarrassment of discussing a condition like vaginismus with a doctor, many women chose to live with the localized pain that only manifested with attempted coitus. After a series of fruitless and agonizing attempts, discouraged couples had to accept the reality of a sexless marriage.[191]

In the summer of 1884, the same year in which Carl Koller and Sigmund Freud conducted their groundbreaking research on the use of cocaine as a local anesthetic, Dr Cazin from Berck-sur-Mer in northern France encountered a vaginismus patient who had been married for six years but had never consummated her marriage. On her wedding night, the woman discovered that she "could not support the advances of her husband. The least touch of her external genitals caused an atrocious pain, degenerating ... into veritable convulsions."[192] Her condition made Cazin's examination a "veritable torture." When she refused to submit to manual dilation under the influence of chloroform, Cazin decided to try a cocaine solution, which he administered topically. This anesthetized the patient enough that Cazin could insert a rubber catheter to administer cocaine into her vagina. The cocaine enabled vaginal penetration. A few months later Cazin reported to the Society of Surgery that five minutes after administering cocaine in this manner "the young woman could endure the sexual rapprochement *without any pain*. From that moment on, for the regular accomplishment of coitus, it was always necessary to turn to preliminary soakings and injections [of cocaine]."[193]

For Cazin's patient, anesthetizing herself with cocaine meant that she could painlessly engage in sex with her husband. While it allowed her to become pregnant and fulfill the duty of motherhood, cocaine eliminated all genital sensation during the sex act, the pleasurable along with the painful. The sexual rapprochement with her husband was an experience she had to endure passively without sensation. It was not a mutual exchange of pleasure. Furthermore, Cazin portrayed the case as a success story, suggesting that he viewed the desensitization of the female sexual organs during coitus as a viable long-term solution, despite the fact that cocaine could only temporarily alleviate pain. Although Michèle Plott has argued that by the 1880s bourgeois marriages had become more self-consciously modern in that they began to recognize the importance of women's sexual needs, the case of vaginismus suggests that the medical community still prioritized reproduction over female pleasure.[194]

When Cazin presented this case to the Academy of Medicine in January 1885, his patient had become pregnant with her first child. Cazin expressed his hopes that childbirth would put a definitive end to the pain and vaginal spasms for which cocaine had provided only transitory relief.[195] He suggested that the expansion of the vaginal canal during childbirth might be enough to overcome her pathological physiological condition permanently in a way that anesthesia could not. The natural pain of childbirth, he hoped, would counteract the pathological pain of vaginismus.

Although doctors discussed vaginismus as a reproductive issue, the women who suffered from this condition explicitly characterized it as an obstacle to sexual pleasure. In 1886, Dr Pierre Garnier received a letter from a thirty-two-year-old French woman living in Egypt. She had been married for over four years, and she had always experienced pain during intercourse. At first her husband could not fully penetrate her, and he sent her to visit a doctor, who examined her with a speculum but found nothing abnormal. After that point her husband could fully penetrate her but the entry was always very painful and made her miserable and discouraged. "My husband can consummate the act entirely, without a drop of blood ever appearing," she explained, "but I only experience suffering without any feeling of pleasure, whereas in [my] dreams, at least once a month, I experience this sensation."[196] The patient framed her complaint not only in terms of the pain she experienced during coitus, but also in terms of the pleasure she did not experience. However, Garnier ignored this last complaint. His proposed solution was washing the painful areas with a cocaine solution before coitus in order to dull sensation.[197] When she had to stop using the cocaine solution because it caused a localized itching and burning sensation, her doctor pre-scribed two to three months of abstinence, after which "relations were less painful."[198] Neither of the medical solutions proposed – cocaine or abstinence – addressed the patient's specific complaint about the lack of pleasure she experienced during sex. As she had submitted to painful sexual relations for four years, her husband's right to sexual pleasure was not questioned. Yet Garnier's response to her complaint demonstrates medical discomfort over the role of female pleasure in conjugal relations.

Cocaine became a common remedy for vaginismus. Many other doctors, including Chéron, Batuaud, Dujardin-Beaumetz, Lejars, and

Doléris, reported success in using cocaine on female patients to facilitate conjugal relations.[199] As it was impractical for a woman to visit a physician before every sexual encounter, Dr Bautaud argued that eventually the patient should be able to administer the cocaine herself to prepare her body for penetration.[200] At a time when iatrogenic morphine addiction was rampant in France, medical professionals usually condemned unsupervised drug use, particularly when it involved sex. However, in this case they made an exception. Significantly, the context in which doctors accepted cocaine as an aid to sexual intercourse was one that treated a physical obstacle to conjugal reproductive sex. Rather than enhancing the pleasurable sensations and intensity of a sexual experience, the medical use of cocaine to treat vaginismus was specifically designed to anesthetize a woman's sexual organs, subordinating female pleasure to the reproductive imperatives of bourgeois conjugality.

France's industrializing pharmaceutical economy gave individuals a wide array of new tools for modifying bodily sensation. While individuals consumed these substances to treat pain, they also deployed psychotropic pharmaceuticals in the pursuit of pleasure. By condemning the asocial, pleasure-seeking elements of psychotropic consumption, doctors reinforced their own authority over the definition of "normal" drug use for therapeutic purposes. In so doing, they simultaneously claimed the right to label psychotropic consumption outside the boundaries of "official medicine" as pathological, bringing these illicit drug practices under the umbrella of their authority as well. However, popular conceptions of psychotropic drugs as aphrodisiacs and their prevalent use among prostitutes and members of the *demimonde* demonstrates the inability of the medical profession to control the context of psychotropic drug use completely. Doctors vilified the recreational use of psychotropic drugs by juxtaposing their moral condemnation of selfish, chemically enhanced sexual pleasure against the tangible ways in which addiction to cocaine, morphine, or opium inhibited an individual's chances of procreation. By debilitating sexual physiology and corrupting desire, doctors argued, psychotropic drugs prevented addicts from fulfilling their reproductive duties to the French nation.

{ 5 }

ECONOMIES
OF PAIN

What might seem to be a dream possible [only] within the
imagination of poets is today realized; science, whose admirable
conquests expand the power of man every day, no longer stops
vanquished in front of pain, and in the same blow it has destroyed
its formidable procession of lamentations, cries, and anguish.
– Dr R.H.J. Scoutetten (1853)

Dr Pierre Nicolas Gerdy, professor of surgical pathology, refused to define pain. As he explained in 1851, "there is no one who does not know it through experience."[1] From the gnawing ache of a decayed tooth to the sharp pain of having it extracted, pain played a significant role in individuals' everyday lives. Over the course of the nineteenth century, psychotropic drugs transformed pain from an experience that was both inevitable and universal to an element of life over which individuals had a degree of control. Laudanum, cocaine, and other psychotropic substances purchased over the pharmacy counter increasingly enabled French citizens to master quotidian bodily suffering. For instances of exceptional pain, like surgical procedures, anesthetic gases offered the most assured means of relief. From 1847 onward, ether and chloroform made the acute, agonizing pain of surgical operations a thing of the past. By inhaling these substances, patients could undergo even the most painful operations blissfully unaware of the surgeon's scalpel carving their bodies.

General anesthesia transformed surgery from an ordeal of speed and brutality into one of calculated precision in which the patient's comfort was a central concern. No longer subject to the pressures of speed, surgeons could attempt more complex procedures and conserve more tissue and functionality. Furthermore, anesthesia enhanced the reputation of the surgeon. By reducing fear and eliminating pain from the experience of surgery, surgeons constructed a new image of themselves as caring healers and skilled practitioners.

In addition to transforming the practice of surgery, the introduction of general anesthesia raised profound questions about the rights of patients. By temporarily severing communications between the mind and the body, the use of anesthetics gave medical professionals incredible power over the vulnerable bodies of their patients.[2] At the same time, by considering and respecting their patients' experiences during procedures and their right to endure otherwise excruciating ordeals in a state free from pain, surgeons acknowledged their patients' subjectivity. Doctors were not only concerned with producing a successful end result from their ministrations. They valued their patients' comfort during the procedures as well. Far from being insentient flesh to be cut, sewn, and manipulated, patients' anesthetized bodies represented a new conception of the surgical experience.

This chapter examines the reconceptualization of pain in the nineteenth century through French anesthetic practices. After examining the impact of surgical anesthesia on the patient as subject, it turns to medical interventions in two gendered acts of suffering for the nation: childbirth and battlefield injury. During the Third Republic, anxieties over the declining strength of the nation placed greater emphasis on the virtues of courage and individual sacrifice in the service of the nation. As Germany's population and material resources outstripped France's considerably, the appeal to the "spiritual" qualities of the French people became even more important for asserting its national strength.[3] Between 1870 and 1914 a growing literature on heroism and the revival of the cult of Joan of Arc lauded courage and self-sacrifice as civic duties of French men and women alike.[4] While men performed this duty as soldiers in the defence of the *patrie*, women could serve France by strengthening its population, offering courageous sacrifices on "the 'battlefield' of motherhood."[5] From the battlefield to the birthing chamber, the use of anesthetic medicines fundamentally transformed the experiences of men and women suffering for the nation. Anesthetic practices during these moments of bodily sacrifice balanced the collective needs of the nation with the subjective experience of the individual.

POSITIONING PAIN

Dr Gerdy framed pain as a universal experience. However, historians of science have demonstrated that pain is a subjective state of being that is deeply embedded within the social and cultural milieu of the individual who experiences it.[6] Until the eighteenth century, Catholic theology provided the dominant framework for understanding pain. Pain served simultaneously as a punishment for sin and a pathway to redemption. By stoically accepting bodily suffering, individuals sought to emulate the sacrifice of Christ. In so doing, they brought themselves closer to God and ensured eternal salvation in the afterlife.[7] During the Enlightenment, however, medical conceptions of pain became secularized. Instead of conceptualizing pain as an issue of sin and divine punishment, doctors began to view pain as a useful sentinel that alerted the individual to a bodily disturbance.[8] Patients dreaded pain, but they had come to accept that doctors and surgeons must occasionally inflict pain in order to heal them.[9] For example, by inflicting the temporary pain of a surgical procedure, a surgeon could relieve the enduring agony of a bladder stone.[10]

Before the introduction of anesthetic gases into surgical practice, doctors only had a few questionably reliable options for alleviating surgical pain. These included nerve compression, cold temperatures to numb the area, intoxication with alcohol, opium, or camphor, or loss of consciousness in a patient. This last one could be accomplished through bleeding, pressure on the carotid artery, mesmerism, hypnotism, or in some cases, a firm blow to the head.[11] Such practices were not employed consistently, and most served merely to diminish rather than eliminate pain.[12] Facing these dubious anesthetic options, a patient's best chance of relief was to find a surgeon with the skill, strength, and speed to complete operations as quickly as possible.

Surgery was a violent, agonizing experience. "To avoid pain by artificial means is a chimera," declared Dr Alfred Velpeau in an 1840 lecture at Charité Hospital. As sharp instruments and pain went hand in hand in the mind of the patient, Velpeau argued that surgeons should focus on "reducing the pain of operations as much as possible" without compromising the integrity of the procedure.[13] Nevertheless, even if the doctor tried to inflict as little pain as possible, the patient's experience of surgical operations before anesthesia was violent and torturous. Restrained on the operating table by cords or strong men, the patient's body and mind rebelled against the scalpel, screaming and struggling against this bodily invasion.[14] In the first few decades of the nineteenth century, perhaps in part to justify their own role, surgeons depicted pain and screaming during surgery as useful indicators of the patient's vitality.[15] However, in 1847, debates over the anesthetic properties of ether and, a few months later, chloroform revolutionized French surgery, reconstructing pain as a cruel and unnecessary element of surgical practice. This anesthetic revolution occurred incredibly quickly. While Velpeau had declared painless surgery to be a "chimera" in 1840, seven years later he became one of surgical anesthesia's most ardent champions.[16]

Anesthesia was amazing. Patients awoke astonished to find their surgery already completed without their having realized it. In fact, patient astonishment became a trope of medical anecdotes of the practice. On 1 February 1847, Dr Philibert Joseph Roux recounted a surgical case at the French Academy of Sciences. He had used ether for a surgery on a patient's abdominal fissures. When the patient awoke after the surgery, Roux decided to trick him. He claimed he had simply performed a test of the anesthesia. He told the patient he would have to put him under again in order to perform the actual surgery. "Great was his surprise and also his satisfaction," Roux explained, "when after a few moments, I let him see a large wound that I had kept hidden."[17] Roux's flair for the dramatic highlighted ether's remarkable effectiveness as an anesthetic. However, it also demonstrated the patient's complete vulnerability. While unconscious, the patient had no awareness of or control over what was being done to his body. Anesthesia endowed the surgeon with incredible authority and power.

The same day that Roux presented his surgical case, a vitriolic debate erupted at the French Academy of Sciences between Velpeau, who championed the use of ether inhalations in surgery, and renowned physiologist Dr François Magendie, whose infamously cruel animal experiments had incited outrage among anti-vivisectionists. The latter criticized the medical community for being imprudent with and over- ly enthusiastic about this new procedure before developing sufficient therapeutic knowledge rooted in animal experimentation.[18] Magendie appealed to a long-standing belief in the utility of pain during surgery.[19] He contended that eliminating a patient's perception of pain deprived the surgeon of useful knowledge during an operation. After all, a fully conscious patient could cry out when the surgeon's scalpel approached an important nerve; an anesthetized "cadaver" could not.[20] The patient's agony communicated vitality. By forcing the patient to cry out, pain could inform the surgeon if he was approaching dangerous territory with his scalpel. For Magendie, pain was a vital communication network between the mind, the body, and the surgeon.

Furthermore, anesthesia seemed ethically dubious to Magendie. He questioned whether it was ethical to submit patients to a state of intoxication that essentially reduced them "to the state of a *cadaver* that one cuts, carves with impunity and without any suffering." The likeness of an anesthetized body to a cadaver was unsettling. A body silenced in such a manner seemed to have lost its humanity through the tempor- ary loss of moral sense and consciousness of its own existence. A body lying on an operating table was mere matter when disconnected from the mind that normally controlled it. Magendie found this state vile and degrading. "For me, and I think that any self-respecting man will share my feelings," he exclaimed, "I would not consent for any reason to let myself be placed in a similar situation, where your body is abandoned, without any defence, in the hands of a surgeon who might be clumsy, incompetent, or inattentive."[21] Highlighting the incredible vulnerability of the anesthetized body, Magendie criticized its objectification. How could a self-respecting subject allow himself to be objectified in such a manner? For Magendie, consciousness was the crucial marker of subjectivity and agency, an essential check on the surgeon's potential incompetence.

Velpeau and other proponents of ether anesthesia understood patient subjectivity in a different manner, prioritizing comfort over conscious- ness. They believed that the humanitarian goal of protecting patients from excruciating pain outstripped the potential utility of that pain to the surgeon. Pain was as much a mental torment as a physical one. The experience of pain was much more than the instantaneous experience of being hurt. The surgical patient's agony surpassed, in both directions, the moment of being cut open. Leading up to the surgery, the patient experienced the fear and anxiety of anticipated pain. This fear of pain tormented patients so much that even a patient with a life-threatening tumour would put off surgery as long as possible.[22] After the immediate agony of the surgery was over, the patient had to live with the torturing memory of the ordeal. Not only did surgical anesthesia relieve the immediate pain and trauma of the operation, but it also served to mitigate patients' fear and anxiety and eliminate their memories of it afterward. Dr Henri Scoutetten, chief physician of the military hospital in Metz, asserted that there could not be a more philanthropic thought than transforming the terrifying and agonizing experience of surgery into a moment of calm.[23] By focusing on the mental torments of surgery, proponents of anesthesia refused to treat patients merely as damaged or pathological bodies in need of repair.

Proponents of anesthesia emphasized the surgeon's compassion. In so doing, they debunked the stereotype of the hard-hearted surgeon indifferent to his patients' pain. "Surgeons are, above all, men like any others," Velpeau insisted, "endowed with as much sensibility as those who accuse them [of hard-heartedness]." However, as they needed to maintain an insensitive appearance to do their jobs, people believed them to be unfeeling. Instead, the emotions that surgeons had to conceal became "the source of anxieties all the more painful, because they must not let them appear."[24] Pain tortured the patient undergoing surgery, but it also denied the humanity of the surgeon, requiring him to conceal his empathy for his fellow human beings. With the aid of ether, both patient and surgeon could experience the surgery without mental anguish. In this state, the surgeon could reconstruct the brutal reputation of his profession as a noble and compassionate one.

While surgeons debated the ethics of anesthesia, other researchers embraced the possibilities it offered for metaphysics. Professor Jacques Lordat of the Montpellier Faculty of Medicine gave a physiology lecture on ether anesthesia in 1847. He hoped to explore what ether could reveal about the alliance between the two powers of human dynamism: the mind and the body.[25] He concluded that man experienced a temporary interruption of the alliance between the "psychic power" and the "vital system" under the influence of ether. Ether divorced the mind from the body. At the same time, however, it also exposed the complex inter-relation of the mind and body in a normal state. Dr Charles Ozanam, writing ten years later, concurred: "Man is not, in fact, a body alone, as the materialists say; neither is he a spirit, a mind, as the philosophers declare; but [rather] a soul united to a body and forming with it a single being."[26] By temporarily uncoupling mind and body, anesthesia ultimately revealed their fundamental interconnection.

Some doctors viewed anesthesia as a suspension of selfhood. Scoutetten argued that chloroform and ether anesthesia provoked "that remarkable state in which the *self* no longer has appreciable con-nections with its own organs or even seems completely suppressed."[27] Consciousness and free will began to disappear first, followed by sensa-tion. As the anesthetized individual's command over his mental faculties and voluntary movements decreased, his being became dominated by instinct, directed by reflexive processes – breathing, reflexive move-ments, blood circulation, and so on – that operated independent of his intellect.[28] Although still alive, the anesthetized individual's mind was no longer able to receive communications from the body. The continuation of physiological functions was the only thing that separated this human shell from a cadaver. Anesthesia fragmented the self. Instinct and reflex directed the organism, not free will or reason.

By temporarily extinguishing free will and consciousness, anesthesia pushed the individual further toward object than subject. During the final stage of anesthesia, there was "neither pleasure nor sorrow: no quality reveals a sensible or intelligent being, and for the surgeon who operates, the patient seems to be a human statue whose substance he dissects or sculpts at will."[29] Anesthetic gases enabled the surgeon to divide his patient, a complex thinking and feeling subject, temporarily into two parts: a material body lying on the operating table, and an immaterial self, resting unperturbed in an ethereal space for the duration of the operation. During this state, "the flesh can be wounded, bruised, div-ided, the patient does not feel it; his mind soars in unknown regions ... Upon awakening no memory, no idea of the progress made; everything is finished, the limb was separated from the torso and the patient asks if the operation will begin soon."[30] The patient's physical body could only be peacefully dismembered in the absence of the conscious self. In a conscious state, pain communicated the trauma of dismemberment to the individual. Without this communication, the self, in a sense, could avoid experiencing the body's trauma. Oblivious to the surgeon's manipulations of his limbs, the patient's mind experienced an ethereal state, distanced from his physical experience.

Surgical anesthesia made pain a matter of choice. It prevented the mind from retaining a memory of the body's physical trauma, leaving the self untouched and whole, even as the body was dismantled and reconfigured under the surgeon's scalpel. On the one hand, anesthesia's temporary Cartesian separation transformed the patient into an object, to be carved, sliced, and stitched. On the other hand, the idea of protecting the patient's mind from the traumatic experience of pain demonstrated a fundamental respect for the individual's status as a subject. Temporarily relinquishing the free will that marked him as a subject enabled the surgical patient to protect himself from pain. Paradoxically, by engaging in what Magendie considered to be the ultimate state of objectification, patients asserted their agency as subjects.

Parisian dentists were quick to capitalize on patients' desire for pain-less surgery. While the members of the Academies were still debating the merits of ether anesthesia, dentists were already advertising their ability to perform tooth extractions "without pain" in the popular press. Mr Marshall, an English dentist who practised on the Faubourg Saint Honoré, advertised his successes with ether anesthesia in La Presse as early as 29 January 1847. While Magendie and Velpeau butted heads over questions of ethics and utility, Marshall presented pain as a matter of patient choice. He hoped to increase business with the possibility of a painless procedure and noted that he used the ether method "each time the patients desire it."[31] Other dentists quickly followed suit. Advertisements from Mr Marshall, M. Cousin on the rue d'Alger, and M. Aussandon at the Palais Royale regularly appeared in La Presse through the month of February while the Academy debates continued.[32] The dreaded ordeal of a tooth extraction had become a trivial process. Pain and anxiety could also be extracted with the aid of a few breaths of ether.

Armed with the knowledge that modern medicine had the power to eliminate pain, patients began to advocate for themselves. They requested, and even demanded, pain relief. After experiencing the painless removal of a cancerous thigh tumour, one of Velpeau's surgical patients declared that he had felt nothing at all. He joyfully exclaimed to the crowded operating theatre, "This here is truly the best method!" Such was his satisfaction that the patient asked his surgeon to repeat the ether inhalations when he changed the bandage if it might be painful.[33] Although anesthesia enhanced the surgeon's power and authority, by eliminating pain it also fostered a respect for the patient as a subject, which in turn endowed patients with a type of agency. Patients began to advocate for themselves by requesting anesthesia even for less invasive procedures, like changing a bandage. Anesthesia, rather than being subject solely to the surgeon's authority, became a negotiation between surgeon and patient.

In the initial months of heady excitement following the introduction of ether anesthesia, doctors published widely on its use in all forms of operations, from the mundane to the truly agonizing, with resounding success.[34] Such was the enthusiasm for ether anesthesia that researchers began to explore other substances that might have similar properties. In March 1847, French physiologist Marie-Jean-Pierre Flourens published animal research on the anesthetic properties of chloroform.[35] However, it was not until November that Scottish obstetrician James Young Simpson first experimented with this new anesthetic on humans.[36] French surgeons followed suit, and within a year most doctors in Paris had replaced ether with chloroform for use in surgical anesthesia.[37]

In July 1848, the sudden death of a young woman forced the members of the Academy of Medicine to face anesthesia's potentially fatal consequences.[38] The patient, Maria Stock, had sustained an injury after being thrown from a carriage. Initially, she refused to let a doctor remove a small fragment of wood that had become lodged deep in her leg. However, after a few days the wound had begun to fester and she consented to its removal on the condition that her surgeon, Dr Gorré, put her to sleep with chloroform. He later noted, "I had no reason not to grant her request."[39] So, he put 15 or 20 drops of chloroform on a handkerchief and placed it under her nostrils. After a few short breaths, she pushed the handkerchief away with her hand and "cried out in a plaintive voice: *I am suffocating.*"[40] She quickly became pale, her breathing became obstructed, and she began to froth at the mouth, all within about a minute.

Gorré removed the chloroform immediately and, believing the situation was temporary, he proceeded to extract the wood fragment from Mlle Stock's leg wound while his colleague attempted to revive her. He then joined his colleague in his efforts. For two hours they tried everything they could think of, splashing water on her face, blowing air into her lungs, and holding ammonia under her nostrils, all to no avail. "This death that we persisted in believing was only apparent was real," Gorré explained, "and it had been so quick, that it was probably already over at the moment when I made the incision."[41] He concluded that the death had been caused by a syncope produced by the sudden ceasing of cerebral function, which he attributed to the chloroform.[42] Ironically, the case seemed to support Dr Magendie's concern over the anesthetized body's resemblance to a cadaver, as it apparently took Gorré and his colleague two hours to realize their patient was deceased.

Gorré's testimony provoked quite a stir at the Academy of Medicine. On the one hand, a surgeon's first duty was to protect the life of his patient. On the other, after months of being able to perform painless surgery, the idea of denying patients anesthesia and forcing them to experience the sharp, agonizing pain of surgery had become untenable. The stakes of the debate were high. Surgeons were reluctant to blame the anesthesia that had revolutionized their practice, even when several other fatalities came to light.[43] "If it were established that chloroform could ... directly or indirectly, compromise the patient's days we would have to renounce it without hesitating," argued Roux, "not only in small operations, but also and even more so in large ones, because the surgeon is never allowed to add to the danger of operations ... [but] it would be imprudent to condemn a method so valuable for a misfortune in which it might not have been involved."[44] The medical community had to decide whether a few inexplicable deaths outweighed the countless benefits of painless surgery to the collective patient experience.

On 25 July, the minister of public instruction transmitted the official statements and reports from the judicial inquiry into Mlle Stock's death to the Academy of Medicine. He requested a medical inquiry into the circumstances of her death. He viewed the question of chloroform's safety to be not only a matter of justice for Mlle Stock but a question of fundamental interest to humanity. Therefore, he emphasized his confidence that the Academy of Medicine would eagerly apply itself to "the resolution of the doubts that still exist over the complete safety of chloroform."[45] Instead of requesting that the Academy inquire into whether chloroform was indeed completely safe, he emphasized the necessity of resolving any doubts over its safety. He implied that chloroform offered such a significant service to humanity that doctors must discover some alternative explanation for the sudden deaths that occurred under its influence. The enormous benefits chloroform offered to surgical patients had made it practically inconceivable to return to surgical procedures without anesthetic.

In response, the Academy of Medicine appointed a commission. The report it presented on 31 October reviewed both the specific medical-legal case of Maria Stock and the potential dangers of chloroform anesthesia in general based on a total of eight reported deaths, only two of which had occurred in France.[46] Vacillating between general claims and particular cases, the commission used a somewhat convoluted logic in its report to mediate between two conflicting tasks. The first was to absolve chloroform as a therapeutic tool, safe when administered by "experienced hands." The second was to absolve the specific practitioner, Dr Gorré, from blame for his patient's death, to avoid setting a dangerous legal precedent. The commission acknowledged that under certain conditions, chloroform was irrefutably fatal. However, in the specific cases it reviewed, rather than attributing death to the toxic action of chloroform or to the incompetence of the surgeon, it emphasized individual idiosyncrasies and contingencies specific to the patients themselves.[47] In general, the commission concluded that chloroform could be administered safely by vigilant and experienced professionals.

The debates in the sessions following the report were heated. The future of anesthesia was at stake. Doctors proposed the use of various apparatuses, procedures, and rules for administering chloroform, all designed to prevent accidents.[48] By emphasizing the expertise and judgment of the practitioner, doctors framed the debate as one of professional freedom as well as medical ethics. Chloroform's benefits to modern surgical practice had become so great over the previous two years that even staunch opponents of the commission's report – who believed that chloroform had killed Maria Stock – did not actually believe that renouncing anesthesia altogether was a feasible solution to prevent further deaths. The report's fiercest critic, Dr Jules Guérin, lambasted the commission for erroneous conclusions, for "closing their eyes to the evidence," and for insufficient knowledge of chloroform's action rooted in animal experimentation.[49] However, even he later proclaimed himself to be one of chloroform's "strongest admirers."[50] Instead of eliminating it, Guérin advocated for additional research into chloroform's effects in various idiosyncratic scenarios in order to protect the public. Eliminating chloroform anesthesia had become unthinkable, even among researchers who believed it to be highly dangerous and potentially fatal.

Although the members of the Academy of Medicine professed to value life above all, they found it difficult to reconcile chloroform's potential dangers in individual cases with the incredible collective benefits it offered surgery in general. One critic dramatically proclaimed, "certainly it's better to expose thousands of men to sharp pains than to bring about the death of a single one."[51] However, this argument did not gain much traction. Returning to surgery without chloroform would have meant a complete reversal of surgical practices that patients had come to expect over the previous two years – practices that had encouraged a reconstruction of the surgeon's image as an empathetic practitioner who was as concerned with the tranquility of the patient's mind as with the rehabilitation of the patient's body. More often, impassioned calls to renounce chloroform immediately if it were responsible for a single death were used hyperbolically by supporters of chloroform anesthesia, who then proclaimed the gas to be completely innocuous when properly administered.[52]

Ultimately, statistics enabled doctors to reconcile the possibility of danger. One surgeon estimated that over the previous two years, medical practitioners on both sides of the Atlantic had used anesthesia in around one hundred thousand cases, while the number of recorded accidents was perhaps eight or ten at the most.[53] Roux, who worked at the Hôtel-Dieu Hospital in Paris, even argued that anesthesia actually increased a patient's chances of surviving by reducing "traumatic exhaustion" and the fear of pain. Before anesthesia, he lost about a third of his patients. After anesthesia, he only lost about a fourth of them.[54] Weighing these "immense services" of surgical anesthesia for thousands against the infinitesimal number of accidents recorded, the choice seemed simple. The consumption of surgical anesthetics in Paris hospitals continued to increase steadily from the mid-1850s to the early 1870s and then dramatically between the early 1870s and 1885 (Figure 5.1).

One point that the Academy did not explicitly discuss in the death of Maria Stock was the fact that the patient herself had specifically

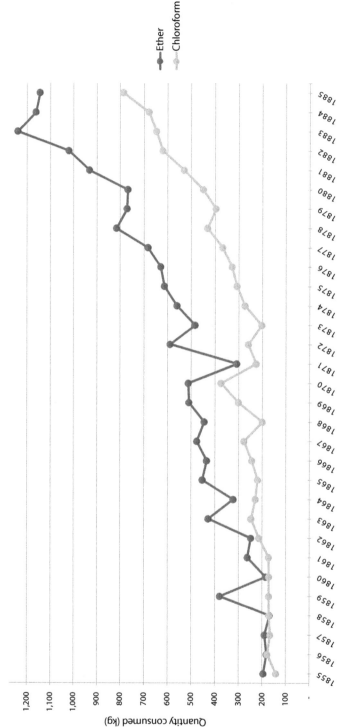

5.1 Ether and chloroform consumed in Paris hospitals between 1855 and 1885 from the Pharmacie Centrale des Hôpitaux de Paris. *Source:* Ether and chloroform statistics from 1855 to 1875 cited in Charles Lasègue and Jules Regnauld, "La thérapeutique jugée par les chiffres," *Archives générales de médecine* (1877): 12; statistics from 1876 to 1885 cited in Bourgoin and Beurmann, "La thérapeutique jugée par les chiffres," *Bulletin général de thérapeutique médicale et chirurgicale* 115 (1888): 159.

requested chloroform. She had done this even though her operation was a relatively minor one. Gorré had agreed to it, as he had "no reason not to grant her request." Other doctors faced similar pressures from patients. Jean Amussat, an opponent of the commission's report who believed chloroform to be highly dangerous, reported two cases in which surgical complications made him wish to avoid using chloroform: the first was a case of ulcerated breast cancer complicated by bronchial catarrh, which increased the risk of respiratory complications; the second was a fibrous uterine tumour complicated by the patient's weakened condition from blood loss and infection. Although these added dangers should have served as counterindications for anesthesia, Amussat noted that "the patients insistently demanded to be shielded from pain." In both cases, he gave in to their demands and administered chloroform. Taking careful precautions, he performed the surgeries without accident.[55] Despite his own reservations, Amussat yielded to pressure and allowed the patients' requests for pain relief to influence his course of treatment.

The debates over the safety of chloroform anesthesia between 1848 and 1849 illustrate a shift in perspective and expectations surrounding the medical infliction of pain and the status of the patient as subject. Despite the potential dangers, instead of banning chloroform, doctors advocated extreme caution. They monitored patients' vital signs during anesthesia, stopping inhalations at any sign of trouble. Just two years earlier, surgeons had performed painful operations as their patients, fully conscious, screamed in agony. By 1848, however, denying a patient relief from such pain had become impossible. The patients themselves would not stand for it.

Patients had come to view freedom from pain during surgery as a right rather than an option. By granting their patients' requests for anesthesia, doctors re-evaluated their surgical priorities to focus on the patient's status as a subject. As medical professionals, surgeons had a duty to protect their patients from harm. However, anesthesia reimagined that duty to encompass a consideration for the quality of a patient's life and his or her right to experience surgery without the trauma of pain – anticipated, experienced, or remembered. Dr Roux empathized with the mindset of a surgical patient. "I dread pain," he admitted, "and if I had to have a surgical operation today, I would very certainly submit myself to chloroform inhalations; I would do it without hesitation as

[I would be] without fear."[56] Anesthesia offered a safe haven from pain and fear. Surgeons used anesthesia to redefine themselves as empathetic professionals. Yet in so doing, they created new patient expectations, empowering patients to advocate themselves.

THE BIRTHING CHAMBER

During the first few months of 1847, as the medical community researched and debated the merits of anesthetic gases for use in general surgery, obstetricians began to research their applications for childbirth. While surgical anesthesia quickly received the almost universal acclaim of French doctors, childbirth anesthesia remained highly contested. Contemporary social, religious, and political ideas about sex difference shaped debates over women's access to childbirth anesthesia throughout the nineteenth century.[57]

Medical debates about the value of childbirth anesthesia were enmeshed within broader debates about the significance of pain. Religious teachings valorized self-sacrifice and the redemptive value of pain, particularly in the case of childbirth. The Catholic Church had long cited the biblical injunction that woman must give birth in pain as a punishment for Eve's original sin.[58] Religious objections to pain relief during childbirth framed many European debates on the subject. In Britain, James Young Simpson published a rebuttal of these arguments in a pamphlet titled "Answer to the Religious Objections Advanced against the Employment of Anaesthetic Agents in Midwifery and Surgery."[59] Yet these religious perspectives on the significance of pain in childbirth persisted in French society, even within the anticlerical climate of the Third Republic. Arguments that women's suffering during childbirth was natural and inevitable remained salient in a culture that continued to associate womanhood with nature and the cyclical process of reproduction.[60] Some conservative physicians attempted to transpose religious arguments that women must give birth in pain onto the medical arguments against anesthesia. In the French medical literature, however, few opponents of childbirth anesthesia seem to have explicitly cited the scriptural sanction that women must give birth in pain as punishment for Eve's original sin. Instead, doctors voiced their objections in medical terms, discussing the potential dangers of anesthesia for mother and child.[61]

Child-bearing and motherhood were politically charged in nineteenth-century France. The French Revolution had eliminated the distinctions of nobility and birth that characterized the social hierarchies of the Old Regime. Thereafter, sexual difference became crucial for maintaining the post-Revolutionary social order.[62] The ideology of separate spheres prevented women from enjoying the political rights of citizenship while at the same time emphasizing that it was their social and civic duty to bear children to strengthen both the family and the French nation. French women were supposed to serve as "republican mothers" charged with the reproductive duty of producing new citizens and educating their children in republican virtues.[63] While secular republicans eschewed religious interpretations of the importance of pain in childbirth, they nevertheless continued to emphasize pain as a natural and inevitable self-sacrifice in the service of reproducing the French nation.[64]

Religious and political perspectives on sex difference continued to shape debates over women's access to childbirth anesthesia throughout the nineteenth century. Nevertheless, during the *fin de siècle*, amid France's mounting demographic crisis, some doctors became more open to the idea. Concerns over France's dwindling birth rates and diminished population provided avenues for physicians to promote therapeutic practices, including anesthesia, that might facilitate or encourage further reproduction.[65] Despite numerous obstacles, some doctors and women in labour pushed back against institutional opposition, apathy, and conservative bias to advocate for the importance of relieving women's suffering during childbirth.

On 19 January 1847, James Young Simpson, an Edinburgh obstetrician, became the first practitioner to administer ether inhalations to a woman in labour.[66] Soon after he published his results, French doctors began to repeat his experiments. Paul Dubois, chair of the childbirth clinic at the Paris Faculty of Medicine, presented one of the earliest French clinical cases of childbirth anesthesia to the Academy of Medicine in February.[67] For Dubois, who had served as the chief *accoucheur* at the Paris Maternité for over twenty years, childbirth anesthesia was relatively uncharted territory. Unlike surgeons experimenting with ether in surgical operations, Dubois had relatively few precedent cases in which ether had been used in obstetrics.[68] Thus it was with great care that he commenced his research to determine whether ether was as harmless to the pregnant body as it was for the body in general. Using ether on women in labour raised many questions, but Dubois focused on two. First, if ether paralyzed voluntary muscular movement, as surgeons had observed, would it also inhibit the uterine contractions that were necessary for labour to progress? Second, even if ether inhalations seemed harmless when administered during labour, would these have secondary consequences for mother and child afterward?[69]

In addition to a dearth of earlier clinical observations, Dubois lacked another resource that his surgical contemporaries could exploit to demonstrate ether's safety. For the male obstetrician, personal experiential knowledge of the effects of ether on the body in labour was impossible. Dubois could not engage in the kind of self-experimentation that many of his surgical colleagues employed to study the general effects of ether anesthesia. Therefore, his research depended upon the pregnant bodies of his clinical patients.

Dubois's first patient was an eighteen-year-old girl who was pregnant with her first child. She came to the Maternité after thirty-eight hours of labour. Her contractions were weakening and becoming farther apart. After dosing her with ergot failed to accelerate the delivery, Dubois determined he would need to use forceps.[70] He decided to administer ether, "which she only accepted with a sort of repugnance and without understanding the purpose."[71] After a couple of tries, he succeeded in producing a snoring sleep. Then he easily inserted the forceps and extracted the infant's head without resistance and without any apparent pain. When the mother regained consciousness, he asked her whether she had given birth, and "as if instinctively, she moved her hands to her belly and responded yes, but assuring me that she did not remember it."[72] Dubois was able to take a more active role in the birth, manually extracting the infant without difficulty. The mother's body offered no resistance to this process, and he even noted that the ether had relaxed her perineal muscles and facilitated the extraction of the child.

After observing the influence of ether on five of his obstetrical patients, Dubois concluded that ether could eliminate the pain of childbirth without hindering the progress of contractions. He also observed that it seemed to have no negative impact on the health of the mother or the child.[73] Although these conclusions seem to suggest that ether could be beneficial for childbirth in general, Dubois inexplicably recommended *against* using it during "natural childbirth," that is, an uncomplicated vaginal delivery. Several of his colleagues at the Academy of Medicine objected to his conclusions. Dubois had acknowledged that ether seemed to be safe for both mother and child, so his research did not seem to support such excessive caution. Instead, Dr Velpeau argued, Dubois's research actually suggested that ether could be used to eliminate pain in all types of deliveries.[74] Nevertheless, as Dubois held prominent positions in Parisian medical institutions, his recommendation for caution seems to have made an impact. French doctors remained skeptical. Later advocates of anesthesia in natural childbirth blamed Dubois's erroneous conclusions for French medicine's resistance to what they viewed to be a safe and valuable practice.[75]

Across the channel, British obstetricians embraced anesthesia. Dr Simpson promoted its use in natural childbirth. He claimed to have used anesthesia in over 1,519 births without accident.[76] In 1853, John Snow administered chloroform to Queen Victoria during the birth of her eighth child. This royal endorsement dramatically increased the popularity of childbirth anesthesia in Britain.[77] In France, however, anesthesia remained controversial. Dubois's erroneous conclusions, general concerns about chloroform's safety, and a lack of consensus on the drug's specific impact on the progress of labour all contributed to doctors' reluctance to use it for natural childbirth.[78]

The one area of obstetrics where French doctors did achieve a level of consensus on the benefits of anesthesia was in exceptional cases that required active medical intervention. Surgical procedures, like the Caesarian section, merited anesthesia.[79] Obstetric practice also sanctioned the use of anesthesia for difficult births that required the use of instruments, like forceps, to manually extract the infant. French midwives were prohibited from using forceps. They were also legally required to summon a doctor to preside over any unusual cases. Therefore, these types of interventions served to distinguish obstetric practice – the purview of male *accoucheurs* – as a profession.[80] During these procedures, the obstetrician's interventions caused the patient additional pain, beyond the typical pains of labour and delivery. Under these circumstances, doctors felt more comfortable administering anesthesia.

By 1870, anesthesia had become standard practice for obstetric surgery. Charles Pajot, a professor of obstetrics at the Paris Faculty of Medicine, stated that in such cases, "the practitioner today no longer really has the right to refuse the benefits of insensibility to women without serious motives."[81] He particularly recommended the use of chloroform for Caesarian sections, embryotomy, and all other serious obstetrical operations.[82] As doctors considered these complications to be pathological, they had a responsibility to offer the same anesthetic relief to women experiencing the agonizing process of Caesarian section that they would to a patient undergoing amputation. Eliminating the exceptional pain of a medical or surgical intervention during childbirth had become a routine practice. However, the same could not be said of relieving the natural pain of childbirth.

The intense debates over whether anesthesia should be administered during natural childbirth divided practitioners into two camps. Opponents viewed anesthesia in natural childbirth as an unnecessary, and sometimes harmful, intervention. Proponents believed that it was their duty to relieve the suffering of their patients regardless of its context. While official obstetric teaching sided with the opponents in denouncing the practice, proponents continued to conduct and publish research throughout the nineteenth century. They rebelled against these establishment proscriptions, citing their patients' right to give birth without pain.[83]

In the early days of obstetric anesthesia, one of the main issues was determining the impact of chloroform on the progress of labour. Physicians were particularly interested in how it affected uterine contractions. Some doctors claimed that chloroform inhalations halted contractions and slowed labour.[84] However, others did not find this to be the case. In 1854, a few rebels published research on the safety of anesthesia during natural childbirth. Dr Houzelot, a surgeon at the General Hospital of Meaux, published twenty observations of chloroform anesthesia during natural childbirth taken from his private clinic. He found no evidence that chloroform had harmed the fetus, increased the risk of accidents, or slowed the progress of uterine contractions.[85] In Paris, Jean Edouard Laborie administered anesthesia to fifteen women at the Maternité. He observed that none of them had experienced any ill effects from the chloroform.[86] Safety, it appeared, was not the problem.

Part of the confusion over the issue of whether chloroform slowed uterine contractions may have been a result of the terminology used to describe them. In common parlance, people and even doctors frequently used the word *douleur* ("pain") interchangeably with "contraction," as thought they were the same concept. One obstetrician chastised the bizarre habit of midwives and obstetricians who, when the contractions were weak, exclaimed, "This will not do, there are no pains!" On the other hand, when the poor woman experienced energetic, agonizing contractions causing her to scream, they enthusiastically said, "Very good, Madame, excellent pain! A few more good pains like this one and it will be over."[87] While frequently conflated, "contraction" and "pain" actually had a causal relationship. Uterine contractions began before the patient felt pain. By placing his hand on her abdomen, the physician could feel the uterus contracting and warn her the pain was coming.[88] Pain was a distinct phenomenon, separate from the actual contraction of the uterus. Proponents of childbirth anesthesia cited this inaccurate conceptual slippage to refute the notion that pain was somehow a necessary physiological element of the birthing process.[89]

By the 1870s, French obstetricians acknowledged that chloroform did not inhibit the progress of labour. They had recorded enough observations of natural childbirth anesthesia to be quite confident of this conclusion. Chloroform had no negative impact on the strength and progress of uterine contractions. Nor did it paralyze the abdominal muscles. It even had several positive indications. For example, doctors found it to be very useful for treating eclampsia, a condition in which the patient's high blood pressure leads to seizures.[90] Even opponents of natural childbirth anesthesia, such as Pajot and J.A.H. Depaul, had to accept that there was no physiological argument against the practice. In fact, the chloroform caused the perineal muscles to relax, which actually facilitated the expulsion of the infant. This could prevent the excruciating side effect of perineal tearing.[91] In 1877, a New York doctor reported that he had administered chloroform to a woman exhausted from a long and arduous labour, expecting that he would need to extract the child manually. However, the chloroform helped the labour along so rapidly that she delivered naturally without recourse to forceps.[92] If anything, then, chloroform seemed to help rather than hinder the natural progress of labour. Nevertheless, despite its potential physiological benefits for natural childbirth, the obstetrics professors at the Faculty of Medicine continued to resist it.

Many doctors viewed the woman in labour as inherently pathological. Women faced the assumption that their bodies were unstable because they were governed by female "periodicity," which manifested at key moments in their reproductive lives: puberty, menstruation, childbirth, and menopause. As Mary Poovey argues in the British case, doctors used chloroform to silence the unruly female body, a product of nature, and bring it back to the ordered realm of culture.[93] Conservative French doctors had a similar attitude. While Pajot generally opposed childbirth anesthesia outside of obstetric surgery, he made one exception. He condoned the use of chloroform for recalcitrant women, "completely unreasonable, deaf to any exhortation," who screamed and carried on in such a wild manner that their "disobedience threatened to compromise the life of the unborn child." Notably, he did not recommend it to relieve the mother's pain, but rather to calm her intractable body out of concern for the safety of her child.[94]

While proponents of natural childbirth anesthesia had greater regard for the suffering of women in labour than conservatives like Pajot, they embraced similar arguments about the inherent pathology of the female condition. They too recommended chloroform for "intellectual unrest."[95] Dr Hippolyte Blot advised the use of obstetric anesthesia for highly nervous women and for women with a history of mental alienation as a precautionary measure.[96] Houzelot treated a patient about to give birth to her sixth child who had a history of difficult deliveries. Her husband warned him to be on his guard, because during labour, "she loses her head, becomes half mad, and *plays the devil.*"[97] Houzelot faced his screaming, agitated patient and determined that her husband was right. He administered chloroform. The patient became calm. Later, she gave birth without pain or any "sign of mental alienation." Houzelot concluded that anesthesia could calm nervous accidents resulting from childbirth. Anesthetics also helped obstetricians to regulate pathological complications following childbirth, including eclampsia, nervous agitation, and puerperal madness.[98] While touting the undoubtable therapeutic benefits of anesthetics, these arguments still played into stereotypes of the female body as inherently pathological and unstable.

The debates over natural childbirth anesthesia hinged on attitudes toward women's subjectivity. The underlying source of opponents' discomfort seems to have been that eliminating labour pains took the parturient mother into consideration as an individual subject at the precise moment when she was performing her biological duty of reproduction. At a meeting of the Society of Surgery in 1854, Dr Forget argued that doctors had to consider interests beyond "maternal individuality" when weighing the pros and cons of obstetric anesthesia. First, they had to consider the health of the child, which should not be compromised without good reason. Then, they had to consider the family, which expected to "accomplish its growth, and often its conservation from the act [of childbirth.]" Finally, they had to consider the interests of society, "which, to maintain and develop itself, requires that the work of reproduction is surrounded by all possible conditions of safety."[99] For Forget, the mother's pain was of secondary importance to the fruit of her labour. Consideration for the child reflected a concern for the health of a new, possibly male, citizen who could preserve the family name. The subjectivity of the mother paled in comparison with the material benefits of the child to the family and to French society more broadly.

Proponents, by contrast, framed natural childbirth anesthesia as a medical duty and a patient's right. "Anesthesia is as legitimate in laborious deliveries as in surgical operations," Houzelot argued, "and we maintain that the doctor acts [according to] morals, logic and law, scientifically speaking, when he offers it to the mother who suffers during parturition." The woman in labour "will almost always receive a notable relief from it, which she can legitimately ask of science, without danger to herself or her child, without either infringing on the rights of nature, or misunderstanding the will of the Creator."[100] By asserting that the relief of pain in childbirth adhered to morality, logic, and science and did not flout divine law, Houzelot constructed natural childbirth anesthesia as an emblem of therapeutic progress. The context of a patient's pain did not change the fact that the doctor's duty was to relieve her suffering.

Proponents of natural childbirth anesthesia viewed pain itself as a pathological symptom to be treated. As with surgical patients, they believed that strong emotions, including fear and anger, caused by suffering diminished the strength of the woman in labour.[101] Doctors frequently witnessed "the painful spectacle of a woman prey to the cruel sufferings of parturition." Administering chloroform was not just a question of combatting pathology; it was a question of compassion. "Under its beneficial influence," argued Dr Bailly, "we see the moans stop, calm is reborn in the body upset by suffering, and, in the interval between uterine contractions, a restorative sleep arises that fortifies the nerves, restores strength, brings back serenity and courage."[102] For Bailly, an ideal childbirth was an experience of calm and tranquility. Not only did chloroform quieten and sooth the parturient mother's agitated, painful body, but it also fortified her mentally. Chloroform enabled her to transcend the physiological disturbances of her body's labour and conform to gendered expectations of stoicism and calm. Furthermore, chloroform facilitated restorative sleep. Bailly and others observed that women relieved of pain during labour seemed to recover more rapidly and completely than those who had experienced pain.[103]

Although proponents believed that women had the right to give birth in the absence of pain, they often justified this argument by appealing to natalist ideas, particularly in the aftermath of France's devastating defeat in the Franco-Prussian War. Writing in 1878, Bailly insisted that childbirth anesthesia was a necessary relief for mothers performing a crucial reproductive service for France. He argued that "chloroform inflicted a resounding rebuttal to the ancient curse of Jehovah; [now] woman gives birth without pain." Unable to believe that anyone would argue against the use of childbirth anesthesia, he questioned how the medical community could deny pain relief to "a mother who will give one more child to her family and her country [patrie]!"[104] Bailly suggested that the act of giving birth to a new child and citizen entitled mothers to freedom from pain. This desire to relieve the suffering of a parturient mother necessitated a consideration of the woman in labour as a subject. The alleviation of pain in childbirth, a process that was naturally a painful one, demonstrates the extent to which the patient's right to freedom from pain had penetrated the therapeutic ideology of medicine in the nineteenth century.[105] Significantly, however, Bailly framed his support for women's individual right to pain relief in the context of her reproductive service to the nation.

The demographic fate of the nation shaped the debates over obstetric anesthesia. Both proponents and opponents appealed to the idea of childbirth as a service to the nation as they debated how the trauma of childbirth might influence the mother-child relationship after birth. Some doctors apparently opposed obstetric anesthesia because, they argued, it could eliminate a woman's "maternal sentiment," making her a less nurturing mother as her children grew up. Jules Chaigneau claimed that, on the contrary, women who experienced the pain of natural childbirth could develop an aversion for their child afterward.[106] By this logic, anesthesia eliminated the memory of agonies endured during labour so that this trauma would not tarnish the relationship of the mother with her child.[107] Therefore, Chaigneau argued, pain relief in childbirth not only encouraged future reproduction but also protected the subsequent bonds of republican motherhood.

Charles James Campbell (1820–1879) was one of the most enthusiastic advocates of obstetric anesthesia in France. Campbell was born in England, but his family moved to France when he was young. He received his medical degree from the Paris Faculty of Medicine in 1849 and later served as the head of its obstetrical clinic from 1853 to 1855."[108] When Simpson visited France to demonstrate his technique of administering chloroform for childbirth anesthesia, Campbell introduced him to the various learned societies and salons of Paris.[109] While some French doctors viewed obstetric anesthesia as part of their medical duty to relieve suffering, the medical community as a whole continued to drag its heels in the 1850s, and this stubbornness frustrated Campbell. "Amid this glacial welcome, the practice of eliminating pain in natural childbirth was going to be brought to an end, and, in France, the old concurrent pain of our species was going to become once more triumphant over the entire obstetric line; but," he quipped, "they had not taken the women into account."[110] Conservative medicine met with resistance from pregnant women who, during the agonies of childbirth, became the champions of their own cause.

Women's experience of childbirth differed significantly based on wealth and social status. Typically, wealthy and bourgeois women of sufficient means would summon a midwife or a doctor-*accoucheur* for a home delivery.[111] Wealthier women who had private home deliveries were far more likely to benefit from natural childbirth anesthesia than poor women.[112] Single, poor, and working-class women could not afford private home deliveries and instead were forced to give birth in a general hospital or maternity hospital, like Paris's infamous Maternité.[113] Given the conservative leanings of French obstetrics and the limited resources of these public hospitals, poor women were far less likely to receive anesthetic to relieve the pain of labour and delivery.[114] However, as hospital maternity wards served as sites for clinical research, some poorer women did have some – albeit limited, experimental, and exploitative – access to childbirth anesthetics.[115]

Childbirth was an agonizing experience accompanied by considerable fear and anxiety. Women knew that death during childbirth was a real possibility. This danger was particularly acute in maternity hospitals before the introduction of antiseptic practices reduced the number of deaths from puerperal fever and other infections.[116] In its worst years, the maternal death rate at the Paris Maternité was as high as one in ten.[117] Women's ignorance of their own bodies further exacerbated their anxieties. In the nineteenth century, mothers prepared their daughters for the marital bed in vague terms, if at all. As women tried "to tame the natural by hiding it," many women experienced sexual intercourse and childbirth for the first time lacking even basic knowledge of these processes.[118] Doctors, however, were quite familiar with seeing women in labour "restless, anxious, constantly emitting groans or harrowing shrieks, and insistently begging to be relieved."[119] Whatever expectations the parturient mother had before childbirth, labour quickly demonstrated that it was an experience defined by pain.

Women in agony began to advocate for themselves. According to Campbell, this assertiveness about pain relief was a foreign import. Foreign women, accustomed to the more liberal use of anesthetics in the English-speaking world, refused to submit to the conservative practices of French obstetrics. Campbell asked, "How could one resist that sort of anesthetic fury which had seized these women, who, coming to Paris … from Edinburgh, would not set out without having a flask of chloroform from Duncan and Flockhart at the bottom of their luggage?" Women who had experienced painless childbirth in Britain or the United States insisted on the same conditions in Paris – they even supplied their own anesthetics. While the conservative male doctors at the Paris Faculty of Medicine eschewed anesthesia during natural childbirth, these foreign women transmitted medical knowledge from the bottom up, standing firm in their refusal to endure what they believed to be unnecessary pain. "It was through their example that the method penetrated and spread little by little in private practice," argued Campbell, until finally, it reached "the French clientele, who ... kept themselves informed of what was happening with the foreign ladies."[120] According to Campbell, the emergence of informal networks through which women transmitted their own knowledge of and experiences with childbirth anesthesia were as, if not more, responsible for the spread of this practice to France than formal, male-centred networks for the exchange of medical knowledge.

Campbell willingly accommodated his patients' requests for pain relief. Early in his career he had worked for Sir Joseph Olliffe, a compatriot of Simpson's who championed the practice of obstetric anesthesia among the Anglo-American community in Paris.[121] Between 1849 and 1873, Campbell attended 1,500 childbirths. Among these, he claimed to have administered ether or chloroform anesthesia 942 times, or in almost two out of every three cases.[122] Rather than administering inhalations when the patient first experienced contractions, Campbell reserved inhalations for the final period of labour, to alleviate the pains of expulsion. He practised intermittent inhalations, which put the patient in a state of partial insensibility and partial consciousness.[123] Campbell was confident in the safety of childbirth anesthesia. Of 1,500 patients over more than twenty-five years, only eleven had died. Campbell attributed their deaths to a variety of pathological complications, including puerperal fever, diphtheria, eclampsia, hemorrhage, cholera, and typhoid fever, and not to anesthesia, which had been administered only in some of the cases.[124]

In natural childbirth, obstetricians faced anesthetic challenges that general surgeons did not. During surgery, anesthesia eliminated the patient's pain and consciousness. It allowed the surgeon to focus more on complex and delicate tasks while the unconscious anesthetized patient lay still on the operating table in a state of near perfect submission. The surgeon's active role contrasted starkly with the passivity of the anesthetized patient. Dr Blot, the former head of the childbirth clinic at the Faculty of Medicine in Paris, described the unique challenges presented by the female body in labour. "Only the surgeon is *active* in operations," he argued; "the obstetrician, on the contrary, must be content in most cases with the role of intelligent observer, paying close attention to direct the efforts of nature ... [therefore] the body, which is completely *passive* during surgical operations, needs to be *active* during the work of childbirth."[125] Unlike the surgical patient, the woman in labour had a duty to perform. Her body could not be entirely objectified and acted upon by the obstetrician, because he could not perform the same work that she could. Her muscles and her contractions moved the process of labour along. Childbirth required her body to be active.

To ensure that the parturient woman could still play an active role in natural childbirth, doctors employed "semi-anesthesia." For this, they administered a lower dose of chloroform, which alleviated the pain of childbirth without causing the woman to lose consciousness during labour. This state in which the conscious subject felt no pain was known by many different names, including "obstetrical anesthesia" and even "anesthesia à la reine," an homage to Queen Victoria's use of chloroform during the birth of her eighth child.[126] One benefit of semi-anesthesia was that doctors could ask the patient what she was feeling and use her responses to inform decisions about care. One of Houzelot's patients, Mme ***, a thirty-one-year-old woman with a nervous constitution, gave birth to her fifth child on 8 September 1852. Houzelot administered chloroform intermittently to calm the pain of her contractions. When she felt a contraction coming, she asked for the chloroform herself. When he asked her later to describe her experience with the chloroform, she recalled,

> I remained completely conscious of everything that took place; I was suffering horribly when you administered the chloroform, which in an instant gave me an indescribable serenity; immediately, I became calm. When the chloroform acted, I saw, I heard, I could move and speak, I was aware of all that was happening around me, and in me, I felt the labour, but I did not suffer nor did I lose consciousness; however, the absence of pain allowed me to push and effectively assist nature. I was mistress of myself, whereas with the pain, I could not control myself.[127]

Chloroform empowered the parturient mother to play an active role in her birth, while relieving her of the physical suffering normally associated with it. Rather than being passive, or overpowered by the pain of contractions, she felt strong and able to push. Taking control of her own body in this way, she felt a powerful sense of self-mastery. After the labour was over, Mme *** exclaimed, "Ah! ... if women knew of the good one feels [with chloroform] they would not want to give birth any other way."[128]

Chloroform, a substance used to eliminate consciousness entirely in surgical operations, paradoxically offered women in labour a powerful tool for exercising their own agency in the process of childbirth. Most doctors who employed semi-anesthesia during childbirth preferred the simplest technology by which to administer the anesthetic agent: a cloth or handkerchief folded into a triangle or a cone and attached at the corners with a pin.[129] While doctors had proposed various different masks and apparatuses for administering ether and chloroform, the simple handkerchief had been in widespread use from the very beginning.[130] In 1848, Dr Sédillot had particularly recommended using a handkerchief for fearful and impressionable patients, who might have been alarmed by a more complex apparatus.[131] Many opponents of natural childbirth anesthesia argued that a shortage of assistants made it impossible to administer anesthesia safely while monitoring the patient's vital signs and the progress of labour.[132] However, proponents of semi-anesthesia argued that with a simple handkerchief, the patient could administer the anesthesia herself by holding the handkerchief a certain distance from her own face.[133] The self-administration of anesthesia ensured that women remained active participants in the birthing process. It also gave them control over their own pain relief.

By the 1880s, as popular awareness of the possibility of giving birth without pain increased, women began to request and even demand anesthesia from their *accoucheurs*.[134] They used their own consent and cooperation as bargaining tools. Medical observations of the use of anesthesia during childbirth document instances in which women took things into their own hands and engaged in small negotiations of power with their male *accoucheurs*.[135] For example, once "Mme H..." got a taste of the "great relief" that chloroform brought her during the birth of her first child, she demanded more of it. Indeed, Chaigneau, her obstetrician, recorded that "she would not consent to push until she was given a sufficient dose of chloroform." Mme H... negotiated pain relief for her active participation in her own childbirth. Chaigneau noted that during the birth of her second child two years later, "like the first time, the patient refuses to push if we stop the inhalations."[136] Mme

H… demonstrated the contested nature of the *accoucheur*'s power over his patients. He depended on her active participation in the labour. She could make things more difficult for him by refusing to cooperate. Women like Mme H…had come to conceptualize the pain of childbirth as a question of choice – and crucially, *their* choice, not the doctor's.

Occasionally, women spoke out quite forcefully about childbirth anesthesia. In 1889, journalist Hugues le Roux wrote about the moral implications of relieving women's pain during childbirth. He argued that a woman did not have the right to risk her own life and that of her child by relieving her suffering using chloroform unless a doctor recommended its use and accepted responsibility for the risk. However, despite this confident assertion, Le Roux concluded the piece enigmatically by quoting a woman who had written to him on the subject. The woman scolded men who stubbornly harped on about a "bible verse that obliges us other poor creatures to tolerate the pains of childbirth without trying to find a remedy." She attested, "There is one man, only one, who has given birth … and he was put to sleep. Reopen the scriptures, if you please. You will see that God, having taken one of Adam's ribs to create Eve, performed this operation while our forbearer was asleep."[137] By pointing out this biblical double standard, she asserted women's right to relief from pain.

Gustave Lebert, a rural doctor in the small commune of Colomby-les-Belles in northeastern France, was a long-time advocate of childbirth anesthesia. He employed it in all cases of childbirth, "normal or abnormal, without exception."[138] Having previously used chloroform for women in labour, in 1880 he began to use ethyl bromide, a chemical compound similar to ether. Highly satisfied with the results, he adopted this new method with zeal.[139]

Lebert wanted to change the minds of doctors in a medical community paralyzed by "false ideas, by fear, by unjust prejudices, by the indifference of many doctors, and especially by routine."[140] He cited a recent case in which he had used ethyl bromide for a particularly difficult delivery in the neighbouring town of Dolcourt. At the onset of each contraction, his patient asked him for relief, which he provided in the form of a few drops of ethyl bromide on a handkerchief. "Oh! I am happy," she exclaimed. "Don't wander off, and give me some more of *that*."[141] Although he eventually had to resort to using forceps to extract the remarkably large infant, thanks to the ethyl bromide the mother experienced no pain during the birth. Moreover, she had sufficiently recovered her strength a month later to walk the fourteen kilometres to Lebert's practice in Colomby.[142]

As a self-avowed partisan of childbirth anesthesia, Lebert emphasized not only the therapeutic benefits of ethyl bromide for women in labour but also the humanitarian benefits of relieving women's fears and anxieties. In 1883, he published a remarkable pamphlet titled "Painless Childbirth through the Use of Ethyl Bromide: Advice for Women on the Verge of Becoming Mothers."[143] Rather than catering to an audience of fellow male obstetricians, Lebert explicitly designed this pamphlet to inform expectant mothers of the efficacy and safety of this new drug for alleviating the agonies of labour.[144] Extolling the merits of his research, Lebert pandered to the women he hoped to reach. "What woman, whatever energy you suppose her to be blessed with, does not dread the moment of birth?" he asked. "Some have had a labour so long, so difficult, have experienced pains so atrocious that the maternal instinct must be very powerful to make them accept its repetition."[145] Lebert worried that the subjective experience of pain during childbirth would make women unwilling to continue reproducing. This was a serious concern amid anxieties over depopulation. By emphasizing the importance of childbirth anesthesia to women, Lebert acknowledged women's status as individual subjects even as he emphasized the importance of their reproductive function in service to the nation.

Lebert's fears echoed the populationist rhetoric of the Third Republic. France's declining birth rates demonstrated that couples were already deliberately limiting family size.[146] Populationists worried that single, independent "New Women" would wreak social destruction by rejecting their reproductive duty to the nation.[147] Paul Robin's neo-Malthusian movement distributed information on birth control techniques in the *fin de siècle* to increase women's access to contraceptive advice.[148] A handful of radical feminists, including Marie Huot and Nelly Roussel, supported the movement and advocated for "freedom of maternity." In the 1890s and 1900s, they called for a "womb strike" to assert women's bodily autonomy and challenge the accepted notion that women were destined for suffering and self-sacrifice.[149]

Roussel had suffered immensely from childbirth.[150] The physical suffering and trauma she experienced during her first two pregnancies motivated her to support the birth control movement. Roussel rejected the perceived necessity or inevitability of motherhood and physical suffering. She published articles and gave public lectures condemning society's apathy toward the suffering of mothers and promoting access to contraception. When in 1904, despite her best efforts, she became pregnant for a third time, she elected to deliver her baby at an "Anesthesiology Establishment" in the wealthy district of Passy in the sixteenth arrondissement. There, Dr Lucas administered a mixture of nitrous oxide and compressed air to relieve the pain of childbirth.[151] Although the birth control measures Roussel so staunchly supported had not succeeded in preventing her pregnancy, she turned to science to alleviate her pain and fear of childbirth. She asserted control over the conditions of her labour, if not the fact of birth itself.

Radical feminists who, like Roussel, publicly championed women's individual autonomy on questions of maternity were rare. The mainstream feminist movement in France tended to celebrate motherhood. Mainstream feminists sought to improve women's status in society by emphasizing complementarity rather than absolute equality with men, to highlight women's unique and essential role as republican mothers.[152] Nevertheless, if most women were unwilling to protest the ideal of motherhood, the medical literature suggests that they might have been more willing to assert themselves in the birthing chamber. In his 1883 pamphlet for expectant mothers, Lebert explicitly encouraged women to advocate for their own pain relief. He advised them to not be afraid to ask for ethyl bromide, to "insist, in a way to force the hand of their doctor if, by routine or by unjustified bias, he refuses to use this means of relief."[153] Lebert presented pain relief as both a patient's right and an obstetrician's duty. Rather than accepting the obstetrician's authority in refusing pain relief, he encouraged women to assert themselves by demanding to experience birth in a manner of their choosing. Lebert believed that expectant mothers could be agents of therapeutic change.

Women in labour advocated for their own pain relief in the birthing chamber, yet the extent to which their efforts shaped therapeutic practices of childbirth anesthesia more broadly is unclear. In general, official obstetric teaching continued to oppose natural childbirth anesthesia throughout the nineteenth century. However, despite this hostility from the medical establishment, clinical research on childbirth anesthesia proliferated from the 1870s onward. Doctors experimented with new anesthetic substances and methods of administration, thereby transforming the maternity ward into a laboratory and blurring the boundaries between clinical treatment and experimentation.

Labouring women in France's maternity hospitals served as guinea pigs in the quest to determine the ideal substances and methods of childbirth anesthesia. Doctors and medical students studied the effects of chloral, opium, morphine, ether, amelyne, ethyl bromide, antipyrine, and nitrous oxide as well as mixed methods that combined chloroform with one or two of these substances.[154] In 1885, on the heels of Carl Koller's discovery of cocaine's therapeutic potential as a local anesthetic, French doctors began to publish their research on the topical use of cocaine in childbirth.[155] Cocaine silenced the agonies of labour. It was so effective that one woman who had screamed in agony before it was administered began to give birth so calmly that her doctor did not realize it was happening. She had to say, "Come, Monsieur, I think it's coming out all on its own."[156] Furthermore, cocaine offered obstetricians a powerful alternative to inhalation anesthesia as, unlike chloroform, it was administered topically. Therefore, it did not pose a risk of asphyxiation. One physician even administered it to his own wife during the birth of their first child, noting that with cocaine "she was not suffering at all."[157]

Cocaine could also relieve the pain of physical complications after birth. Doctors used it to perform sutures after perineal and cervical tearing. It could also be used to numb the pain of cracked nipples caused by breastfeeding.[158] One of Dr Herrgott's patients had such painful nipple fissures that she "could not give the breast without screaming." After the topical application of cocaine, however, she could nurse her child without pain.[159] Popular health and hygiene guides for new mothers also recommended this practice, to spare young mothers unnecessary suffering.[160] Cocaine not only relieved pain during childbirth but helped the new mother to recover from the physical damage of parturition and enabled her to nourish her child in relative comfort.

The sheer volume of research on different substances to relieve the pain of childbirth in *fin-de-siècle* France suggests that doctors considered obstetric pain relief to be a project worthy of scientific inquiry. While some researchers were compassionate practitioners who championed the right of women to give birth without pain, most were pragmatists who hoped to inspire reluctant women to reproduce in service of the French nation. Doctors experimented on the bodies of poor women in maternity hospitals to develop new knowledge about the possibilities for childbirth anesthesia. Aside from this experimental context, poorer women rarely had access to pain relief.[161]

Wealthier women who employed *accoucheurs* for private home deliveries were in a far stronger position to advocate for themselves. Still, these individual negotiations of power in the birthing chamber do not seem to have translated into a systematic shift in therapeutic practice. Proponents of natural childbirth anesthesia depicted the power to alleviate the pain of childbirth – which women had endured for millennia – as an indication of scientific progress.[162] However, French obstetrics as a whole remained obstinately conservative. At the turn of the twentieth century, labouring women and proponents of natural childbirth anesthesia continued to clash with obstetricians who were reluctant to conceive of women in labour as subjects rather than objects of reproduction.

THE BATTLEFIELD

In the nineteenth century, French citizenship was associated with the twin, gendered pillars of soldiering and mothering. After 1870, the sting of military defeat and the mounting population crisis amplified nationalist rhetoric. Male citizens had a duty to defend the fatherland through military service. Female citizens had a duty to support this mission by increasing the population. While radical feminists like Roussel criticized repopulationists for treating women like "machine[s] for turning out cannon-fodder," military service had been a fundamental duty of male citizenship since the Revolution.[163]

Military service was particularly important for citizenship in the French nation. With the *levée en masse* in 1793, the French government established the world's first nationwide conscript army.[164] In the Revolutionary era, supporters of obligatory military service as a fundamental duty of citizenship hoped that it would encourage civic virtue and physical prowess in the image of the citizen-soldiers of Greece and the Roman Republic.[165] However, the reality differed dramatically. While the Jourdan Law established systematic military conscription in France in 1798, exemptions, special dispensations, and the practice of paying to send a substitute in one's stead enabled men of means to avoid this obligatory military service for much of the nineteenth century. After France's humiliating defeat during the Franco-Prussian War of 1870, however, the Third Republic worked to make military service a truly universal obligation of male citizenship. In 1873 it abolished the practice of substitution, and by 1889 it had put an end to special dispensations and exemptions.[166] Amid anxieties over a crisis of masculinity, stagnant birth rates, and the decadence of modern civilization, *fin-de-siècle* military rhetoric emphasized the importance of soldiering not only for reinvigorating and strengthening the physical prowess of male bodies but also for reinforcing the masculine virtues of courage, honour, discipline, and self-sacrifice in the service of the French nation.[167]

The introduction of battlefield anesthesia transformed the soldier's experience of suffering for the nation. During the Napoleonic Wars, battlefield surgery had been a grizzly, agonizing affair for surgeons and soldiers alike. Speed was one of the surgeon's only tools of mercy.[168] The legendary Napoleonic military surgeon Baron Dominique Jean Larrey reputedly could perform as many as two hundred amputations in a single day.[169] In the mid-nineteenth century, the introduction of inhalation anesthesia to battlefield surgery precipitated therapeutic progress. Surgeons moved beyond the straightforward amputations characteristic of Napoleonic battlefield surgery to perform increasingly sophisticated and conservative surgical procedures.[170] Between the Crimean War and World War I, anesthetic practices, like surgical procedures, advanced considerably. The introduction of new substances for local anesthesia, including cocaine and ethyl chloride, and new procedures, including spinal anesthesia and mixed inhalation anesthesia, reflected a desire to find the optimal solution for individual pain in a context of mass casualties.

In battlefield surgery, the surgeon had to navigate between his duty to each individual patient and the needs of the army as a whole. Triage – from the French *trier*, meaning "to choose" or "to sort out" – held that wounded soldiers should be prioritized according to the gravity of their injuries and the urgency of their need for treatment.[171] The introduction of anesthesia in battlefield surgery represented a basic respect for the soldier as an individual subject even within the collective group of the military. Military doctors came to believe that the soldier, after enduring the fear and agony of shrapnel or bullets ripping through his body, had a right not to experience a second round of flesh-tearing agony as the surgeon attempted to remedy the destruction of war.

French military surgeons experimented with chloroform for the first time in a major conflict during the Crimean War (1853–56), during which France and Britain joined forces with the Ottoman Empire to check the imperialist ambitions of Russia.[172] In 1854, the allies began a year-long siege of the Russian naval base at Sevastopol, on the Black Sea. Auguste Marroin, a naval medical officer, treated the wounded during the siege. He remarked that chloroform "was employed everywhere" to treat gaping projectile wounds. With it, doctors could perform amputations and treat dislocated limbs, "without the least impact."[173] After a bloody naval assault on the Russian fortress in October, Gaspard Scrive, chief physician of the French Armée d'Orient, treated 110 wounded. He performed twenty-two amputations of legs, arms, and fingers, noting that "chloroform was constantly employed."[174] In Crimea alone, Scrive estimated that chloroform had been administered to over 20,000 wounded soldiers, and Lucien Baudens held that it have been used in over 30,000 cases in the Armée d'Orient as a whole.[175] For the first time, surgeons could approach a seemingly endless succession of battlefield surgeries by systematically employing an anesthetic agent to protect wounded soldiers from further suffering.

At first Scrive feared that chloroform would diminish wounded soldiers' already weakened vital forces, so he meticulously measured the chloroform administered using a special apparatus. However, his fears dissipated rapidly. "Far from adding to the general stupor of the patient," he found, chloroform "favourably excites the depleted nervous system [and] raises the circulatory movement [that had been slowed] and weakened by the general commotion, all while destroying the irritating and difficult feeling of pain."[176] So, surgical pain relief was the main but not the only physiological benefit of administering chloroform to a wounded soldier in a weakened state. Doctors even used chloroform on seriously wounded soldiers after surgery to relieve pain while changing their bandages.[177]

With the promise of painless surgery, soldiers no longer had to fear the surgeon's knife. "In the past, we often had to waste a long time in making the wounded understand the need for painful operations," Dr Quesnoy observed, but "today, certain not to suffer, they submit without resistance."[178] Without the fear of suffering, wounded soldiers were far more cooperative with amputations.[179] This tractability among soldiers sped up the process of battlefield surgery. While anesthesia reduced the individual soldier's fear and anxiety about surgery, it also made the surgeon's job easier.

Anesthesia's psychological benefits extended beyond the individual soldier. Some doctors argued that it improved the troops' morale more broadly. On naval ships, it was impossible to isolate the wounded from the rest of the sailors, and before anesthesia the whole ship would hear the "piercing screams" of wounded sailors enduring amputation.[180] By silencing the suffering bodies of the wounded, chloroform strengthened the able-bodied by sheltering them from the second-hand experience of pain.

Pain relief became a humanitarian issue. French surgeons administered anesthesia to their own troops and enemy combatants alike. Scrive claimed that almost 4,000 wounded Russian prisoners of war experienced surgical anesthesia, adding, "It was a touching sight to see their profound astonishment at our good remedies." As a sign of their immense gratitude, "these good people betrayed by the luck of battle ... embraced us, their hands red with their blood, and looked up to heaven devoutly and gave thanks for the benefits of our Samaritan compassion."[181] On the one hand, by portraying French surgeons as benevolent and compassionate in their willingness to relieve the pain of their enemies, Scrive presented the French Army as a noble, moral, and superior force. On the other hand, he implied that the agony of surgery was a fate that no soldier, regardless of nationality, should have to endure. Just as pain was a universal experience of all wounded combatants, so too was the succour of anesthesia.

This humanitarian impulse to relieve suffering led surgeons to administer anesthesia even in hopeless cases. Scrive found it difficult to stand by and watch an inoperable patient in agony as he slowly bled to death. He recalled the pleading screams of a dying captain whose face "reflected the most sublime expression of a supreme struggle of the powerful vitality of youth against a destructive agent stronger than it." All who witnessed this agonizingly slow spectacle of death were moved to tears.[182] Regarding inoperable cases, Scrive argued that instead of condemning the dying soldier to "atrocious pain," the surgeon should use chloroform to "cushion [his] painfully exalted sensibility until the end of life."[183] If surgical intervention could not prevent the soldier's death, anesthesia at least gave the surgeon the power to control its context. Rather than being forced to watch passively as a soldier slowly died in agony, the surgeon could perform a "charitable *chloroformisation*" to ease the suffering of his final moments.[184] The relief of soldiers' pain had become the surgeon's noble duty.

The primary disadvantage of battlefield anesthesia seems to have been the time it took to administer. Dr Léon Legouest claimed that it took about ten minutes of inhalations before most people reached a state of anesthesia and that for some it took fifteen or twenty minutes. In a battlefield hospital, with huge numbers of wounded in need of urgent attention, this delay was a problem. On 8 September 1855, French forces successfully assaulted the Russian fortifications on Malakoff Hill, breaking the year-long siege of Sebastopol. This attack left the five French ambulances with 4,472 French and 554 Russian wounded. Two days later, all the wounded had been bandaged, but surgeons had performed only 350 of the 550 serious operations deemed necessary. Doctors finally finished operating on the remaining wounded three days after those patients had sustained their injuries. Legouest found this delay unacceptable. It put patients at a higher risk for complications. Before anesthesia, Baron Larrey had recorded that most operations at the Battle of Eylau in 1807 were performed within twelve hours. Legouest argued that without chloroform all the operations from the assault on Malakoff Hill could have been performed in two days instead of three.[185]

Nevertheless, Legouest did not suggest returning to surgery without anesthesia, as such a practice had become unthinkable. In spite of the delay, which could have killed or severely harmed the soldiers waiting for surgery, Legouest declared, "the benefits of anesthesia cannot be denied to our soldiers, who never fail to clamour for them, and it's up to our surgeons to familiarize themselves with the quickest and surest means of administering chloroform."[186] In this case, the right of the individual soldier to undergo surgery without pain overrode the needs of the group. The surgeon's duty was not only to fix the wounded soldier's damaged body but to do so in a manner that respected the soldier's right to be unconscious for that process, protecting his mind from further trauma while his body was mutilated once more, albeit in a restorative fashion.

In the sixty years between the Crimean War and World War I, practices and techniques of military surgery advanced considerably. Anesthesia enabled surgeons to perform longer and more delicate procedures than ever before. Military surgeons became much more conservative with their surgeries, performing fewer amputations and preserving as much functional tissue as possible.[187] It also enabled them to operate on abdominal and chest wounds, which had been considered inoperable at the beginning of the nineteenth century. Furthermore, the introduction of Joseph Lister's antiseptic techniques to French medicine in 1869 reduced the likelihood that a patient who survived surgery would later die of infection.[188] Military surgeons used antiseptic techniques sporadically in the Franco-Prussian War (1870–71) and then more consistently in later conflicts.[189]

During the Franco-Prussian War, chloroform remained the most popular anesthetic among military surgeons.[190] Armand Sabatier, chief surgeon of the Ambulance du Midi, frequently used chloroform, not only during operations but also for painful exploratory examinations.[191] When a surgeon felt particularly confident in the skills of his aids, he could have them perform *chloroformisation d'attante*, the practice of anesthetizing a second patient shortly before the end of the first operation so that this second patient could be placed on the operating table immediately after the first operation had finished.[192] In this manner, surgeries could be performed with a factory-like efficiency. Unfortunately, when facing a constant stream of casualties, the most vital medicines usually ran out first. Just Lucas-Championnière, a young doctor who served with the Armée de la Loire, complained that his ambulance had "only 1,500 gr. of chloroform [remaining], but 18 kg, of cucumber pomade."[193] Between August and October of 1870, the Prussian armies besieged the fortified city of Metz, hoping to starve the French Army into surrendering. Toward the end of the siege, the chief physician, Dr Grellois, recalled that "the most essential medicines were lacking … we were even about to run out of chloroform."[194] The French Army's depleted supplies of medicines during the war seem to have been exacerbated by shortages during the siege of Paris.[195]

Doctors also administered new analgesic medicines to relieve the pain of wounded soldiers while they waited for treatment. Doctors carried small Pravaz syringes in their pockets to offer rapid and immense relief to suffering soldiers. The famous "flying ambulances" provided first aid on the battlefield and evacuated wounded soldiers for further treatment. Although the nightly administration of different potions and pills for a large number of wounded required more personnel than were available, with "a short tour of the surgeon or an aid" they could administer morphine injections to all the patients each evening.[196] Morphine injections were convenient and effective, so the Ambulance du Midi used them liberally. "Every night," Sabatier recalled, "one of us distributed the benefits of sleep and forgetfulness in this manner to those unfortunates tortured by pain and dominated by a profound sadness."[197] Sabatier constructed the relief of pain through morphine as a humane act of service to the individual. He recognized that the pain of being wounded went far beyond the physical suffering following an injury. Morphine also enabled wounded soldiers to cope with the emotional turmoil of war.

This act of mercy transcended nationality. Wounded soldiers called out to the doctor administering injections. Sabatier remembered one cruelly mutilated German soldier's expression of joy at receiving his injection from the French ambulance: the soldier exclaimed, "Das ist so schön!" (That is so nice!).[198] It was difficult to estimate "the sum of the pain that was spared by a doctor who, the evening of a battle, went from one wounded man to another, equipped with his small syringe in one hand, and a flask filled with a concentrated solution of morphine in the other."[199] Sabatier's reliance on morphine was not exceptional. The Anglo-American branch hospitals established around the Battle of Sedan also administered it liberally. As one American doctor explained, "no one was allowed to suffer pain" if morphine – that "precious boon" to humanity – was available to relieve it.[200] Out of compassion, surgeons administered morphine to soothe the physical pain and relieve the mental anguish of wounded men devastated by the state of their mutilated bodies.[201]

In the years following the Franco-Prussian War, doctors proposed various strategies for relieving pain on the battlefield itself. The *Officers' Practical Medical Guide*, published in 1876, praised the hypnotic action of chloral, which had recently been introduced into medical practice, and recommended its use for alleviating pain in cases of moderate wounds.[202] The guide noted that chloral "pearls" were included along with bandages, scissors, tongs, and tourniquets in a small kit called the "battlefield pharmacy." This kit also included instructions in capital letters, which were designed to be easily legible for a semi-literate soldier to understand so he could provide first aid to his officer.[203] After 1884, cocaine injections enabled doctors to alleviate pain locally during minor interventions on the battlefield.[204] While triage dictated that doctors had to prioritize the most serious injuries, military medicine increasingly sought to relieve soldiers' pain while they waited for treatment.

On the eve of World War I, military surgeons had many more anesthetic options than did their predecessors a half century before. The 1857 edition of the French military's *Pharmaceutical Formulary* included only very basic *materia medica* for relieving pain, including ether, chloroform, morphine, and opium.[205] In contrast, in 1917 the *Pharmaceutical Formulary* included many more options for anesthetic and analgesic medicines, including ethyl chloride, cocaine, heroin, novocaine, and stovaine. These medicines were contained in ampoules, small hermetically sealed glass vials designed to facilitate syringe injections and prevent volatile anesthetic gases from evaporating.[206] With this diverse arsenal of drugs, military doctors and surgeons could tailor their treatments to the particular needs of a patient. They were able to administer general and localized anesthesia for surgery and a variety of analgesic remedies to treat pain during recovery. Nevertheless, while cocaine and other methods of local anesthesia for minor operations entered into the military surgeon's medicinal arsenal, chloroform remained the primary general anesthetic used by the French military during the war.[207]

Anesthetic drugs were crucial tools of military medicine during World War I. Owing to advances in sanitation, hygiene, and inoculation, fatal injury outstripped disease as the leading cause of death for combatants for the first time in a major conflict.[208] The French government recognized the vital importance of anesthetic drugs to military medicine. Thus, in 1914 it began to conserve its supply of drugs by restricting exports of chemicals used to manufacture chloroform and other pharmaceuticals. For the duration of the war, Professor Auguste Behal of the Paris Pharmacy School served as director of the Office of

Chemical Products and Pharmaceuticals, a temporary office attached to the Ministry of Commerce and Industry. Its mission was to take stock of the chemicals and pharmaceuticals in France, to measure and increase their production, to manage provision and distribution, and to restrict exports of vital chemical and pharmaceutical products.[209]

The medical forces on the Allied side were organized into three evacuation zones behind the trenches. The first, the "zone of advance," extended a few miles behind the front line and included first aid stations, mobile surgical units, field hospitals, and divisional ambulances.[210] At first aid posts, medical officers determined how far a soldier would be evacuated from the front based on the severity of his wounds. Those with less serious injuries remained close to the front lines so they could return to their posts as soon as they were able. Those with more serious injuries were evacuated farther back.[211] The overwhelming volume of wounded soldiers together with the wet, muddy conditions made it difficult for stretcher-bearers to carry the wounded to first aid posts. Uneven terrain, cratered from shell fire, prevented them from using carts to help with transportation. The muddy ground meant that often six or even eight stretcher-bearers had to struggle to carry a single wounded man.[212] Soldiers frequently had to treat their own wounds using the packet of field dressings each soldier carried. Many waited hours and sometimes even days to be found and evacuated.

Before the war, the medical community had discussed strategies for relieving a soldier's pain during this waiting period. In 1906, *La Presse médicale* published a short article on a new anesthetic technique known as the "Schleich mix": a combination of ether, chloroform, and ethyl chloride. Carl Ludwig Schleich, the German surgeon who developed this new method, suggested that soldiers should carry small metal casings containing his mixture and a piece of gauze as part of their equipment on the battlefield. He hoped this would enable wounded soldiers to anesthetize themselves in the long hours of waiting for stretcher-bearers to arrive.[213] Later that year, the French Surgical Congress acknowledged that the ability of soldiers to anesthetize themselves in this manner would be of real value.[214] It is unclear whether French soldiers carried these types of anesthetics with them on the battlefield; however, it is unlikely that German soldiers did. In his memoirs, Schleich bitterly noted that his "humane and perfectly practical idea" of soldiers practising "self-narcosis" while waiting for relief had been rejected because some had claimed "the soldiers might drink the mixture!"[215] Although self-narcosis might not have taken place on the battlefields of World War I, the medical enthusiasm for the proposal before the war reinforces the idea that the medical community was actively considering new ways to spare the wounded soldier any pain beyond that which he incurred under enemy fire.[216]

First aid posts were often situated in dugouts in the rear line of trenches. Stretcher-bearers transported wounded soldiers to these first aid posts, where a doctor and one or two aids diagnosed and bandaged their injuries.[217] Situated close to the front lines, first aid posts were dangerous places. They served primarily as stations for preparing wounded soldiers to move on to a hospital that was better equipped to treat their injuries.[218] Only in the most important first aid posts could doctors perform emergency amputations. Except in the most desperate cases, they did not use chloroform anesthesia for these emergency procedures. It was too time consuming and dangerous, because it incapacitated wounded soldiers who might need to be quickly evacuated.[219] Instead, surgeons turned to other substances.

Ethyl chloride, an anesthetic gas prepared by combining ethyl alcohol with hydrogen chloride, became a popular anesthetic for minor procedures at the turn of the twentieth century. It worked quickly, producing unconsciousness within a few seconds of inhalation. It also did not last long after the inhalations ceased, so the patient would regain consciousness quickly after the procedure. While most surgeons used it for quick, relatively minor interventions, in 1915 French surgeons at the No. 18 temporary hospital on the Western Front began to use ethyl chloride systematically for more serious procedures, including disarticulations, amputations, and resections.[220] Ethyl chloride offered considerable advantages for battlefield surgery close to the front lines. Compared with chloroform, which took longer to administer, ethyl chloride enabled the surgeon to move more quickly from operation to operation, allowing him to treat more patients. Furthermore, as the patient would awaken soon after the inhalations ceased, this method of anesthesia did not leave the surgeon with large numbers of unconscious patients in recovery in the event of an evacuation.[221]

While they might practice emergency amputations, doctors at first aid posts would not attempt more complex procedures. Thanks to anesthesia and antiseptic practices, abdominal wounds no longer meant a death sentence under normal conditions. On the battlefield, however, the surgeon had a duty to try to save as many soldiers as possible, and abdominal interventions were still highly dangerous operations that offered little chance of success. Dr Demmler argued, "Certainly, it is cruel not to yield to the sentiments of humanity that push us toward these bold attempts. But is the surgeon right to attempt an operation that he knows must be almost fatally useless, while a multitude of other soldiers are assured of their salvation or relief of their suffering, if they are rescued in a timely manner?"[222] The seriously wounded – those suffering from abdominal, chest, and head injuries – had to be transported down the lines to more permanent hospital facilities, which were better equipped for serious surgical interventions.

Wagons, dogcarts, and small motorized ambulances transported the wounded from the first aid posts and field hospitals near the front to the second evacuation zone, known as the "intermediate zone," which began about seven miles behind the front lines.[223] This zone contained the French hospitals of evacuation (HOE) and British casualty clearing stations. In these evacuation hospitals, doctors conducted another triage of patients to determine which ones could be cured in a short amount of time, which were stable enough to be evacuated, and which patients should not be evacuated because of the severity of their injuries.[224] Surgeons then conducted the initial rounds of surgery. Anesthesia eased soldiers' agony even in relatively minor procedures. Henri Vignes, stationed at the French HOE at Bouleuse in the Marne, administered morphine injections before surgery to relieve pain and employed a wide variety of local and general anesthetics for surgical interventions including chloroform, ethyl chloride, ether, cocaine, novocaine, and stovaine, either alone or in combination. He found these anesthetics remarkably effective in relieving his patients' pain.[225]

Wounded soldiers deemed stable enough to evacuate from the HOE travelled by road, water, and rail to the third and final zone, the "zone of the interior," which was the farthest from the front line.[226] It contained the base hospitals, which were permanent medical facilities located in fixed structures such as hotels or *châteaux* and designed for more advanced surgical procedures. Often by the time soldiers reached the second and third evacuation zones they were covered in mud, suffering from shock and anemia. However, as one frontline surgeon put it, "in spite of all this, a wounded man evacuated to the rear represents several victories of the activities of the health services on the front."[227]

The pace and intensity of the war and the incredible violence of new weapons technologies made battlefield surgery incredibly intense. In July 1915, Henry Reynès supplied a brief account of his experiences during "nine months of intensive surgery" as a *médecin-major (2me classe)* at the temporary hospital at Verdun. The report gave only a general sense of his activities. Personally, he had treated seven hundred patients and performed two thousand anesthesias, and he noted that his patients had tolerated the anesthesia remarkably well. Reynès demonstrated the type of conservatism that had become common in military surgery. For example, only in cases "where all hope of conservation was impossible" did he perform amputations. He lamented that "the intensity of our activity at the front does not allow us to provide more comprehensive works or statistics."[228]

Army corps hospitals situated in *châteaux*, schools, or other appropriate buildings ten to twenty kilometres from the front had the equipment and medications needed for serious surgery.[229] Divisional field hospitals near the front lines often had only rudimentary surgical materials, as their primary role was "to warm up, bandage, [and] feed the wounded, inject anti-tetanus serum and morphine, and review bandages and fracture apparatuses." The army corps hospitals, in contrast, had a large number of surgical instruments and anesthetic medicines, including "ampoules of morphine, ampoules of novocaine for lumbar anesthesia (Leclerq), trioxymethylene tablets, anti-tetanus serum, flasks of adrenalin for adding to artificial serum or a cocaine solution."[230] With this arsenal of medicines, surgeons in the army corps hospitals could perform more complex procedures, including operations conducted under spinal anesthesia.

Spinal anesthesia was a new procedure, introduced at the turn of the twentieth century, which combined elements of general and local anesthesia. Spinal anesthesia involved injecting a solution of cocaine, stovaine, or novocaine into a patient's spine to produce insensibility in the lower half of the body.[231] The patient would remain conscious during the procedure. Spinal anesthesia offered several potential advantages for military medicine. Chloroform inhalations were labour intensive. They took time and skills to administer, and without careful monitoring of a patient's vital signs, there was a risk of asphyxiation. Spinal anesthesia could be administered quickly. With lumbar injections of novocaine, Laventure argued, "an intelligent well-trained aid can anesthetize a good number of wounded in advance."[232] This kind of rapid anesthesia enabled the surgeon facing huge numbers of casualties and personnel shortages to work more quickly, shortening the time between wounding and surgery to increase a soldier's chances of survival. Furthermore, some proponents argued that spinal anesthesia was safer than chloroform because the patient did not run the risk of syncope or asphyxia and it could be used on patients in weakened conditions.

Despite these advantages, in practice the contingencies of war made a delicate procedure like a spinal puncture dangerous on the battle-field.[233] Battlefields were filthy. In such conditions, a lumbar puncture ran a high risk of infection. Furthermore, although patients remained conscious during spinal anesthesia, they were still paralyzed from the waist down. Dr Anathese Demmler argued that this created the same mobility problem as chloroform anesthesia because in neither case could soldiers evacuate themselves during an emergency. While working in a French mobile surgical hospital near Ypres, American nurse Ellen La Motte observed one such operation. The surgeons used spinal anes-thesia because the patient was nearly dead and his chances of survival would have diminished greatly under general anesthetic.[234] In spite of the hopelessness of the case, the surgeons ensured that the wounded soldier felt no pain as they made one last futile attempt to save his life.

The processes that military medical manuals recommended for administering anesthesia reflected a broader concern for the subjective experience of the individual patient.[235] Medical officers recognized that the trauma and shock of being wounded could put a soldier in a fragile mental state before his operation. Therefore, in addition to instruc-tions on preparing the equipment for anesthesia, a pre-war technical manual for *maître-infirmiers* (master-nurses) included instructions for the emotional preparation of the patient before an operation. "One must reassure him by explaining the purpose of these preliminaries," it explained, "and by offering words of encouragement."[236] Pierre Picard, a medical student who served as a surgeon during the war, similarly argued it was important to prepare the wounded soldier psychologically before surgery. As a soldier was often upset and worried about the surgery, "we must explain to him what we are going to do to him, but also what we expect of him." Procedures for administering anesthesia also reflected a consideration for the wounded soldier's fragile mental state. To avoid upsetting the patient or causing shock, surgeons introduced the anesthetic mask gradually, telling the patient to "breathe deeply to be quickly put to sleep," which he did willingly.[237] By soliciting the patient's cooperation to breathe deeply, rather than forcing the mask upon him, this procedure made the patient feel safe and as though he retained a degree of control over the situation, even as he was about to lose consciousness.

The incredible volume of casualties during World War I kept medical personnel extremely busy. As a result, detailed observations of surgeries from this conflict are rare. However, by examining journals, essays, and novels written by nurses and surgeons, it is possible to catch a glimpse of how anesthesia influenced the individual wounded soldier's experiences. Although contingencies of war sometimes made it necessary for doctors to perform procedures without recourse to anesthetic, the idea of allowing a soldier to suffer unnecessarily during medical treatment had become abhorrent. Mme Emmanuel Colombel, a Red Cross nurse stationed in Arras in 1914, recalled the horrors of the operating room and shortages of both time and supplies. She was appalled when a surgeon, in order to conserve their limited supply of chloroform, attempted to remove a piece of shrapnel that was embedded in the leg bone of a wounded soldier without anesthesia.[238] Amid the brutal pace of surgeries in an operating room that was in continuous use, the surgical team had no time to clean or clear the room. Colombel remembered her feet sliding on the soldiers' blood as buckets brimmed over and blood-soaked sheets littered the floor.

Colombel experienced an overpowering need to relieve the suffering of the individual soldier within this factory-like process of continuous surgery, conducted in an impersonal and mechanical fashion. As her "poor wounded [patient]" shrieked in agony, the surgeon cut into his flesh to extract the shrapnel. When she requested that they give him chloroform, the doctors "all continued to move about without hearing me, saying that too little chloroform remained; that we were saving it for great circumstances. [The surgeon] said 'this thing here is really holding on, give me a pair of surgical tongs to pull it all out, fast.'" At this point, Colombel's compassion for the soldier's suffering won out: "I took it upon myself to grab the flask of chloroform and quickly put it on a handkerchief, under the nose of my wounded patient, saying, 'Breath deep, deep.'"[239] However callous the surgeon may have seemed, his desire to conserve the limited supply of chloroform for more serious cases reflected his concern for the larger needs of the military as a whole, according to the principles of triage.[240] Colombel nevertheless blatantly disregarded his orders, refusing to stand by while her patient screamed in agony. She respected the patient as an individual and took it upon herself to relieve his suffering rather than saving anesthetic for more "worthy" future cases. In this moment, by placing the immediate needs of the individual over the abstract needs of an anonymous collective, Colombel interrupted the mechanisms of the impersonal and endless carving of bodies and interjected a moment of compassion into the grim operating chamber.

While many accounts of life in the trenches focused on the anonymity of total war and the regularity of death, mangling, and destruction, the pain of being wounded was a highly personal experience for the individual patient. Georges Duhamel (1884–1966) served as a military doctor on a mobile ambulance during the war. He wrote a novel, *La vie des martyrs, 1914–1916*, that revealed deeply personal experiences of wounded soldiers on the front. Rather than remaining anonymous, the wounded soldiers he described had names, faces, and histories. Duhamel's literary depiction of wounded soldiers vividly portrayed not only their physical agony but the depth of their emotional trauma.

One wounded soldier called Derancourt had been wounded and taken captive in Germany. He returned from Germany with several other captives: "fifteen or twenty good men who had a good dozen legs between them."[241] Derancourt had a long blond moustache and was covered with scars from injuries that had healed during his captivity. His leg had been amputated at the thigh, but it would not heal properly. He was distant and reserved. He did not laugh much. He never talked about himself or complained about his hardships. When the medical aids laid him on the operating table so that they could try to make something useful out of his raw leg stump, he appeared self-possessed, watching them prepare him for surgery with apparent indifference. However, when they placed the compress of chloroform under his nose, after a few deep inhalations "something strange happened: Derancourt began to sob in a terrible manner and to speak of all the things of which he never spoke. Contained for months and months, the pain spread or rather burst out into desperate, hopeless lamentations."[242] Chloroform opened the floodgates.

In the state of liminal consciousness before chloroform took its full effect, Derancourt felt the crushing emotional toll of being wounded at war. He described the long-drawn-out agony of the experience: how he had lain seriously injured on a battlefield close to his hometown of Longwy in northeastern France; how his father had come from the town to try to rescue him, only to perish at his side; how for nine days and nights, sprawled alongside his father's corpse, he had drifted in and out of delirium, sustaining himself by sucking on dew-covered grass in the mornings; and how he had suffered as a captive in Germany, worrying about his wife and children left without resources in a land invaded.[243] Chloroform broke through the mental barriers he had erected to cope with such extreme misery. Duhamel described it as "the collapse under a light shock, of a will too tightly wound. Derancourt had, for months, fortified himself against despair and, all of a sudden, he yielded, he abandoned himself with heartrending words and tears. The flood suddenly withdrew, revealing the bottom of the horrible and tormented seas." Acting first on the will that had retained stoic composure in the face of prolonged misery, chloroform reawakened the feeling self that had been desensitized by the destruction of war. His surgeons stood "gaping, with tight throats, imbued with sadness and respect," before administering more chloroform to render him entirely unconscious.[244] While chloroform brought on the deep sleep that allowed surgeons to reconstruct his mangled body, it also exposed the magnitude of his emotional torment.

When wounded soldiers had little hope of survival, doctors and nurses could administer anesthetics to ease their suffering in their final moments.[245] At the outbreak of the war, Mary Borden, a wealthy American heiress, donated money to build a French Army field hospital in the Belgian zone. She also served as a nurse at a large French field hospital in the Somme. At the field hospitals, nurses injected morphine to relieve the suffering of dying patients. La Motte, one of her colleagues at the hospital in Belgium, recalled the agonized screams of dying soldiers in the night. For those men, she explained, "only death could bring relief from such a pain as that, and only morphia, a little in advance of death, could bring partial relief."[246] Borden recalled caring for a terribly wounded soldier, whom she described as a "monstrous thing." His head was unrecognizable and his limbs "seemed to be held together only by the strong stuff of the uniform." As she gazed in horror at the soldier's mangled body, the chief surgeon came over and said, "Give him morphine … a double dose. As much as you like … In cases like this if I am not about, give morphine, enough, you understand."[247] Relieving a soldier's excruciating pain took priority over the protocols of morphine administration. The chief surgeon authorized Borden, a volunteer nurse without formal medical training, to administer morphine in his absence to relieve the intense agony of fatal wounds and provide comfort and relief during the patient's last moments. Furthermore, as he seemed to suggest, morphine could be used to hasten a merciful death for cases beyond hope of recovery.

This desire to spare the courageous wounded from further pain and suffering extended beyond the operating room to the process of rehabilitation. Raw surgical wounds seeped, oozed, and clung to dressings, which made the process of changing a bandage excruciating. Like Scrive a half century before, medical personnel during World War I recognized the benefits of changing bandages on serious wounds under the influence of anesthesia. In January 1916, several months prior to the main thrust of the ten-month Battle of Verdun, Maurice Savariaud advocated for the use of ethyl chloride to anesthetize patients while changing the bandages on their amputated limbs, to spare the patients additional pain.[248]

Soldiers who had suffered limb injuries often faced subsequent complications during convalescence caused by the immobilization of their fractures in fixed apparatuses or bandages. These including muscle atrophy, joint rigidity, and ankylosis, a stiffening caused by an abnormal fusion of the bones. To rehabilitate muscle atrophy and joint stiffness and to restore functionality to the limbs, doctors used "mechanotherapy." This treatment relied on movement – either exercises performed by the soldier or manipulations of the limb using external force – to improve kinesthetic function.[249] During the first year of the war, Edmond Delorme treated hundreds of joint cases, many with anesthesia. While anesthesia was not always necessary, Delorme often found it to be beneficial for these painful interventions. Yet soldiers did not always cooperate. Some refused anesthesia and chose the "sharp but temporary pain" of "de-stiffening." Others – those either less brave or prone to malingering – rejected anesthesia as a way of trying to avoid the procedures altogether. In response to this stubbornness, Delorme explained, "most often I begin my 'de-stiffenings' without anesthesia, but I conduct them very slowly and at the first pain then I propose the anesthetic, which is accepted without resistance."[250] In this manner, Delorme respected a soldier's right to choose pain relief himself, making anesthesia a choice rather than a medical imposition.

If a patient preferred to be unconscious for the procedure, he administered chloroform or ether as a general anesthetic. However, as the procedures for "de-stiffening" were relatively quick, he most often used kelene (ethyl chloride) or somnoforme. These fast-acting anesthetics were particularly useful for patients who had bad memories of chloroform from the battlefield. He made a point of telling them he was using the same substances that dentists used to pull teeth.[251] Delorme's account of his procedures for anesthetizing joint patients during rehabilitative procedures reflected a careful consideration of his patients' mental states. He presented anesthesia as a choice instead of an imposition from above. The patients had the power to prevent pain if they wished to do so, but they also had the right to refuse anesthesia. Taking their fears and past encounters with chloroform into consideration, Delorme also ensured that the anesthetic he used was one they might find less upsetting. If a patient elected not to be anesthetized, Delorme tried to distract him during the painful manipulations.[252] In November 1915, Delorme estimated that he had returned over a thousand patients' joints to flexibility in this manner, noting the great social and functional gain for both the patient and the state.[253]

On the battlefield, soldiers sacrificed their bodies to defend the French nation. The physical and emotional trauma of trench warfare left a lasting impression on them. However, anesthesia minimized the subsequent trauma of rehabilitation. Both military surgery and the rehabilitation of wounded soldiers were designed to restore their bodies to functionality and productivity.[254] In recognition of wounded soldiers' sacrifice on the battlefield, military surgeons tried to prevent them from experiencing further pain and trauma on the operating table. Battlefield anesthesia revealed a profound concern for the subjective experience of the wounded soldier that often conflicted with triage and the needs of the army as a whole.

The introduction of general anesthesia revolutionized surgical practice and reconceptualized the role of the surgeon. Through the use of anesthesia, the surgeon redefined himself as a skilled practitioner who not only restored patients' bodies to healthy functionality but also relieved their pain. However, the surgeon's power over pain was a double-edged sword. General anesthesia simultaneously enhanced and constrained medical authority. Patients' recognition of the medical profession's ability to control pain enhanced the authority of surgeons and obstetricians. At the same time, it also empowered patients to advocate for themselves, requesting, even demanding, pain relief regardless of the practitioner's professional opinion.

During the nineteenth century, anesthesia both constructed and undermined the patient as subject. By considering the patient's comfort and right to experience surgical operations in the absence of pain, doctors acknowledged the patient's subjectivity. However, the state of unconscious anesthesia artificially and temporarily separated the conscious mind from the physical body. In a sense, this process paralyzed the patient's subjectivity, transforming his or her body into an object to be cut open, exposed, operated upon, and sewn back together. In childbirth as in battlefield surgery, anesthesia fragmented the experience of suffering for the nation, locating it increasingly within the body rather than the mind. While the postpartum mother and the wounded soldier experienced the bodily disruption and transformation of these acts of national suffering, anesthesia enabled them to protect their minds from the experience and memory of it.

CONCLUSION

During the nineteenth century, psychotropic drugs enabled French citizens to realize new levels of control over their own minds and bodies. Doctors administered chloroform during surgery to eliminate pain and consciousness. Mothers used laudanum to sooth their infants' colic. Prostitutes sold cocaine to enhance their clients' pleasure and desire. Countless acts of psychotropic consumption transformed the everyday lives of French citizens and contributed to the emergence of a new modern French medicine. As psychotropic drugs became increasingly available and reliable with the industrialization of pharmaceutical production, the relief of pain became an expectation, one that citizens came to view as a fundamental individual right. An injection of morphine could rapidly and efficiently dispel a wide variety of bodily ailments. In France's psychotropic society, the modern individual was no longer subjected to the distress and agony of a body in pain. Reliable commodities and new therapeutic regimens normalized the chemical enhancement of modern life.

Although individuals could use psychotropic substances to exercise unprecedented control over bodily sensation, psychotropic power proved difficult to contain. The making of knowledge about drugs was somewhat haphazard, fuelled by curiosity and conducted through trial and error. Self-experimentation enabled researchers to produce crucial medical knowledge about how psychotropic drugs affected the human mind and body. Yet, by exploring the ruptures and distortions of the mind-body connection, psychotropic self-experimenters revealed the extent to which individual free will was connected to the physiological imperatives of the body. Nowhere was this more apparent than in judicial cases of morphine addiction, in which addicted defendants were not considered legally responsible if they were suffering from the agonies of withdrawal. Addiction was an unanticipated consequence of public confidence in the capacity of drugs to relieve pain, modify conscious-ness, and stimulate desire.

To mitigate the potential dangers of psychotropic medicines, doctors appealed to their own specialized knowledge and expertise about the drugs' therapeutic effects. In so doing, they positioned themselves as gatekeepers of these psychotropic drugs in order to enhance their own status as professionals. However, individuals consumed these substances both within and beyond the boundaries of "official medicine." Practices of self-medication and unanticipated iatrogenic addiction demonstrated that these psychotropic substances frequently eluded the professionals who sought to control them.

In the twentieth century, French drug legislation created new legal distinctions between licit and illicit consumption. The Poisonous Substances Law of 1916 ushered in a new age of drug regulation in which these substances were no longer regulated simply as poisons, as they had been during the nineteenth century. The 1916 legislation classified particular psychotropic drugs as *stupéfiants* (narcotics), whose primary social threat was the nefarious spread of chemical addiction.[1] Under this new system of regulation, doctors' and pharmacists' legal monopoly over the prescription and distribution of psychotropic pharmaceuticals took on a new significance. Beginning with the 1916 legislation, medical sanc-tion became the distinguishing factor between the legal consumption of opium, morphine, and cocaine for therapeutic purposes and the illegal consumption of the same substances for other reasons.

Advances in pharmacological research changed the landscape of pain management in the early twentieth century. Mass-produced as-pirin gradually replaced laudanum and other opiate-based remedies in family medicine cabinets. Beginning in 1903 with the introduction of Véronal (barbital), barbiturates offered doctors new options for treating insomnia and nervous conditions. Pharmacists also developed a new series of supposedly less addictive patent medicines designed to replace morphine and cocaine for treating intense pain, including Pantopon, Spasmalgine, and Stovaïne.[2] Despite the introduction of these new substances, opiates and cocaine remained reliable and essential tools for managing pain after World War I. While the 1916 law codified nar-cotic addiction as an undesirable social pathology, doctors still had the freedom to prescribe opiates and cocaine for therapeutic purposes. The evolution of therapeutic practice was gradual. Although the 1916 law authorized doctors as the arbiters of legal drug consumption to stem the tides of drug addiction, iatrogenic addiction resulting from medical treatment continued to be a significant problem in the interwar period.[3]

Twentieth-century drug laws vaunted medical expertise as the vanguard against addiction. The French drug law of 1970, which is still in effect today, instituted harsher penalties for the "recreational" consumption of psychotropic drugs, in the wake of the famous student protests in 1968. French authorities constructed the drug addict as a product of a deviant counterculture.[4] In recent years, however, perceptions of addiction have shifted. The prescription opioid epidemic in the United States has complicated the image of the drug addict associated with the twentieth-century "War on Drugs." Therapeutic overconfidence and intentionally misleading pharmaceutical advertising have led millions of American patients to become addicted to OxyContin and other prescription opioid pain relievers.[5] Although France has significantly lower opiate consumption and fewer deaths from opioid overdose every year than the United States, researchers have observed that medical prescriptions for strong opiates, like morphine, fentanyl, and oxycodone, increased by 74 per cent between 2004 and 2015.[6] According to National Health Insurance statistics, 17.1 per cent of French residents were reimbursed for some kind of opioid pain reliever in 2015.[7] Iatrogenic addiction continues to be a problem. Between 2000 and 2015, France saw a 128 per cent increase in hospitalizations related to prescription opioids.[8] Twentieth-century drug legislation demonized the deviant behaviours of heroin addicts while sanctioning drug consumption under the supervision of a medical prescription. However, the overprescription of opiate pain relievers in France, in the United States, and across Europe has starkly illustrated that the "addict" is not solely a product of illicit, back-alley drug deals. Rather, addiction is also a product of the pharmaceutical industry and the medical establishment.

France is still a psychotropic society. Individuals treat pain, anxiety, depression, insomnia, and other psychosomatic disorders with a plethora of psychotropic pharmaceuticals. Buttressed by an authority rooted in claims of scientific expertise, the medical profession continues to monopolize control over the legal consumption of psychotropic drugs. However, in practice, psychotropic consumption continues to exceed the power and authority of medical therapeutics. Practices of self-medication and self-experimentation continue to subvert medical control over the definition and circulation of psychotropic drugs in society. Amid contemporary debates over the benefits of medical marijuana[9] and the dangers of prescription drug addiction,[10] distinctions between "medical" and "recreational" drugs have become incredibly muddled. Furthermore, recent news reports have highlighted the continued uncertainties and risks involved in psychotropic drug research. In January 2016, five volunteers in a French clinical trial experienced serious side effects from a new pain and anxiety drug, which left one of them with permanent brain damage.[11] While the substances may have changed, the elusive nature of psychotropic power has not. Despite scientific advances and modern regulations, psychotropic drugs continue to transcend the boundaries of medical control.

NOTES

INTRODUCTION

1 On pharmaceutical industrialization, see Faure, "Les officines pharmaceutiques françaises"; N. Sueur, "La Pharmacie Centrale de France"; Mory, "Dorvault."

2 On changing conceptions of pain in the nineteenth century, see Rey, *Histoire de la douleur*.

3 Although other psychotropic substances – including nitrous oxide (laughing gas), chloral, and potassium bromide – appear intermittently, I have chosen to focus on these six substances because of their importance to therapeutic research, anesthesia, and pain management in the nineteenth century.

4 Yvorel, *Les poisons de l'esprit*; Padwa, *Social Poison*; Guba, *Taming Cannabis*; Retaillaud-Bajac, *Les paradis perdus*. On the history of psychotropic drugs in Britain and America, see Courtwright, *Dark Paradise*; Parssinen, *Secret Passions*; Hickman, *Secret Leprosy*. On psychotropic drugs in literature, see Mickel, *Artificial Paradises*; Hayter, *Opium*.

5 In this body of scholarship, the examination of the therapeutic use of narcotic drugs serves primarily to highlight the medical origins of addiction in the late nineteenth century, rather than to shed light on the significance of these substances in transforming therapeutic practices or the experience of everyday life. There are a few notable exceptions. While David Guba's book *Taming Cannabis* focuses on the ways in which France constructed an image of cannabis as a dangerous "Oriental" substance, he takes the medical history of cannabis seriously. He has a fascinating chapter on the short-lived attempts of doctors and pharmacists to "civilize" and medicalize cannabis for use in French medicine as a treatment for cholera and plague in the 1840s. See Guba, "'A Drug Not to Be Neglected': Medicalizing Hashish in France, 1810–50," in *Taming Cannabis*, 106–49. Virginia Berridge's research on opium in nineteenth-century Britain is a prime example of the medical-recreational combination study; see Berridge and Edwards, *Opium and the People*. Although *Drugging France* is not a sweeping social history, it examines psychotropic drugs in therapeutic practices, considering the drugs as technologies of the self and the entangled power relationship between individuals and psychotropic material commodities.

6 Ackerknecht, *Medicine at the Paris Hospital*; Porter, *Greatest Benefit*, 306–20. On Paris as the pre-eminent centre of science at the turn of the nineteenth century, see Gillispie, *Science and Polity*; Ben-David, "Rise and Decline." In the second half of the nineteenth century, Germany's early embrace of laboratory research produced competing centres of scientific research. While Joseph Ben-David and other earlier scholars argued that French science reached its zenith during the Napoleonic Empire and then declined over the course of the nineteenth century, more recent historical scholarship has challenged this image of a "decline" in French science. These revisionist scholars emphasize that earlier arguments about French science's decline both embraced French scientists' own anxieties about French science when compared with Germany's robust scientific productivity (which were exacerbated by the humiliating defeat in the Franco-Prussian War of 1870) and overlooked the continued dynamism and productivity of French scientific research. Tresch, *Romantic Machine*, 17–19; Fox, *Savant and the State*, 50–51, 279–84.

7 Lawrence Brockliss and Colin Jones demonstrate that some elements of France's new clinical medicine in the early nineteenth century traced their roots back to the Enlightenment. However, the major shift in medical education came after the institutional disruptions of the French Revolution. Brockliss and Jones, *Medical World*, 370–479; Belhoste, *Paris Savant*.

8 Ramsey, "Public Health in France," 48–51.

9 Weiner and Sauter, "City of Paris." While the Crown had funded the Academy of Sciences and the Royal Academy of Medicine through royal patronage under the Old Regime, the revolutionaries dissolved them with the Allarde law of 1791. Napoleon reorganized the Academy of Sciences under the Institute de France in 1803. The reconstituted Faculty of Medicine served as an advisory body for the French government under Napoleon. Finally, in 1820, the Restoration government established the Royal Academy of Medicine, to advise the government on matters of public health. Ramsey, "Public Health in France," 49, 55. For more on the Academy of Sciences, see Hahn, *Anatomy of a Scientific Institution*; Crosland, *Science under Control*. On the Academy of Medicine, see Weisz, *Medical Mandarins*; Weisz, "Constructing the Medical Élite."

10 Some of the most significant diagnostic techniques associated with Paris's new clinical medicine were percussion and auscultation, facilitated by R.T.H. Laennec's introduction of the stethoscope in 1816. This allowed doctors to listen for internal indications of disease, making it possible to investigate pathology on living bodies rather than through postmortem dissection. Ackerknecht, *Medicine at the Paris Hospital*; Porter, *Greatest Benefit*, 306–20.

11 Galenic humoral theory, which dominated French medicine in the early modern period, began to give way to vitalist and iatromechanical theories of health and disease in the eighteenth century. Brockliss and Jones, *Medical World*, 411–33.

12 Warner, *Therapeutic Perspective*, 85–7.

13 The "bacteriological revolution" did not occur overnight. Acceptance of the

new germ theory was still contested in the early 1880s, and even when it became more widely accepted between the mid-1880s and 1890s, doctors frequently combined germ theory with some of the older environmental elements of miasma theory, particularly to explain disease outbreaks. Barnes, *Great Stink of Paris*, 36–48, 105–39. On Pasteur and the bacteriological revolution, see Latour, *Pasteurization of France*; Faure, *Histoire sociale de la médecine*, 169–83; Salomon-Bayet, *Pasteur et la révolution pastorienne*. On the earlier miasma theory of disease, see Kudlick, *Cholera in Post-Revolutionary Paris*, 75–81; Ackerknecht, "Anticontagionism"; Cooter, "Anticontagionism."

14 Quinine was one exception. Doctors had been using cinchona bark (of which quinine is a derivative) to treat malarial fevers since the seventeenth century; however, while they observed it was effective, they did not understand why. Porter, *Greatest Benefit*, 233, 450–61; Lesch, *First Miracle Drugs*.

15 The Ventôse Law instituted a medical monopoly among doctors with medical degrees and *officiers de santé*. The *officier de santé*, a position established in response to the relative scarcity of rural physicians, earned a less prestigious and less expensive degree than a medical doctorate – a practice that effectively created a two-tiered medical system in France. Doctors resented competition from the *officiers de santé*, who devalued their services by charging lower fees, and eliminating this inferior degree was one of the primary objectives of medical professionalization in the nineteenth century. France did not eliminate the *officier de santé* degree until 1892. "No. 2436. – Loi … du 19 Ventôse"; "No. 2676. – Loi … du 21 Germinal."

16 On medical professionalization in France, see Ramsey, "Politics of Medical Monopoly"; Weisz, "Politics of Medical Professionalization"; Nye, "Honor Codes."

17 For more on the social history of medicine in France and the competition doctors faced from irregular practitioners, see Ramsey, *Professional and Popular Medicine*; Ramsey, "Medical Power"; Léonard, *La vie quotidienne*; Ackerman, *Health Care*; Faure, *Les français et leur médecine*; Faure, *Histoire sociale de la médecine*.

18 Cole, *Power of Large Numbers*, 1–10.

19 Coleman, *Death Is a Social Disease*.

20 Early hygienists like Louis Villermé adopted Pierre Louis's "numerical method," using statistics to study broad population trends. La Berge, *Mission and Method*, 49–81; Coleman, *Death Is a Social Disease*, 124–48; Cole, *Power of Large Numbers*, 55–85. For more on the emergence of public health in France, see Ackerknecht, "Health and Hygiene"; Hildreth, *Doctors, Bureaucrats, and Public Health*.

21 Baker, "Scientism." On the turn toward empiricism in Enlightenment medicine, see Brockliss and Jones, *Medical World*, 433–8.

22 La Berge, *Mission and Method*, 1–2; Cole, *Power of Large Numbers*, 6, 11, 16–19; Coleman, *Death Is a Social Disease*, 237–8; Ramsey, "Public Health in France," 45.

23 Ellis, *Physician-Legislators*; Steffen, "Medical Profession."

24 Cole, *Power of Large Numbers*, 2–4; McLaren, *Sexuality and Social Order*, 9–27.

25 Doctors and social reformers alike used the concept of degeneration to classify numerous seemingly unrelated social pathologies, such as alcoholism, hysteria, impotence, criminality, decadence, anarchism, and morphine addiction, under a comprehensive scientific theory of national decline in which individual deviance threatened the collective fate of the population. Nye, *Masculinity*, 75–7; Yvorel, *Les poisons de l'esprit*, 78–85; Pick, *Faces of Degeneration*, 42–3, 222–3, 230; Nye, *Crime, Madness and Politics*, 12, 119–24, 232; Offen, "Depopulation, Nationalism, and Feminism"; Stewart, *For Health and Beauty*.

26 Foucault, *History of Sexuality*, 139–46. Recent scholarship on gender and sexuality in *fin-de-siècle* France has examined the ways in which the embodied nature of the liberal subject, understood as both sexed and gendered, disrupted perceptions of a stable social order founded upon the abstract notion of the autonomous self, guided by reason and free will. Surkis, *Sexing the Citizen*; Forth, *Dreyfus Affair*.

27 While the French government had encouraged *départements* to create programs to provide medical care for the poor and indigent in the mid-1850s, these piecemeal efforts were not required and access to care varied widely in different areas. Ramsey, "Public Health in France," 48–52, 67–8. For a detailed examination of medicine and the individual right to health care in the French Revolution, see Weiner, *Citizen-Patient*.

28 The 1893 medical assistance law required French *départements* to provide medical care for the indigent. Ramsey, "Public Health in France," 76–79; see also Faure, "La médecine gratuite"; Hildreth, "Medical Rivalries."

29 On positivism and science, see Mandelbaum, *History, Man, and Reason*, 1–20; Jennings, "Positivism, Science, and Philosophy," in *Revolution and the Republic*, 344–87.

30 On the significance of military service to male citizenship, see Weber, *Peasants into Frenchmen*, 298, 333, 336. On the significance of motherhood as a civic duty for French women, see Fuchs, *Poor and Pregnant*, 35–98; Offen, *Debating the Woman Question*, 86–93, 249–67.

31 The revolution of 1848 toppled the July Monarchy of King Louis-Philippe d'Orleans (1830–1848) and established the Second Republic (1848–1852). However, this short-lived republic came to an abrupt end when its popularly elected president, Louis-Napoleon Bonaparte, proclaimed himself emperor of France. He ruled during the Second Empire (1852–1870) until his defeat in 1870 during the Franco-Prussian War. The Third Republic (1870–1940) that followed was France's longest regime of the nineteenth century.

32 Accampo, "Class and Gender," 99.

33 In the late eighteenth century, theories of children's domestic education shifted to emphasize freedom and self-control as a way of producing virtuous and autonomous liberal subjects to serve the nation as citizens. Popiel, *Rousseau's Daughters*, 4–7, 9–10; see also Offen, *Debating the Woman Question*, 18, 53–9.

34 Landes, *Women and the Public Sphere*; Scott, *Only Paradoxes to Offer*, 10–11, 35; Jennings, *Revolution and the Republic*, 23–5, 53–4, 81.

35 Surkis, *Sexing the Citizen*, 4, 127.

36 Goldstein, *Post-Revolutionary Self*, 11–12, 140, 324–5. Jan Goldstein notes that except for the twelve-year period following Louis-Napoleon Bonaparte's coup d'état in 1851, the unified Cousinian self was a core tenet of the French *lycée* philosophy curriculum from 1832 until 1925, when the *programme* (syllabus) abandoned the term *moi* for the more flexible term *personalité* ("personhood" or "personality"), which left the question of unity more ambiguous. Goldstein, "Neutralizing Freud," 78.

37 Goldstein, *Post-Revolutionary Self*, 8–11, 156–7.

38 Goldstein demonstrates that while everyone had a unified self in theory, bourgeois men demonstrated the "capacity for reflection" that they used to distinguish themselves from "unselved" women and working-class men by practising "interior observation," which revealed a self identified with activity and will. Goldstein, *Post-Revolutionary Self*, 11, 161, 165–79, 172, 200–1.

39 As several scholars note, the particularity and individuality of embodied subjects exposed the instability of abstract political ideals. Surkis, "Carnival Balls"; Scott, "French Universalism." On free will and criminal responsibility in classical jurisprudence, see Wright, *Between the Guillotine and Liberty*, 109–28; Harris, *Murders and Madness*, 2–5, 16–17. On individual autonomy and republican citizenship, see Déloye, *École et citoyenneté*.

40 Olsen, "Material Culture after Text"; Hodder, *Entangled*; Hodder, "Entanglements."

41 Tiersten, *Marianne in the Market*; Spary, *Eating the Enlightenment*; Spang, *Invention of the Restaurant*; Auslander, *Taste and Power*; Williams, *Dream Worlds*; Cohen, *Household Gods*; Rappaport, *Shopping for Pleasure*; Shannon, *Cut of His Coat*; Whitlock, *Crime, Gender*; Styles and Vickery, *Gender*; Berg and Clifford, *Consumers and Luxury*; Richards, *Commodity Culture*.

42 Rey-Debove and Rey, *Le Nouveau Petit Robert*, s.v. "psychotrope."

43 The historiography of alcohol in France has focused on wine's incredible national, economic, and cultural significance. On wine, see Brennan, *Burgundy to Champagne*; Dion, *Histoire de la vigne*; Plack, "Drinking and Rebelling"; Plack, "Liberty, Equality, and Taxation"; Guy, *When Champagne Became French*; Paul, *Science, Vine, and Wine*; Heath, *Wine, Sugar*. On the cultural history of alcohol consumption, see Haine, *World of the Paris Café*; Brennan, *Public Drinking*; Brennan, "Towards the Cultural History." As with addiction in the history of drugs, alcoholism has loomed large in the historiography of alcohol in France. Patricia Prestwich's classic work on alcoholism and the anti-alcohol movements in France, *Drink and the Politics of Social Reform*, demonstrates that France's high per capita

consumption of alcohol, the great economic and regional significance of wine production, and the powerful French alcohol lobby produced an anti-alcohol movement in France that was less absolute in its opposition to alcohol consumption than in Britain and the United States. In France, doctors, politicians, and the alcohol lobby tended to distinguish between hygienic beverages like wine, beer, and cider, considered central to French national and regional identities, and cheap industrial alcohol, like absinthe, viewed as a scourge that was precipitating the degeneration of the French population. In contrast to Britain and the United States, where abstinence was a prominent goal of temperance societies, the French anti-alcohol movement focused more on the quality of the alcohol (hygienic wine versus the dangers of industrial distilled spirits) and emphasized moderation in consumption rather than complete abstinence. For more on alcoholism and degeneration, see Barrows, *Distorting Mirrors*, 43–72; Barnes, *Making of a Social Disease*, 138–62.

44 A detailed analysis of the use of alcohol in medical therapeutics is beyond the scope of this particular project, but it would be a useful direction for future scholarship.

45 The "stupéfiants" category encompassed opium, cocaine, morphine, and hashish. The French Law of 12 July 1916 was the first piece of legislation that prohibited non-medical consumption of this new category of substances in order to protect the public from the dangers of addiction. The French term "stupéfiants" is often misleadingly translated into English as "narcotics," although the substances included in this classification do not all qualify as narcotics in the pharmaceutical sense. Although the law restricted the non-medical consumption of opium, morphine, cocaine, hashish, and their derivatives, doctors still could, and did, prescribe these substances for therapeutic purposes. "No. 10090. – Loi … du 12 Juillet 1916."

46 "No. 12,115. – Loi … [du] 19 Juillet 1845"; Griolet, Vergé, and Bourdeaux, *Code d'instruction criminelle*, 625–7.

47 France actually regulated the distribution of opium and other psychotropic drugs as poisons and placed them under medical control long before they were regulated in Britain and the United States. In Britain, the distribution of opiates was first regulated by the 1868 Pharmacy Act; in the United States, the first opium regulations were the 1909 Smoking Opium Exclusion Act and the 1914 Harrison Narcotic Act. This later British and American drug legislation reflects the shifting logic of drug regulation. The British legislation was justified in part by concerns that the working classes were using opium as a "stimulant." The US legislation, enacted even later, was informed by concerns over opium addiction. Berridge and Edwards, *Opium and the People*, xxvii–xxviii, 113–22; Courtwright, *Dark Paradise*, 1.

48 Even then, the 1916 law only prohibited the social use of these substances.

49 The French terms used to describe earlier instances of what would come to be called "addiction" were *besoin* (need), *dépendance* (dependence), and *accoutumance* (habituation, dependence). When doctors began to

understand and classify drug addictions in the late 1870s and early
1880s, they did so in terms of the specific drug, labelling the problem
morphinomanie (1880), *cocaïnomanie* (1886), or *opiomanie* (1909). The
general term *toxicomanie* only emerged at the end of the nineteenth
century. The anglicized terms *addiction* (1979), *addict* (1985), and *addictif*
(1983) were introduced into the French language in the late twentieth
century. Rey-Debove and Rey, *Le Nouveau Petit Robert*, s.vv. "besoin,"
"dépendance," "accoutumance," "morphinomanie," cocaïnomanie,"
"opiomanie," "toxicomanie," "addiction," "addict," "addictif."

50 Detailed written accounts of the subjective experience of psychotropic
consumption are relatively rare. However, I incorporate the voices of
individual consumers whenever possible using letters, journals, accounts
of self-experimentation, poems, paintings, and novels to access the broad
spectrum of everyday experiences of psychotropic drug consumption.

51 This approach is part of the historiographical trend of writing the history
of medicine from "the patient's view," inspired by Roy Porter's 1985 article,
"The Patient's View."

52 In 2013, France spent 26.8 billion euros on pharmaceuticals. Three
analgesic substances – paracetamol, ibuprofen, and codeine – were the top
three active substances in terms of quantity sold in French pharmacies
in 2013, comprising 20.1 per cent of the total market (excluding hospital
consumption). Several other analgesics, hypnotics, anesthetics, and
antidepressants featured among the top thirty medicines sold in terms of
quantity. Agence national de sécurité du médicament, *Analyse des ventes*,
6, 13–14.

53 Office Parlementaire d'Évaluation des Politiques de Santé, *Rapport sur le
bon usage*, 17, 58, 357.

54 "France's Drug Addiction."

CHAPTER ONE

1 Deschamps, *Étude comparative des codex français*, 6, 10–11; *Code des
médicamens* (1818).

2 *Codex: Pharmacopée française* (1837); *Codex medicamentarius* (1866); *Codex
medicamentarius* (1884); *Codex medicamentarius gallicus* (1908).

3 Berridge and Edwards, *Opium and the People*, xxii; Courtwright, *Forces of
Habit*, 31–3; Booth, *Opium*, 15; Davenport-Hines, *Pursuit of Oblivion*, 30–9.

4 Berman, "Persistence of Theriac"; Fonssagrives, "Opium," in Dechambre,
Dictionnaire encyclopédique (1881), 136–265, 154–6.

5 Sebastian, *Dictionary of the History of Medicine*, 32; Berridge and Edwards,
Opium and the People, xix.

6 Fonssagrives, "Opium," 149–50.

7 Direction Générale des Douanes, *Tableau général du commerce*.

8 Berman, "Drug Control," 8–9; Millant, *La culture du pavot*, 25.

9 Chevallier, *Notice historique*, 19; Pécarrere, *Traité sur l'opium*, 10.

10 Aubergier, *Mémoire sur l'opium indigene*, 11. The adulteration of foodstuffs was quite common. While the Ministry of Commerce technically set and enforced quality standards, it did not have the resources for systematic testing and enforcement. France passed its public health law banning adulterated food and agricultural products in 1905. Ellis, *Physician-Legislators*, 196–200; Zylberman, "Making Food Safety."

11 Bouchardat, "De la valeur de l'opium indigène," *Bulletin générale de thérapeutique médicale et chirurgicale* (1853): 10–16, 12.

12 Chevallier, *Notice historique*, 6.

13 Aaslestad and Joor, *Revisiting Napoleon's Continental System*.

14 Bouchardat, "De la valeur," 10.

15 Spary, *Feeding France*, 268–314.

16 Bouchardat, "De la valeur," 10; Belon, *Les observations*, 405. Early advocates of domestic opium cultivation included Savary des Bruslons (1748), Schroder (1767), the Abbé Rozier (1793), and Dubuc (1801). Chevallier, *Notice historique*, 7–9.

17 Professor Alphonse Chevallier of the Paris Pharmacy School cited over twenty French experimenters, naturalists, and scholars who debated this issue in the early nineteenth century, in addition to experiments in Britain, Italy, Switzerland, and Germany. Chevallier, *Notice historique*, 18. On Britain, see also Berridge and Edwards, *Opium and the People*, 11–17.

18 Chevallier, *Notice historique*, 19; Berthé, *Lettre*, 2.

19 By mid-century M. Guilliermond's process for isolating morphine was generally accepted as the standard method. He dissolved 15 grams of opium in 60 grams of alcohol, filtered it, and discarded the residue. He then dissolved the tincture with 40 grams of alcohol and placed the mixture in a flask containing 4 grams of ammonia. Twelve hours later, dark morphine crystals formed in the bottom of the flask. He washed these with water several times to remove the *méconate* ammonia; finally, to obtain pure morphine, he decanted the crystals in water to remove the narcotine. Decharme, *Mémoire sur l'opium indigène*, 19–20. For detailed descriptions of the various other processes used to determine the levels of morphine contained in a given sample of opium, see Barret, "De la morphimétrie."

20 Vauquelin, "Examen de l'opium indigène, et reclamation en faveur de M. Séguin, de la découverte de la morphine et de l'acide méconique," *Annales de chimie et de physique* 9 (1818): 282–6.

21 Lamarque's experiments were cut short in 1830 by the July Revolution, and his death in 1832 prevented further experimentation. J.-B. Caventou, "Notice pour servir à l'histoire et à la récolte de l'opium indigène," *Bulletin de l'Académie de médecine* 9 (20 February 1844): 472–81, 474; "Sur la culture du pavot somnifère en Algérie et sur la qualité de l'opium qui a été récolté," *Bulletin générale de thérapeutique médicale et chirurgicale* (1843): 431–2.

22 H. Baillon, "Pavot (Botanique)," in Dechambre, *Dictionnaire encyclopédique* (1885), 727–30.

23 Aubergier, *Mémoire sur l'opium indigène*, 10.

24 Ibid., 14.

25 Bouchardat, "De la valeur," 10–16.

26 Ibid., 14.

27 Ibid., 15.

28 Sessions, *By Sword and Plow*, 19–66.

29 Davis, *Resurrecting the Granary*; Davis, "Restoring Roman Nature"; Sessions, *By Sword and Plow*, 208–32.

30 Payen, "Rapport sur les communications de MM. Hardy, Liautaud, et Simon, relatives à l'opium d'Algérie," *Comptes rendus des séances de l'Académie des sciences* 17 (23 October 1843): 845–53, 847.

31 Caventou, "La récolte de l'opium indigène," 476.

32 Davis, "Restoring Roman Nature," 63–4.

33 Payen, "Rapport sur les communications," 847–8.

34 Chevallier, *Notice historique*, 17.

35 Payen, "Rapport sur les communications," 852.

36 Payen, "Rapport supplémentaire sur l'opium d'Alger," *Comptes rendus des séances de l'Académie des sciences* 18 (12 February 1844): 238–40.

37 The ambiguity of the results stemmed from the small samples tested, possible inconsistencies in the chemical analysis of samples, the likely adulteration of the commercial samples used as controls, possible inconsistencies between the types of poppies cultivated, and the difficulty of maintaining accurate results when opium loses weight rapidly through evaporation.

38 "Correspondance," *Comptes rendus des séances de l'Académie des sciences* 17 (27 November 1843): 1247. The reports from the Academy of Sciences appeared in the *Moniteur Algérien* in instalments between May and June 1845. "Rapport sur les communications de MM. Hardy et Simon, relatives à l'opium d'Algérie," *Moniteur Algérien* 14 (30 May, 10 June, 13 June 1845), 686, 688, 689.

39 Ministère de la Guerre, *Catalogue explicatif*, 90–2, 195.

40 Barrows, "Alcohol, France, and Algeria," 530; Todd, "Algeria, Informal Empire Manqué," 80, 86, 91, 104–10.

41 These agricultural tariffs were later reduced and then ultimately eliminated during the Second Empire. Barrows, "Alcohol, France, and Algeria," 529–30; Roughton, "Economic Motives," 365–70; Isnard, "Vigne et colonisation," 213.

42 Decharme, *Mémoire sur l'opium indigène*, 14.

43 Before the late nineteenth-century "wine boom," colonial agricultural producers focused on the production of cereals, like wheat, which did not need as much capital to produce. Davis, *Resurrecting the Granary*, 94.

44 To incentivize French settlers to cultivate wine, the colonial government offered cheap loans, financial subsidies, and virtually free land that had been confiscated from indigenous populations under the 1873 Warnier Law. France

also used protective tariffs to defend the nascent industry against foreign competition. Barrows, "Alcohol, France, and Algeria," 533–5. On the Algerian wine industry, see also White, *Blood of the Colony*; Studer, "The Same Drink?"; Znaien, "Drinking and Production Patterns."

45 Wild poppies grew abundantly in Algeria, particularly in wheat fields. Poppy heads were used in indigenous medical remedies and wet nurses also deployed them frequently as sedatives. Battandier, *Algérie*, 9; "El-Thebib."

46 Decharme, *Mémoire sur l'opium indigène*; Bénard, *Résumé des expériences*; Bénard and Collas, "Opium indigène, son extraction du pavot-oeillette," *Bulletin général de thérapeutique médicale et chirurgicale* 58 (1860): 427–32.

47 Statistics cited in Bénard and Collas, "Opium indigène," 429.

48 Ibid.

49 In 1853, Bénard's sample was 14.75 per cent morphine, and in 1854 it was 16 per cent. Ibid., 431. Aubergier in Auvergne and Odeph, a pharmacist in Champlitte (Haute-Saone), also found *pavot à oeillette* to contain similarly high levels of morphine. Decharme, *Mémoire sur l'opium indigène*, 17; Alphonse Odeph, "Culture de l'opium indigène," *Union pharmaceutique* (March 1862): 84–8, 86.

50 Bénard and Collas, "Opium indigène," 431.

51 A hectare is 10,000 square meters and a hectoliter is 100 liters. Ibid., 428.

52 Ibid., 431.

53 Ibid., 429–31.

54 Decharme, *Mémoire*, 30.

55 Odeph, "Culture de l'opium indigène."

56 Odeph, *Abrégé pratique*.

57 Guibourt, *Mémoire sur le dosage*, 16, 30, 58.

58 Berthé, *Lettre*, 2.

59 Berthé, *Note*; Berthé, *Examen critique*, 2–3.

60 Guibourt, *Mémoire sur le dosage*, 42. Indian opium had relatively low morphine content so the British exported it for sale in China instead of trying to sell it as pharmaceutical-grade opium in Europe. Parssinen, *Secret Passions*, 11.

61 Guibourt, *Mémoire sur le dosage*, 16, 30.

62 Berthé, *Du titrage de l'opium*, 5–6.

63 Millant, *La culture du pavot*, 30–2.

64 *Codex medicamentarius* (1866), 70. Ordinary Smyrna opium had to contain at least 10 per cent morphine before drying. Fonssagrives, "Opium," 149.

65 *Codex medicamentarius* (1866), 70–1.

66 Direction Générale des Douanes, *Tableau général du commerce*.

67 After 1914, Turkish opium imports to France ceased because the Ottoman Empire was allied with the Central Powers in World War I. As Virginia Berridge has noted, Turkey was also the primary supplier of opium for Britain in the nineteenth century. Despite Britain's role in the Opium Wars in the Far East, between 80 and 90 per cent of British opium imports came from Turkey between 1827 and 1869. Berridge and Edwards, *Opium and the People*,

3–4, 273. For statistics on Britain's role in the international opium trade, see Parssinen, *Secret Passions*, 10–14.

68 C.O. Harz, "Opium Production in Europe," *Pharmaceutical Journal* 3 no. 2 (9 September 1871): 223–5, 223.

69 "Mission d'études de l'acclimatation dans les colonies françaises de nouveaux végétaux (pavot à opium, caoutchouc, gutta percha, vigne du Japon) de Édouard Raoul, pharmacien de la Marine (1885/1891)," 50 COL 77, Archives National d'Outre Mer, Aix-en-Provence (hereafter cited as ANOM).

70 "Note sur la nécéssité de l'introduction de nouvelles cultures dans les colonies françaises," n.d., 50 COL 77, ANOM.

71 Dispatch from 29 April 1886, 50 COL 77, ANOM.

72 From 1897 onward, the main source of the French colonial budget in Indochina came from indirect taxes on opium, salt, and rice alcohol. Descours-Gatin, *Quand l'opium finançait*, 267.

73 "No. 2676. – Loi … du 21 Germinal." For more on the 1803 Germinal Law and a discussion of pharmaceutical training, see Faure, *Les français et leur médecine*; Faure, *Histoire sociale de la médecine*, 41–9.

74 "No. 2676. – Loi … du 21 Germinal," 122–4, 126.

75 Deschamps, *Étude comparative*; Daston and Galison, *Objectivity*, 16–17.

76 A "gros" is an old unit of mass, equal to ⅛ ounce. Jourdan, *Code pharmaceutique*, 555.

77 *Codex: Pharmacopée française* (1837), 451.

78 "Pilules de cynoglosse opiacées," in *Codex medicamentarius* (1866), 554–5. This recipe remained essentially unchanged in both the 1884 and 1908 versions of the Codex; see *Codex medicamentarius* (1884), 485; *Codex medicamentarius gallicus* (1908), 480.

79 Daston and Galison, *Objectivity*, 37–9.

80 "No. 2676. – Loi … du 21 Germinal," 127.

81 Some pharmacists were rumored to simply substitute different ingredients when they did not have the right ones on hand. N. Sueur, "La Pharmacie Centrale de France," 83–5.

82 Faure, "Les officines pharmaceutiques françaises"; Faure, "Officines, pharmaciens, et medicaments"; N. Sueur, "La Pharmacie Centrale de France."

83 Faure, "Officines, pharmaciens, et medicaments," 34.

84 Julien, "Un empire industriel"; Valentin, "Jean-Antoine-Brutus Ménier."

85 Valentin, "Jean-Antoine-Brutus Ménier," 368–9.

86 Ibid., 375–6.

87 Ibid., 378. See also Ménier et Cie, *Prix courant général* (1845); Ménier et Cie, *Prix courant général* (1854).

88 Ménier et Cie, *Prix courant général* (1854), 5.

89 Ménier et Cie, *Prix courant général* (1845), 20, 38, 44, 47, 54, 57, 59.

90 Ménier et Cie, *Prix courant général* (1854), 6.

91 Valentin, "Jean-Antoine-Brutus Ménier," 378–82.

92 Ramsey, *Professional and Popular Medicine*; Ramsey, "Medical Power";

Léonard, *La vie quotidienne*; Ackerman, *Health Care*; Faure, *Les français et leur médecine*; Faure, *Histoire sociale de la médecine*.

93 N. Sueur, "La Pharmacie Centrale de France," 82.

94 Mory, "Dorvault," 81.

95 N. Sueur, "La Pharmacie Centrale de France," 84.

96 Mory, "Dorvault," 83–4.

97 Julien, "Un empire industriel," 180–2.

98 N. Sueur, "La Pharmacie Centrale de France," 85.

99 Faure, "Les officines pharmaceutiques françaises," 678.

100 Dorvault, *Catalogue pharmaceutique* (1877).

101 Rey, *Histoire de la douleur*, 78–9. On the early history and production of ether, see Zimmer, *Histoire de l'anesthésie*, 17–26.

102 "Chloroforme," in Dechambre, *Dictionnaire usuel*, 317–18; Rey, *Histoire de la douleur*, 195–7.

103 For an account of the specific debates over ether anesthesia in the Academy of Medicine, see *Bulletin de l'Académie de médecine* 12 (12 January–23 February 1847): 262–411.

104 Flourens, "Note touchant l'action de l'éther sur les centres nerveux," *Comptes rendus des séances de l'Académie des sciences* 24 (8 March 1847): 340–4.

105 *Codex medicamentarius* (1866), 277–8.

106 *Codex medicamentarius* (1884), xiv–xv.

107 *Codex medicamentarius* (1884), 173–5, 175.

108 "Ether rectifié du commerce," in *Codex medicamentarius* (1884), 210–13; *Codex medicamentarius gallicus* (1908), 245–7.

109 Derosne, Séguin, and German pharmacist Friedrich Wilhelm Sertürner all published papers on this alkaloid independently between 1803 and 1806, although Sertürner is frequently credited with its discovery. Fonssagrives, "Morphine (Thérapeutique)," in Dechambre, *Dictionnaire encyclopédique* (1875), 493–516, 493–4. In 1817, Sertürner named the substance "morphium," after Morpheus, the god of dreams. Lesch, *Science and Medicine*, 137.

110 The history of the hypodermic syringe is somewhat contested. Charles-Gabriel Pravaz, a French orthopedic surgeon, and Alexander Wood, a Scottish physician, are both independently credited with its invention, though the syringe became known in France as the Pravaz syringe. Writing in the 1890s, Dr Ernest Chambard traced the early origins of the morphine injection to Dr Lafargue de Saint-Émilion, who used needles covered with morphine to penetrate the skin in the 1820s and 1830s, and Dr Rynd, a surgeon from Dublin who injected medical substances under the skin using a hollow needle attached to a bottle in 1844. Chambard, *Les morphinomanes*, viii.

111 Jourdan, *Code pharmaceutique*, 387–9; *Codex: Pharmacopée française* (1837), 133–4; *Codex medicamentarius* (1866), 239–40.

112 *Codex medicamentarius* (1884), 171, 239–41; *Codex medicamentarius* (1908), 423–6.

113 "Coca (Botanique)," in Dechambre, *Dictionnaire encyclopédique* (1876), 161–3.

114 "Cocaïne," in Dechambre, *Dictionnaire usuel*, 374–5.

115 Duncum, *Development of Inhalation Anaesthesia*, 39–40; Rey, *Histoire de la douleur*, 212–14; Gootenberg, *Andean Cocaine*, 9–10, 22–6.

116 *Codex medicamentarius* (1884), 48, 413–14, 525–6, 603–4, 609, 626.

117 Chauveau, "Les origines de l'industrialization," 631, 629–30.

118 Aubergier, *Des préparations d'opium indigène*; N. Sueur, "Les spécialités pharmaceutiques."

119 Ramsey, "Academic Medicine," 28.

120 Faure, "Officines, pharmaciens, et medicaments," 36.

121 On the rise of similar "patent remedies" in Britain, see Berridge and Edwards, *Opium and the People*, 123–31.

122 Faure, "Officines, pharmaciens, et medicaments," 35.

123 Faure, "Une pharmacie lyonnaise," 311.

124 Chauveau, "Les origines de l'industrialization," 637.

125 "Gouttes blanches de Gallard," in *Formulaire des pharmaciens français*, 145; "Gouttes noires anglaises," in *Codex medicamentarius* (1866), 388.

126 Dehaut, *Manuel de médecine*, 696–8. Dr Clertan also sold chloroform "pearls." A pharmacist could purchase a box of thirty "pearls" wholesale from the PCF for 1.75 francs. Dorvault, *Catalogue pharmaceutique* (1877), 181.

127 Ibid., 149–208.

128 Chauveau, "Les origines de l'industrialization," 637.

129 Ibid., 628.

130 "No. 2436. – Loi … du 19 Ventôse," 567–76; "No. 2676. – Loi … du 21 Germinal," 121–9.

131 Berman, "Drug Control," 3–14; Chast, "Les origines."

132 "No. 2436. – Loi … du 19 Ventôse," 121–9.

133 Yvorel, *Les poisons de l'esprit*, 103.

134 "No. 12,115. – Loi … du 19 Juillet 1845"; see documents in DB 441 and DB 442, Archives de la Prefecture de Police de Paris.

135 "Police médicale: Vente des Poisons. – Les articles 34 et 35 de la loi du 21 Germinal an XI s'appliquent à toutes les substances réputée vénéneuses, bien qu'elles n'y soient pas nominativement specifiées," *Gazette médicale de Paris* 3, no. 1 (14 November 1846): 904.

136 See Articles 5, 6, and 9 of the 1846 Ordinance: Griolet, Vergé, and Bourdeaux. *Code d'instruction criminelle*, 625–7.

137 See Article 11 of the 1846 Ordinance: ibid., 627.

138 "Tableau des Substances Vénéneuses annexé à l'ordonnance du 29 Octobre 1846. – Rapport et décisions de la Société de pharmacie à ce sujet, *Bulletin général de thérapeutique médicale et chirurgicale* 32 (1847): 126–32.

139 Ibid., 131.

140 Ibid., 128.

141 On the history of drugging infants and children with opiate "soothing syrups" like Godfrey's Cordial in British industrial areas, see Parssinen, *Secret Passions*, 42–58. While pharmacists may have liked to believe that the

administration of opiates to children was an English practice, there are some indications that it was also popular in France, particularly in the industrial areas of the Nord. "Épicier condamné pour vente des pavots," *Répertoire de pharmacie* 3, no. 22 (1910): 368–9.

142 "Rapport et décisions de la Société de pharmacie," *Bulletin général*, 129–30.

143 Ibid., 131.

144 "Décret du 8 juillet 1850," in Griolet, Vergé, and Bourdeaux, *Code d'instruction criminelle*, 627.

145 "Chapitre XI. Alcalis végétaux," in *Codex: Pharmacopée française* (1837), 133–42.

146 See also Black, "Doctors on Drugs."

147 Sussman, "Glut of Doctors"; Goldstein, *Console and Classify*, 147–51.

148 I use the term "bourgeois" here not in the Marxist sense but rather to describe the post-Revolutionary social elite whose power was defined not by nobility but by wealth, sociability, and shared values. C.E. Harrison, *Bourgeois Citizen*, 3–9. On the difficulties of defining the bourgeoisie as a cohesive social group in the early nineteenth century, see Maza, *Myth of the French Bourgeoisie*.

149 "No. 2436. – Loi ... du 19 Ventôse," 567–76.

150 Sussman, "Glut of Doctors," 288.

151 Despite stauch opposition by doctors and the efforts of the Medical Facultés to monopolize medical education, the inferior *officier de santé* degree was not abolished until 1892. Weisz, "Politics of Medical Professionalization," 5, 22.

152 Ibid., 6; Ackerman, *Health Care*, 32–59.

153 Jégo cited in Léonard, *La France médicale*, 220–1.

154 Pichon, *Morphinisme*, 457.

155 On the use of opiates to treat incurable illness, see Szabo, *Incurable and Intolerable*, 136–58.

156 Payen, "Rapport sur les communications," 845.

157 Curator Roger Gounot, who organized an exhibition of Maurin's work in 1978 at the Musé Crozatier du Puy, believes the lithograph was conceived as a design for a menu. Gounot, *Charles Maurin*, 39, pl. 20, no. 67.

158 Truffles had an erotic reputation in the nineteenth century, which, coupled with the patient's exposed body, suggests that the doctor might have profited from the situation in more ways than one. On truffles and eroticism, see Rosario, *Erotic Imagination*, 6–7.

159 Faure, "Officines, pharmaciens, et medicaments," 33.

160 George Weisz notes that these statistics were virtually unchanged in 1881. Weisz "Politics of Medical Professionalization," 6.

161 Ackerman, *Health Care*, 20–58.

162 "No. 2676. – Loi ... du 21 Germinal," 127–8.

163 Faure, *Les français et leur médecine*, 49–54.

164 *Bulletin commercial* 1, no. 6 (1873): 138.

165 Faure, *Les français et leur médecine*, 50.

166 "Épicier condamné pour vente des pavots."

167 Faure, *Les français et leur médecine*, 49–54.

168 Dorvault, *Catalogue pharmaceutique* (1877).

169 Ibid., 166.

170 Léonard, "Femmes, religion et médecine."

171 Schmitt, "La pharmacie hospitalière."

172 Faure, *Les français et leur médecine*, 53–4.

173 Léonard, "Femmes, religion et médecine," 898.

174 Bataille cited in Ackerman, *Health Care*, 42. Jacques Léonard also notes that many nuns refused to uphold the poisonous substances legislation of 1846. Léonard, "Femmes, religion et médecine," 897, 907. Jack Ellis cites a doctor in Haute-Marne who complained that a *curé* in Musseau dispensed opium tinctures illegally purchased from a sympathetic pharmacist. The doctor also complained that the *curé* treated twice as many patients as he did. Ellis, *Physician-Legislators*, 69.

175 Cited in Schmitt, "La pharmacie hospitalière," 231.

176 Ackerman, *Health Care*, 42.

177 *Manuel des soeurs*, 150.

178 Ibid., 1.

179 Ibid., 141–2.

180 Ibid., 219–20.

181 Ibid., 227–8.

182 Ibid., 294.

183 Ibid., 294–5.

184 For more on the social history of *morphinomanie* in France, see Yvorel, *Les poisons de l'esprit*, 111–44; Bachmann and Coppel, *La drogue*, 142–57.

185 Black, "Doctors on Drugs." On morphine addiction in America, see Courtwright, *Dark Paradise*, 42.

186 Dalbanne, *Essai sur quelques accidents*; Terrail, *De la morphine*; Jouet, *Étude de morphinisme chronique*; Pichon, *Le morphinisme*.

187 Chambard, *Les morphinomanes*, 8.

188 Degoix, *Maladies et médicaments*, 13.

189 Pichon, *Le morphinisme*, 459–60.

190 For comparison, the maximum daily dose of morphine hydrochloride recommended for adult consumption in the 1908 French Codex was 0.08 grams. *Codex medicamentarius gallicus* (1908), 896.

191 "Le morphinisme devant les tribunaux," *La Semaine médicale*, 10 May 1883, 98–9; A…-V…, No. 25117, 15 May 1883, D1U6 5994, Archives de la Ville de Paris.

192 On the progressive regulation of psychotropic drugs as poisonous substances in France, see Retaillaud-Bajac, *Les paradis perdus*, 30–8; Chast, "Les stupéfiants"; Padwa, *Social Poison*, 87–91, 115–16, 130–3.

193 These included meetings in Shanghai (1909), the Hague (1912–19), and Geneva (1925, 1931). Padwa, *Social Poison*, 86–91.

194 "No. 10090. - Loi … du 12 Juillet 1916."

195 Ackerknecht, *Medicine at the Paris Hospital*; Porter, *Greatest Benefit*,

306–20.

196 Ackerknecht, *Medicine at the Paris Hospital*, 18–19; Bouchardat, *Nouveau formulaire magistral*, 19.

197 Mollet and Pradeau, "La pharmacie centrale," 39.

198 Charles Lasègue and Jules Regnauld, "La thérapeutique jugée par les chiffres," *Archives générales de médecine* (1877), 14.

199 Bourgoin and Beurmann, "La thérapeutique jugée par les chiffres." *Bulletin général de thérapeutique médicale et chirurgicale* 115 (1888): 145–62, 207–22, 160.

200 L. Grimbert, "La thérapeutique jugée par les chiffres," *Bulletin de l'Académie de médecine* 81 (29 April 1919): 540–50, 542, 544.

201 Weiner, *Citizen-Patient*; Weiner "Le droit de l'homme."

202 Weiner, *Citizen-Patient*, 10.

203 Ackerman, *Health Care*, 109, 119.

204 Faure, "La médecine gratuite," 597; Ramsey, "Public Health in France," 67–8.

205 Léonard, "Femmes, religion et médecine," 890.

206 Faure, "La médecine gratuite," 597.

207 Ramsey, "Public Health in France," 77–9; see also Hildreth, "Medical Rivalries."

208 "No. 27052. – Loi … du 15 Juillet 1893," 841.

209 Faure, "La médecine gratuite," 603.

210 Ramsey, "Public Health in France," 79; Ackerman, *Health Care*, 58.

211 Statistics from the *Statistique du personnel médical et pharmaceutique de France et d'Algérie* cited in Chauveau, "Les origines de l'industrialization," 633.

212 Faure, "Officines, pharmaciens, et medicaments," 37.

213 Powdered morphine hydrochloride had to be mixed with water for subcutaneous injection. Pharmacie Centrale de France et Maison Ménier réunies, *Bulletin commercial: Anexe de l'Union pharmaceutique* 1, no. 1 (1873): 12; *Bulletin commercial: Journal des intérêtes scientifiques, pratiques et moraux des pharmaciens* 27, no. 1 (1899): 4.

214 Ackerman, *Health Care*, 58; Léonard, *La France médicale*, 216–17.

215 Private papers cited in Léonard, *La France médicale*, 216.

216 Le Roux, *Le chemin du crime*, 196–7.

217 Ackerman, *Health Care*, 3, 20–30; Faure, *Les français et leur médecine*, 62–8.

218 Berlanstein, *Working People of Paris*, 104–5.

219 Ménier et Cie, *Prix courant général* (1845), 110–12.

220 Cavaillès, *Guide pratique*, 34–6.

221 Vermot, *Petit guide de la santé*, 787–8.

222 Cavaillès, *Guide pratique*, 3, 33–42.

223 Ibid., 21, 25, 28.

224 Dehaut, *Manuel de médecine*.

225 Vermot, *Petit guide de la santé*.

226 Lescure, *La médecine du peuple*.

227 Dehaut, *Manuel de médecine*, 210, 288, 356, 408, 430–2, 434; Lescure, *La médecine du peuple*, 40, 66–7.

228 Dehaut, *Manuel de médicine*, 616.
229 Ibid., 266, 636; Lescure, *La médecine du peuple*, 26–7.
230 Lescure, *La médecine du peuple*, 6, 29, 37.
231 Dehaut, *Manuel de médicine*, 537.
232 Cavaillès, *Guide pratique*, 27.
233 Dehaut, *Manuel de médicine*, 476.
234 Ibid., 173, 212.
235 Ibid., 477.
236 Ibid., 316, 356, 406, 469.
237 Ibid., 130, 390; see also Lescure, *La médecine du peuple*, 62–3.
238 Dehaut, *Manuel de médicine*, 151, 202, 316, 469, 808.
239 Ibid., 202, 438.
240 Ibid., 438.
241 Vermot, *Petit guide de la santé*, 11.
242 Lescure, *La médecine du peuple*, 2, 60, 62, 79

CHAPTER TWO

1 On the history and ethics of self-experimentation, see Strickland, "Ideology of Self-Knowledge"; Schaffer, "Self Evidence"; Luauté, "Contexte historique"; Carroy, "Observation"; Chamayou, *Les corps vils*, 139–61; Herzig, *Suffering for Science*; Altman, *Who Goes First?*, 53–105; Foster, *Ethics of Medical Research*; Jonas, "Philosophical Reflections."

2 Daston and Galison, *Objectivity*, 200–1, 207–10, 217–27. Appropriately cultivating one's sensibility – understood as both physical sensation and moral sentiment – through focused attention and reasoned reflection would lead to enlightenment. If cultivated to excess, however, sensibility could lead to pathology, excessive emotion, and disorder. Riskin, *Science in the Age of Sensibility*, 1–2; Vila, *Enlightenment and Pathology*, 1, 80–8.

3 Immanuel Kant is commonly associated with this vision of the unified wilful self in nineteenth-century Europe. However, Jan Goldstein has demonstrated that the specific vision of the unified self that Victor Cousin institutionalized in the *lycée* philosophy curriculum in France during the July Monarchy also drew extensively on the philosophy of Maine de Biran (1766–1824), who viewed the unified self, cultivated through introspection, as a remedy for the political turmoil brought on by the Revolution. Goldstein, *Post-Revolutionary Self*, 10–12, 129–38; Daston and Galison, *Objectivity*, 33, 201–2, 205–10; Tresch, *Romantic Machine*, 51–3, 66–7. On the reception of Kant's philosophy in France, see Kopper, "La signification de Kant."

4 Daston and Galison, *Objectivity*, 202, 228; Goldstein, *Post-Revolutionary Self*, 10–12.

5 Shapin and Schaffer, *Leviathan and the Air-Pump*; Gower, *Scientific Method*, 21–62.

6 Daston and Galison, *Objectivity*, 203, 227.

7 Ibid., 37-9.

8 Ibid., 196-9, 203; Foucault, *Technologies of the Self*.

9 For more on Davy's self-experimentation, see Davy, *Researches, Chemical and Philosophical*; Golinski, "Humphry Davy"; Bergmann, "Humphry Davy's Contribution"; Rey, *Histoire de la douleur*, 169-75.

10 I have adjusted the spelling for the sake of clarity, changing *f* to *s* when appropriate. Davy, *Researches, Chemical and Philosophical*, 460-1.

11 Fourcroy, Vauquelin, and Thénard, "Mémoire sur la nature comparée du gaz oxide d'azote ou de l'oxide nitreux de M. Davy, et du gaz nitreux," *Mémoires de l'Institut des sciences, lettres, et arts* 6 (1806): 312-31, 328.

12 Ibid., 329, 330.

13 Schaffer, "Self Evidence," 334, 338.

14 *Bulletin de l'Académie de médecine* 12 (23 February 1847): 295-396.

15 Davy, *Researches, Chemical and Philosophical*, 465.

16 For an account of this event, see Elizabeth Whitman Morton, "The Discovery of Anesthesia: Dr W.T.G. Morton and His Heroic Battle for a New Idea. – How Painless Surgery Began Fifty Years Ago," *McClure's Magazine* 7 (September 1896): 311-18.

17 Rey, *Histoire de la douleur*, 183.

18 Altman, *Who Goes First?*, 58-9.

19 "Lettre de M. Wells," *Bulletin de l'Académie de médecine* 12 (23 February 1847): 394-5.

20 Altman, *Who Goes First?*, 60-1. Roselyn Rey suggests that Wells's preference for nitrous oxide likely worked against him. After his letter was read aloud, Dr Orfila recalled what negative experiences Vauquelin and Thénard had had with it and described his own unpleasant experience. Wells committed suicide with chloroform shortly before the Société médicale de Paris sent a letter acknowledging his discovery in January 1848. Rey, *Histoire de la douleur*, 183.

21 Morton, "Discovery of Anesthesia," 313.

22 Zimmer, *Histoire de l'anesthésie*, 65-141.

23 Crosland, *Science under Control*, 242-9, 383.

24 *Comptes rendus des séances de l'Académie des sciences* 24 (18 January 1847): 74-6.

25 Malgaigne, "Emploi d'éther," *Bulletin de l'Académie de médecine* 12 (12 January 1847): 262-4.

26 *Bulletin de l'Académie de médecine* 12 (19 January 1847): 283-4.

27 *Bulletin de l'Académie de médecine* 12 (26 January 1847): 301.

28 Velpeau, "Physiologie. – Sur les effets de l'éther," *Comptes rendus des séances de l'Académie des sciences* 24 (1 February 1847): 129-34, 133.

29 *Bulletin de l'Académie de médecine* 12 (26 January 1847): 299-310.

30 *Comptes rendus des séances de l'Académie des sciences* 24 (1 February 1847): 139.

31 Société des médecins allemands à Paris, "Recherches et expériences sur l'inhalation de l'éther sulfurique," *Gazette médicale de Paris* 3, no. 2 (6 February 1847): 101–3, 101.

32 Ibid., 101–2.

33 They determined that sensibility, pulse, and respiration increased at the beginning of the experiment. As the perception of pain decreased, the pulse also decreased, although it always remained higher than normal. Ibid., 103.

34 Ibid., 101.

35 Daston and Galison, *Objectivity*, 115–90.

36 Ibid., 210.

37 Strickland, "Ideology of Self-Knowledge," 456; Schaffer, "Self Evidence," 330, 334–7.

38 Schaffer, "Self Evidence," 339, 344, 347, 350.

39 Société des médecins allemands à Paris, "Recherches et expériences," 101.

40 Ibid., 102.

41 Roux, "Physiologie: Communication relative aux effets de l'éther introduit par la respiration," *Comptes rendus des séances de l'Académie des sciences* 24 (25 January 1847): 89–91, 91.

42 Société des médecins allemands à Paris, "Recherches et expériences," 103.

43 Roux, "Physiologie," 91.

44 *Bulletin de l'Académie de médecine* 12 (26 January 1847): 308.

45 *Comptes rendus des séances de l'Académie des sciences* 24 (8 February 1847): 203.

46 *Bulletin de l'Académie de médecine* 12 (26 January 1847): 303–6, 303.

47 *Bulletin de l'Académie de médecine* 12 (9 February 1847): 355.

48 Strickland, "Ideology of Self-Knowledge," 459–60; Tresch, *Romantic Machine*, 78.

49 *Bulletin de l'Académie de médecine* 12 (9 February 1847): 350–5, 350.

50 Gerdy, "Effets des inhalations d'éther," *Gazette médicale de Paris* 3, no. 2 (1847): 96–7.

51 Ibid.

52 Daston and Galison, *Objectivity*, 242–6.

53 Gerdy, "Effets des inhalations d'éther," 96.

54 *Bulletin de l'Académie de médecine* 12 (26 January 1847): 304–5.

55 Goldstein, *Post-Revolutionary Self*, 161.

56 Ibid., 8–12, 155–65; Daston and Galison, *Objectivity*, 33, 201–2, 205–10.

57 When France introduced a national *lycée* system for girls in the early years of the Third Republic, educators did not include the philosophy course in the new curriculum for *lycéennes*. Goldstein, *Post-Revolutionary Self*, 11–12, 192, 322–4.

58 *Bulletin de l'Académie de médecine* 12 (26 January 1847): 305.

59 Several other doctors also experimented with ether during their own tooth extractions. *Comptes rendus des séances de l'Académie des sciences* 24 (8

February 1847): 204; *Bulletin de l'Académie de médecine* 12 (2 March 1847): 413-17, 416.

60 *Bulletin de l'Académie de médecine* 12 (2 February 1847): 326.

61 Ibid.

62 Ibid., 327.

63 Ibid., 326–7.

64 Sauvet had been inspired by Jacques-Joseph Moreau's self-experimentation with hashish (examined in the next section on hashish experimentation) and was determined to discover whether deep inhalations of ether might produce a similar state of "artificial madness."

65 J.J. Sauvet, "De l'inhalation de l'éther, et de ses effets psychologiques. – Expérimentation personnelle," *Annales médico-psychologiques*, no. 10 (1847): 467–70, 467.

66 Ibid.

67 Ibid., 468.

68 He had read and was inspired by Moreau's work *Hashish and Mental Illness* and thought that ether could produce a similar state. Perhaps these expectations influenced his visions and hallucinations. Gautier's "Club des Hachichins" had already been published by this time.

69 Sauvet, "De l'inhalation de l'éther," 469.

70 Ibid., 469, 470.

71 Flourens, "Note touchant l'action de l'éther sur les centres nerveux," *Comptes rendus des séances de l'Académie des sciences* 24 (8 March 1847): 340-4.

72 Simpson, *Account of a New Anaesthetic Agent*, 6–7.

73 *Comptes rendus des séances de l'Académie des sciences* 25 (13 December 1847): 887–9; Zimmer, *Histoire de l'anesthésie*, 237–8.

74 Eugène Souberian, director of the Pharmacie Centrale des Hôpitaux de Paris, who had also been one of the original discoverers of chloroform in 1831, rushed to present his process for purifying chloroform for anesthetic use in response to surgeons who were impatient to use it. *Comptes rendus des séances de l'Académie des sciences* 25 (29 November 1847): 799–801.

75 Gerdy, "Emploi du chloroforme dans les hôpitaux. Hôpital de la Charité," *Gazette des hôpitaux* 9, no. 140 (27 November 1847): 583–4, 583.

76 Ibid., 584.

77 Ibid.

78 "Hôtel Dieu – M. Blandin," *Gazette des hôpitaux* 9, no. 140 (27 November 1847): 584.

79 *Bulletin de l'Académie de médecine* 12 (30 November 1847): 427.

80 *Comptes rendus des séances de l'Académie des sciences* 25 (13 December 1847): 887–91.

81 *Comptes rendus des séances de l'Académie des sciences* 25 (29 November 1847): 806.

82 Aubert-Roche, *De la peste*, 212–49.

83 Ibid., 211.

84 This was long before the popularization of the germ theory of disease and the discovery of the plague bacillus at the end of the nineteenth century. Aubert-Roche was an anticontagionist who believed that the plague was a nervous disease caused by toxic miasmas from unsanitary environments. As hashish stimulated the nervous system, he believed it would be an effective treatment for the plague. On Aubert-Roche's plague research, see Guba, *Taming Cannabis*, 123–8.

85 Said, *Orientalism*, 123–30.

86 Polo, "Of the Old Man," 48–51; Daftary, *Assassin Legends*, 133.

87 Daftary, *Assassin Legends*, 1–7.

88 Théophile Gautier, "Le Club des Hachichins," *Revue des deux mondes* (February 1846): 520–35, 523.

89 Lewis, *Assassins*, 11–12; Daftary, *Assassin Legends*, 1–7, 35.

90 Guba, "Antoine Isaac Silvestre de Sacy."

91 Aubert-Roche, *De la peste*, 212. He is likely referring to La Fontaine's poem "Le chameau et les Batôns flottants."

92 Ibid., 212–13.

93 Ibid., 213.

94 Aubert-Roche claimed to have cured seven out of eleven plague patients with hashish. He explained that he chose the direst cases to treat with hashish as a matter of ethics, as he did not know what its effects on a sick person would be. Ibid., 214–15, 248.

95 "Notice sur le Hachisch," *Journal de chimie médicale, de pharmacie et de toxicologie* 6 (1840): 447–50.

96 Moreau, *Mémoire sur le traitement des hallucinations*, 15; Moreau, *Du hachisch*, 92.

97 Dowbiggin, *Inheriting Madness*, 55.

98 Moreau, *Mémoire sur le traitement des hallucinations*, 14.

99 Moreau, *Hashish and Mental Illness*, 1, 17.

100 Moreau, *Mémoire sur le traitement des hallucinations*, 18.

101 Ibid.

102 On hashish in French-occupied Egypt, see Guba, *Taming Cannabis*, 49–82.

103 Davenport-Hines, *Pursuit of Oblivion*, 92–3. Edmond Courtive notes that he tested samples of several different Algerian hashish preparations, including *madjoun* and *dawamesk*, and also tried samples of Cannabis indica and Cannabis sativa preparations cultivated in the gardens of the Paris Pharmacy School, some of which were grown from Algerian seeds. Courtive, *Haschish*, 19, 35.

104 Tresch, *Romantic Machine*, 2, 5.

105 Brière de Boismont, "Expériences toxicologiques sur une substance inconnue," *Gazette médicale de Paris* 8, no. 18 (2 May 1840): 278–9. Brière de Boismont was a prominent alienist who ran a private asylum out of his

home in Montmartre. Although he attended this gathering to witness the effects of hashish on others, he was a vocal opponent of hashish. He viewed it, through the lens of Sacy's Assassins legend, as a dangerous Oriental drug that compromised sanity. Guba, *Taming Cannabis*, 156–61. For more on Brière de Boismont, see Hewitt, *Institutionalizing Gender*, 67–91.

106 Brière de Boismont, "Expériences toxicologiques."

107 Ibid., 279.

108 Foucault, *Technologies of the Self.*

109 Goldstein, *Post-Revolutionary Self*, 165–79, 200–1.

110 This metaphor comes from Abrams, *Mirror and the Lamp*, 11–14, 21–3, 30–46, 57–69.

111 Rey-Debove and Rey, *Le Nouveau Petit Robert*, s.v. "kif." French spellings of *kif* vary. For consistency, I use "kif" throughout.

112 Théophile Gautier, "Feuilleton de la Presse," *La Presse*, 10 July 1843, 2.

113 Indeed, the comparison of hashish intoxication to madness is a trope that reappears in descriptions of self-experimentation with hashish throughout the nineteenth century, likely as a result of Moreau's research on the subject.

114 Gautier, "Feuilleton de la Presse."

115 Ibid.

116 For more on the Hashish Eaters' Club, see Hayter, *Opium*, 151–61.

117 French spellings of the word *dawamesk* vary. For continuity, I use "*dawamesk*" throughout.

118 Boissard to Gautier, 27 October 1845 (letter no. 713), in Lacoste-Veysseyre, ed., *Correspondance générale*, 292–3. Boissard also mentioned Moreau in another invitation; see Boissard to Gautier, 16 December 1845 (letter no. 740), in Lacoste-Veysseyre, ed., *Correspondance générale*, 315–16.

119 Goldstein, *Post-Revolutionary Self*, 11.

120 Tresch, *Romantic Machine*, xiv.

121 Gautier, *Baudelaire*, 155.

122 Baudelaire, *Oeuvres complètes*, 220.

123 Honoré de Balzac to Madame Hanska, 23 December 1845, in Balzac, *Lettres à Madame Hanska*, 3:112. Balzac wrote to Mme Hanska again on 6 January 1846, claiming that he took hashish as a means of ensuring that he could destroy himself if he ever lost her love.

124 Ibid., 154.

125 Gautier, *Baudelaire*, 155.

126 Baudelaire had a complicated relationship with drugs, and scholars have debated whether or not to take his writings condemning hashish at face value. Guba, *Taming Cannabis*, 175–84.

127 Baudelaire, *Oeuvres complètes*, 376.

128 Ibid., 222.

129 Dupouy, "Charles Baudelaire, toxicomane et opiomane," *Annales médico-psychologiques* 11 (1910): 353–64. See also Hilton, *Baudelaire in Chains*.

130 Gautier, "Le Club des Hachichins," 529.
131 Given their mixed feelings about hashish, it is likely that Baudelaire and Balzac acted as *voyant* on occasion.
132 Gautier, "Le Club des Hachichins," 529.
133 Ibid., 530.
134 Ibid., 523.
135 Keller, *Colonial Madness*, 124–5.
136 As Bonnie Smith demonstrates, psychotropic drug use was one of several strategies that Romantics used to "decenter" their identities by drawing on elements from non-Western cultures. Others incorporated non-Western thought and philosophy into their work or explored tantrism. Smith, "Decentered Identities."
137 Courtive, *Haschish*, 9.
138 Gautier, "Le Club des Hachichins," 522.
139 Ibid., 530.
140 Ibid., 535.
141 Ibid., 523.
142 Gautier, *Baudelaire*, 155.
143 Jules Giraud, "L'art de faire varier les effets du hachich," *L'Encéphale* (1881), 418–25; Bosc, *Traité théorique et pratique*; Jules Claretie (1840–1913), "Haschichomanie," in the revue *Fantasio* (1913). In 1849, Gustave Flaubert and Maxime du Camp toured the Middle East, where they experimented with hashish and opium. Davenport-Hines, *Pursuit of Oblivion*, 93. Other hashish users in the literary world included Charles Cros, Stanislas de Guaita, Adolphe Retté, and Alfred Jarry. Yvorel, *Les poisons de l'esprit*, 144.
144 Several of them, including Auguste Voisin, Benjamin Ball, and Charles Richet, went on to conduct other drug research later in their careers. Arveiller, "Cannabis."
145 Courtive presented his research in September of 1847, but because of his bad health, he was unable to defend it or publish it until April of 1848. Courtive, *Haschish*, 7, 19; Arveiller, "Le Cannabis en France," 466–7; Siegel and Hirschman, "Edmond de Courtive"; Guba, *Taming Cannabis*, 135–41.
146 Courtive, *Haschish*, 5.
147 Ibid., 19.
148 Ibid., 22.
149 Courtive, "Sur le haschisch," *Journal de pharmacie et de chimie* 3, no. 13 (1848): 427–41, 429.
150 Courtive, *Haschish*, 23.
151 Riskin, "Defecating Duck."
152 Courtive, *Haschish*, 35–6.
153 Ibid., 37–8.
154 Ibid.
155 Ibid., 39.

156 Ibid., 40.
157 Ibid., 40–7.
158 Ibid., 47.
159 See Guba, *Taming Cannabis*, 150–87.
160 Snelders, Kaplan, and Pieters, "On Cannabis," 464–6.
161 Guba, *Taming Cannabis*, 142–6.
162 Doctors and colonial officials viewed the "hashish madness" they observed in the local Arab populations as a sign of their inherent "Oriental savagery" and a threat to French civilization. Reports of Algerian Muslims who committed violent crimes under the influence of hashish, published in Parisian newspapers in the 1850s and 1860s, contributed to hashish's decline in medical therapeutics. Ibid., 18, 148, 172, 188, 200–9.
163 Charles Richet, "Les poisons d'intelligence. I. L'alcool. Le chloroforme," *Revue des deux mondes* 19 (1877): 816–40; Richet, "Les poisons d'intelligence. II. Le Hachich. L'opium. Le café," *Revue des deux mondes* 20 (1877): 178–97.
164 Richet, "Les poisons d'intelligence. I. L'alcool," 820.
165 Richet, "Les poisons d'intelligence. II. Le Hachich," 178.
166 Ibid., 179.
167 Richet, "Les poisons d'intelligence. I. L'alcool," 822.
168 Richet, "Les poisons d'intelligence. II. Le Hachich," 180, 181.
169 Ibid., 181–2.
170 Ibid., 186.
171 Ibid., 197.
172 Giraud, "L'art de faire varier."
173 Sometime around 1912, Giraud published a monograph titled *Testament of a Hashish Eater*, which may have been intended for a broader audience, although it was reviewed in *Journal de magnétisme et du psychisme éxperimental*. Giraud, *Testament d'un haschischéen*.
174 Giraud, "L'art de faire varier," 418–19.
175 Ibid., 422.
176 Ibid., 418–19, 421.
177 Ibid., 421, 419.
178 Ibid., 423, 424.
179 Bosc, *Traité théorique et pratique*.
180 Ibid., 10, 12, 13.
181 Ibid., 14. The original text was written in the formal first-person plural (*nous*). For clarity, I have translated the passage here using the first-person singular.
182 Claretie's 1913 article "Haschichomanie," printed in the revue *Fantasio*, was translated into English and published in the *New York Times*: "Famous French Author Tries Hashish and Describes Weird Effects: Jules Claretie, Academician, Recently Took the Drug Purely for Curiosity's Sake and Had Friends Make Detailed Notes of His Actions under Its Influence," *New York Times*, 8 June 1913, 18.

183 Benjamin, *On Hashish*, 2, 19–22.
184 Baudelaire, *Artificial Paradises*, 74–5.
185 On Baudelaire's laudanum addiction, see Hilton, *Baudelaire in Chains*.
186 See Mickel, *Artificial Paradises*; Hayter, *Opium*; Smith, *Gender of History*, 14–36; Smith, "Decentered Identities"; Yvorel, *Les poisons de l'esprit*, 31–48.
187 Sertürner, "Analyse de l'opium: De la morphine et de l'acide méconique, considéré comme parties essentielles de l'opium." *Annales de chimie et de physique* (1817): 21–42, 27–8.
188 A French *grain* was approximately 53 milligrams. Rey-Debove and Rey, *Le Nouveau Petit Robert*, s.v. "grain (poids)."
189 Sertürner, "Analyse de l'opium," 28–9.
190 Black, "Doctors on Drugs."
191 Writing in 1877, Richet did not conceptualize opiate addiction in the modern sense; rather, he viewed opium abuse as a nefarious habit of Chinese and Indian people comparable to alcoholism in Europe. Richet, "Les poisons d'intelligence. I. L'alcool," 821.
192 Richet, "Les poisons d'intelligence. II. Le Hachich," 191.
193 Ibid.
194 Chambard, *Les morphinomanes*, 59.
195 Ibid., 62.
196 Pichon, *Le morphinisme*.
197 Jules Christian, "Discours au nom de la Société médico-psychologique," *Annales médico-psychologiques* 7, no. 17 (1893): 285, 328–9; Yvorel, *Les poisons de l'esprit*, 127.
198 An earlier version of this case study was published as part of an article in *Social History of Medicine*; see Black, "Doctors on Drugs." I would like to thank Oxford University Press and the Society for the Social History of Medicine for permission to reprint it here in this revised and expanded form.
199 Artières, *Journal d'un morphinomane*, 7.
200 Ibid., 2 October 1880, 9.
201 Ibid., 20 October and 9 November 1880, 9.
202 Ibid., March 15, 1889, 46–7.
203 Ibid., 22 August 1883, 20.
204 Ibid., 14 March 1888, 38–9.
205 On opium in French Indochina, see Descours-Gatin, *Quand l'opium finançait*.
206 Artières, *Journal d'un morphinomane*, 20 February 1883 and 8 May 1886, 18, 35.
207 Ibid., 9 July 1884, 21.
208 Ibid., 11 January 1885, 27.
209 Ibid., 15 March 1885, 29.
210 Ibid., 2 April 1885, 30.

211 Ibid., 17 April 1886, 34.
212 Ball, *La morphinomanie*, 23–4.
213 Artières, *Journal d'un morphinomane*, 5 September 1882, 13.
214 Ibid., 7 October and 9 October 1892, 72–3.
215 Ibid., October 13, 1892, 74–5.
216 Ibid., 20 November 1888, 41.
217 Ibid., 9 November 1884, 24–5.
218 Ibid., 4 June 1886, 35.
219 Ibid., 29 November 1885, 31.
220 Ibid., 30 December 1887, 36.
221 Fauchier, *Contribution à l'étude*, 12.
222 Ibid., 17–18. The original quote was written in the formal first-person plural (*nous*). For clarity, I have translated the passage here using the first-person singular.
223 Ibid., 18–19.
224 Ibid., 18–19, 20.
225 Ibid., 20, 21.
226 Ibid., 20–1.
227 Ibid., 21–2.
228 Ibid., 22.
229 Ibid., 24.

CHAPTER THREE

1 Hewitt, *Institutionalizing Gender*, 9–11; Goldstein, *Console and Classify*, 278.
2 Weiner, *Citizen-Patient*, 9, 59–68; Goldstein, *Console and Classify*, 41–2. For more on the "Great Confinement" of undesirables within the institutions of the Hôpital Général in the seventeenth century, see Foucault, *Madness and Civilization*, 38–64.
3 Condillac cited in Goldstein, *Console and Classify*, 92–3.
4 Ibid., 109.
5 On the relative relationship between normal and pathological, see Canguilhem, *Normal and the Pathological*; L. Sueur, "La fragile limite."
6 Goldstein, *Console and Classify*, 42–3.
7 Esquirol's statistics cited in Hewitt, *Institutionalizing Gender*, 5.
8 While "alienist" was a term commonly used in the nineteenth century, I also use "psychiatrist" and "asylum doctor" at various points to describe these specialists in the study and treatment of mental illness. "No. 7443. – Loi sur les Aliénés du 30 Juin 1838." See also L. Sueur, "Les psychiatres français"; Hewitt, *Institutionalizing Gender*, 5, 43–4, 163–4; Goldstein, *Console and Classify*, 276–321.
9 Hewitt, *Institutionalizing Gender*, 5.
10 Goldstein, *Console and Classify*, 276–8.

11 Ibid., 51.

12 Weiner, *Citizen-Patient*, 256–71; Goldstein, *Console and Classify*, 60, 64–119, 207; Hewitt, *Institutionalizing Gender*, 34–6, 60; Harsin, "Gender, Class, and Madness"; Quétel and Morel, *Les fous*, 231–72.

13 Asylums continued to restrain unruly patients in the nineteenth century, but they adopted more "humane" methods, including the straitjacket and solitary confinement. Harsin, "Gender, Class, and Madness," 1054; L. Sueur, "Les psychiatres français," 301. See also L. Sueur, "La violence."

14 Weiner, *Citizen-Patient*, 247–77; Goldstein, *Console and Classify*, 108–9.

15 Goldstein, *Console and Classify*, 263–7; Quétel and Morel, *Les fous*, 67–140. On the controversy surrounding the cold shower treatment, see Hewitt, *Institutionalizing Gender*, 43–66.

16 Pinel, *Traité médico-philosophique*, 40.

17 Ibid., 105, 245.

18 There were some cases in which even opium was ineffective. Pinel observed a manic patient who was experiencing the most violent epileptic attacks and appeared close to death. Pinel took advantage of the intervals between attacks to administer opium, but he saw no diminution in the intensity of the patient's symptoms. The patient died in frightening convulsions five days later. Ibid., 272.

19 Hewitt, *Institutionalizing Madness*, 63, 163–4; Dowbiggin, *Inheriting Madness*, 17–18; Postel and Quétel, *Nouvelle histoire*, 433.

20 Rech, "Des effets du hachisch sur l'homme jouissant de sa raison et sur l'aliéné," *Annales médico-psychologiques* (1848): 3.

21 Berthier, "Essais sur les propriétés hypnotiques du hachisch dans les maladies mentales," *Journal des maladies mentales* (1868): 434.

22 Ripa, *Women and Madness*; Hustvedt, *Medical Muses*; Didi-Huberman, *Invention of Hysteria*; Appignanesi, *Sad, Mad, and Bad*; Wilson, *Voices from the Asylum*; Matlock, "Doubling Out." Two notable exceptions that focus on the experience of male patients are Hewitt, *Institutionalizing Gender*, and Micale, *Hysterical Men*.

23 Hewitt, *Institutionalizing Gender*, 24; Goldstein, *Console and Classify*, 48, 52.

24 Hewitt, *Institutionalizing Gender*, 170–1. Prestwich's study of admissions statistics at Sainte-Anne Asylum between 1873 and 1913 demonstrates that men were actually admitted at higher rates than women. However, as men were more likely to be admitted for alcoholism, they tended to be released sooner after a period of detoxification. Women tended to be admitted for depression, which doctors found responded slowly to treatment, so women tended to stay in asylums for longer. Prestwich, "Family Strategies," 803.

25 Hewitt, *Institutionalizing Gender*, 120–1.

26 This seems to reflect the research agenda of particular doctors who worked in segregated asylum wards rather than an assumption that certain drugs would be more effective for one gender. For example, Moreau de Tours,

arguably the strongest proponent of hashish as a therapeutic agent, worked at Bicêtre where he had regular access to male patients to serve as clinical subjects. Charcot and Voisin were both at Salpêtrière, where they administered morphine to female patients. Certain drugs were also considered particularly effective in treating conditions that were more prominent among one gender. For example, doctors found opiates and morphine useful for treating depression, which was more commonly diagnosed among female patients. Prestwich, "Female Alcoholism," 326.

27 Ackerknecht, *Medicine at the Paris Hospital*, 15–22, 191–4; Weiner, *Citizen-Patient*, 177–84; Porter, *Greatest Benefit*, 306–20.

28 Moreau, *Mémoire sur le traitement des hallucinations*. For more on self-experimentation as a research methodology, see chapter 2.

29 For more on Moreau de Tours's psychopharmacological research, see Ledermann, "Pharmacie."

30 Moreau, *Mémoire sur le traitement des hallucinations*, 5.

31 Moreau, *Traité pratique de la folie névropathique*, 180.

32 Moreau, *Hashish and Mental Illness*, 206.

33 Ibid., 211.

34 The patient did experience another incident of hallucinations, but these were dissipated with another dose of hashish. L. du S., "Hallucinations de la vue et de l'ouïe. Intermittence. Traitement par le haschisch. Guérison," *Annales médico-psychologiques* (1856): 579–82.

35 Moreau, *Mémoire sur le traitement des hallucinations*, 6, 13.

36 Berthier, "Essais sur les propriétés hypnotiques," 435.

37 Auguste Voisin tried to use hashish to treat the hallucinations and agitation of a melancholic dipsomaniac patient in 1872, but it produced no noticeable change in the patient's state. Auguste Voisin, "Nouvelles observations sur le traitement curatif de la folie par les injections sous-cutanées de chlorhydrate de morphine," *Bulletin général de thérapeutique médicale et chirurgicale* (1876): 115.

38 This research revolutionized surgical practice as it allowed doctors to eliminate patients' pain during procedures. On the anesthesia debates of 1847 in the Academy of Sciences and the Academy of Medicine, see Rey, *Histoire de la douleur*, 180–95; Zimmer, *Histoire de l'anesthésie*, 95–107.

39 Moreau, "Influence des inspirations éthérée sur les affections convulsives," *Union médicale*, no. 3 (1847), reproduced in *Annales médico-psychologiques*, no. 10 (1847): 133–6; Moreau, "De l'action de la vapeur d'éther dans l'épilepsie," *Gazette des hôpitaux*, 1 April 1847, reproduced in *Annales médico-psychologiques*, no. 12 (1848): 237–44.

40 Moreau observed this a few times with four of his patients. Moreau, "De l'action de la vapeur d'éther," 240–1.

41 Ibid., 239.

42 Ibid., 238.

43 Falret, "Inspirations d'éther dans l'aliénation mentale," *Annales médico-psychologique* (1847): 285–6.

44 Académie des sciences, Séance du 14 Juin 1847, "Traitement de l'épilepsie par l'étherisation," *Annales médico-psychologiques* (1847): 146–7.

45 Desterne, "De l'hystérie chez l'homme. – Du traitement du paroxysme hystérique par le chloroforme," *Annales médico-psychologiques* (1849): 419–23. On early theories of male hysteria in France, see Micale, *Hysterical Men*, 58–76.

46 Binder, *Des indications de l'opium*, 4.

47 In 1854, Dr Forget of Strasbourg used opium to cure a young woman of delicate and nervous constitution who suffered from delirium that had become aggravated into "prolonged and furious mania." "Délire violent. – Guérison par l'opium," *Annales médico-psychologiques* (1855): 666–7.

48 Sauvet, "Répertoire d'observations inédites. – Manie durant depuis six mois. Emploi de l'opium. – Guérison rapide. (Bicêtre, service de M. Moreau)," *Annales médico-psychologiques* (1845): 312–14.

49 Michéa, *De l'emploi des opiacés*, 4.

50 Ibid., 6.

51 Baillarger, "Manie. – Influence des règles. – Emploi de l'opium. – Guérison," *Annales médico-psychologiques* (1855): 555–6.

52 Hewitt, *Institutionalizing Gender*, 10, 23–4.

53 Baillarger, "Manie," 556.

54 He claimed that the last three patients he had observed who were treated with prolonged baths had succumbed.

55 Michéa, *L'emploi des opiacés*, 7. For more on the early history of cerebral congestion, see Román, "Cerebral Congestion."

56 Binder, *Des indications de l'opium*, 32.

57 Ibid., 33.

58 L.V. Marcé, "Observation de mélancholie traitée et guérie par l'opium à haute dose," *Annales médico-psychologique* (1857): 230.

59 Ibid., 232, 234.

60 Ibid., 235.

61 Legrand du Saulle, "Recherches cliniques sur le mode d'administration de l'opium dans la manie," *Annales médico-psychologiques* (1859): 2.

62 On everyday life in French asylums, see Ripa, *Women and Madness*.

63 For example, fewer than 25 per cent of the patients admitted to the French asylums in 1874 were cured. Dowbiggin, *Institutionalizing Madness*, 17–19, 140–1. Didi-Huberman cites an even lower cure rate for Salpêtrière in 1862: 9.72 per cent. Didi-Huberman, *Invention of Hysteria*, 15.

64 Legrand du Saulle, "Recherches cliniques," 18–20.

65 Ibid., 21.

66 Ibid., 22.

67 E. Dumesnil and A. Lallier, "De l'association de la digitale à l'opium contre l'excitation dans diverses formes d'aliénation mentale," *Annales médico-psychologiques* (1868): 70–6; Dr Henne, "De l'emploi de l'opium dans le traitement des psychoneuroses," *Annales médico-psychologiques* (1871): 304–5.

68 Legrand du Saulle, "Recherches cliniques," 24.
69 Auguste Voisin, "Du traitement curatif de la folie par le chlorhydrate de morphine," *Bulletin general de thérapeutique médicale et chirurgicale* (1874): 49–54, 115–22, 154–64, 202–14, 296–309, 52.
70 Hildenbrand, "Injections médicamenteuses hypodermiques chez les aliénés," *Annales médico-psychologiques* (1869): 279–83; Krafft-Ebing, "Note sur le traitement des maladies mentales par les injections sous-cutanées de morphine," *Annales médico-psychologiques* (1870): 147–8; Dr Tigges, "Injections sous-cutanées de morphine chez les aliénés avec sensations péripheriques anormales (Dysphrenia neuralgica)," *Annales médico-psychologiques* (1871): 303.
71 Hildenbrand, "Injections médicamenteuses hypodermiques," 282.
72 Tigges, "Injections sous-cutanées," 303.
73 Krafft-Ebing is best known for his 1886 book on sexual deviance, *Psychopathia sexualis*. When he published his findings on the therapeutic value of morphine injections, he was still a young psychiatrist, having only qualified as a doctor in 1863.
74 Krafft-Ebing, "Note sur le traitement," 147.
75 Ibid., 148.
76 Pichon, *Le morphinisme*, 467.
77 Auguste Voisin was the nephew of Esquirol's student Félix Voisin.
78 A. Voisin, "Du traitement curatif."
79 A. Voisin, "Nouvelles observations," 62; A. Voisin, *Leçons cliniques sur les maladies mentales et sur les maladies nerveuses* (1883): 684–762.
80 A. Voisin, "Du traitement curatif," 49. He published additional observations on the curative treatment of madness with morphine in 1876 and then republished his research as part of his *Leçons cliniques sur les maladies mentales et sur les maladies nerveuses* (Clinical lessons on mental pathology) in 1883.
81 A. Voisin, "Du traitement curatif," 210.
82 Ibid., 211.
83 Voisin believed that it was not advisable to use morphine in cases of inflammatory madness, epileptic madness, or any form of madness accompanied by general paralysis. Ibid., 212–13.
84 Ibid., 209, 214.
85 Ibid., 115.
86 It is unlikely that this was a sign of addiction as the dose and frequency are both too low.
87 A. Voisin, "Du traitement curatif," 203.
88 Ibid., 208–10.
89 Calvet's thesis from 1876 was one of the first on chronic morphinism in France. German doctors had begun to research this condition a few years prior. Calvet, *Essai sur le morphinisme*.
90 A. Voisin, "Du traitement curatif," 303.

91 A. Voisin, "Nouvelles observations," 5.

92 The new observations from 1876 included only successful cures. This might indicate a desire to normalize morphine as a treatment for madness or that Voisin's ability to determine which cases would benefit most from the use of morphine had improved.

93 A. Voisin, "Nouvelles observations," 58–9.

94 Ibid., 5.

95 Ibid., 4.

96 He does not explain why he attempted to use this morphine-wine treatment first. It is possible he was experimenting with alternative forms of administration as a clinical experiment, though given his enthusiasm for injected morphine it is surprising.

97 A. Voisin, "Nouvelles observations," 10.

98 Ibid., 10–11.

99 A. Voisin, Leçons cliniques, 715–20.

100 Ibid., 737.

101 Ibid., 738.

102 Ibid., 281–9.

103 Ibid., 283–5, planche VII ("Folie haschischique"), photographic plates follow page 766.

104 Guba, Taming Cannabis, 21, 33, 110, 112, 164, 200–4.

105 A. Voisin, Leçons cliniques, planche VIII ("Aliénés traitées et guéries par la morphine"), photographic plates follow page 766.

106 Goldstein, Console and Classify, 323; Micale, Hysterical Men, 5, 9–10.

107 Lasègue cited in Goldstein, Console and Classify, 324.

108 Micale, Hysterical Men, esp. chap. 3 ("Charcot and La Grand Hystérie Masculine"); Goldstein, Console and Classify, 322.

109 For more on Charcot's classification of these four stages, see Didi-Huberman, Invention of Hysteria, 115; Micale, Hysterical Men, 151–2; Hustvedt, Medical Muses, 21–2; Goldstein, Console and Classify, 326–7.

110 Goldstein, Console and Classify, 337, 343–5, 375.

111 Bourneville and Regnard, Iconographie photographique (1878), 103–8.

112 Célina Marc is referred to in the Iconographie as "M...."; Bourneville and Regnard, Iconographie photographique (1877), 110.

113 Hewitt, Institutionalizing Gender, 76.

114 Bourneville and Regnard, Iconographie photographique (1877), 153.

115 Feelings of suffocation along with a laundry list of other symptoms usually preceded her hysterical attacks. Ibid., 120.

116 Ibid., 121.

117 Ibid., 135.

118 Ibid., 136–7.

119 For more on Blanche's "career" as a hysteric at Salpêtrière, see Hustvedt, Medical Muses, 33–141.

120 Bourneville and Regnard, *Iconographie photographique* (1879), 13.

121 Ibid., 34–5.

122 Ibid., 22, 35; Hustvedt, *Medical Muses*, 57, 61.

123 She appears as "Observation VI"; Terrail, *De la morphine*, 43–4.

124 Daniel Jouet claimed that Dr Levinstein was the first to distinguish between *morphinisme*, a group of somatic accidents resulting from morphine intoxication, and *morphinomanie*, a sort of "obsessive *vésanie*" comparable to dipsomania. Jouet, *Étude de morphinisme chronique*, 5–6, 23.

125 One of the earliest studies was Dr Levinstein's "Die Morphiumsucht," *Berliner Medizinische Gesellschaft* (1875).

126 Calvet, *Essai sur le morphinisme*, 1.

127 Ibid., 54.

128 Dalbanne, *Essai sur quelques accidents*. See also Black, "Doctors on Drugs."

129 Even Auguste Voisin, the greatest proponent of the curative value of morphine, occasionally used it to restrain patients and control episodes of violence. A. Voisin, "Du traitement curatif," 204–5.

130 Chambard, *Les morphinomanes*, 7.

131 Pichon, *Le morphinisme*, 457.

132 Chambard, *Les morphinomanes*, viii.

133 Pichon, *Le morphinisme*, 456.

134 Dalbanne, *Essai sur quelques accidents*, 11.

135 Ibid., 11.

136 Terrail, *De la morphine*, 24–5, 37–9.

137 Chambard, *Les morphinomanes*, 7n1.

138 Bourneville and Regnard, *Iconographie photographique* (1879), 92.

139 See chapter 4: "Sex and Drugs."

140 Out of 120 cases of morphine addiction (66 men and 54 women), Dr Pichon found that almost 50 per cent had some personal connection to medicine either professionally (e.g., doctors, pharmacists, midwives, medical students, nurses) or socially (e.g., the wives of doctors and pharmacists). Pichon, *Le morphinisme*, 16; Black, "Doctors on Drugs."

141 "De la morphinomanie," *Bulletin de la Société de thérapeutique* (1883): 29.

142 Dr Dujardin-Beaumetz suggested that the widely disparate results of research on morphine and hysteria could be attributed to diagnostic error.

143 Terrail, *De la morphine*, 7–8, 26, 22–3, 21.

144 Charcot began his Tuesday lessons in 1882. Goetz, Bonduelle, and Gelfand, *Charcot*, 243; Charcot, *Leçons du mardi à la Salpêtrière*.

145 Ball, *La morphinomanie*, 31–2.

146 Ball mentioned that she was one of the patients he had spoken about at the beginning of his lessons – in all likelihood the female hysteric to whom he introduced morphine in the first place.

147 Ball, *La morphinomanie*, 32.

148 Jouet, *Étude de morphinisme chronique*, 25.

149 At the time Jouet recorded her case, she had decreased her dose to between eleven and twelve injections per day.

150 Jouet, *Étude de morphinisme chronique*, 44.

151 Ibid., 44–5.

152 Ibid., 46.

153 Ibid., 47–8.

154 Gaudry, *Du morphinisme chronique*, 8–9.

155 Pichon, *Le morphinisme*, 387.

156 Gaudry, *Du morphinisme chronique*, 9.

157 Pichon, *Le morphinisme*, 402.

158 Ibid., 387.

159 Erlenmeyer cited in Pichon, *Le morphinisme*, 389.

160 Doctors also attempted to use hypnotic suggestion and the moral treatment to cure addiction, but these methods met with limited results.

161 For more on the treatment of morphine addiction in France, see Yvorel, *Les poisons de l'esprit*, 221–41. For example, see the case study of M. K…, who initially took up to 2 grams of morphine at a time but managed over the course of a year to reduce his dose to between 5 and 15 centigrams per day, only to experience a crisis and relapse to higher doses again. Another attempted cure achieved the same results and the patient died a year later from an illness unrelated to his morphine addiction. Calvet, *Essai sur le morphinisme*, 55–64, esp. 63. Victor Neveu-Dérotrie claims it is much more likely to see a recidivist *morphinomane* than one who has been cured. Neveu-Dérotrie, *De l'hystérie consécutive*, 32.

162 Regnier, *Essai critique sur l'intoxication*, 158–9.

163 Pichon, *Le morphinisme*, 430.

164 Yvorel, *Les poisons de l'esprit*, 223–4.

165 Ibid., 226.

166 Purportedly, the first doctor to prescribe cocaine as a treatment for morphine addiction was Dr Bentley in 1878. Courtois-Suffit and Giroux, *La cocaïne*, 14; Chambard, *Les morphinomanes*, 144.

167 Chambard, *Les morphinomanes*, 144.

168 Psychiatrists began to identify *névroses* in the 1870s. They distinguished these from cases of full-fledged insanity, classified as *maladies mentales*. Jan Goldstein has argued that psychiatrists appropriated the study and treatment of nervous disorders to develop outpatient care, expanding the psychiatry's professional reach beyond the sequestered patients of mental asylums. Goldstein, *Console and Classify*, 334, 337.

169 Durkheim, *On Morality and Society*, 152.

170 Ibid., 161. On the influence of Durkheim's sociology in *fin-de-siècle* France, see Surkis, *Sexing the Citizen*, 125–83.

171 Pichon argues that this "loss of moral temperament" that Fournier

described in his treatise on cerebral syphilis also is found in *morphinomanes.* Pichon, *Le morphinisme*, 282.

172 Ibid., 283.

173 Gaudry, *Du morphinisme chronique*, 24.

174 Neveu-Dérotrie, *De l'hystérie consécutive*, 18; Terrail, *De la morphine*, 30.

175 Jules Voisin was Auguste Voisin's cousin. His father, Benjamin Voisin (1804–1868), was the brother of the famous aliéniste Félix Voisin (1794–1872), uncle to both Jules and Auguste.

176 J. Voisin, "Morphinomanie et hystérie," *Bulletins et mémoires de la Société médicale des hôpitaux de Paris* (2 May 1890): 367–75, 368.

177 Ibid., 368–9.

178 Chambrin, *Contribution à l'étude des accidents.*

179 Neveu-Dérotrie, *De l'hystérie consécutive*, 70.

180 Dr Regnier also argued that a "good number of *fous* become victims of this habit." Regnier, *Essai critique sur l'intoxication*, 8; Neveu-Dérotrie, *De l'hystérie consécutive*, 70.

181 Neveu-Dérotrie, *De l'hystérie consécutive*, 22.

182 Dowbiggin, *Inheriting Madness*, 116–43.

183 Regnier, *Essai critique sur l'intoxication*, 49.

184 Lefèvre, *Contribution à l'étude de la morphinomanie*, 89.

185 Charles Lefèvre, "De l'internement des morphinomanes," *Annales de psychiatrie et d'hypnologie dans leurs rapports avec la psychologie et la médecine légale* (1891): 88–91, 88.

186 Paul Brouardel also complained of France's lack of special asylums for treating addiction in his 1906 medical-legal study of morphine, opium, and cocaine. Brouardel, *Opium, morphine et cocaïne*, 74. For an example of the expensive private institutions, see Piouffle, *La cure des toxicomanes.*

187 Lefèvre, "De l'internement des morphinomanes," 89.

188 Prestwich, "Family Strategies," 799–800; Hewitt, *Institutionalizing Gender*, 9, 92–9, 120–1.

189 Prestwich, "Family Strategies," 804–10.

190 Hewitt, *Institutionalizing Gender*, 93, 95–6; Weiner, *Citizen-Patient*, 249–53.

191 Lefèvre, "De l'internement des morphinomanes," 90.

192 Ibid.

193 Ibid, 91.

194 This section is a revised and expanded version of my article "Morphine on Trial: Legal Medicine and Criminal Responsibility in the *Fin de Siècle*," published in *French Historical Studies* in 2019. I would like to thank Duke University Press and the Society for French Historical Studies for their permission to reprint it here.

195 Although the *distribution* of psychotropic drugs without a medical prescription was prohibited under the 1845–46 poisonous substances legislation, the French government did not criminalize the *consumption* of

drugs until 1916. Even then, the law did not criminalize individual private consumption but only drug usage "in society." "No. 10090. – Loi ... du 12 Juillet 1916." On the criminalization of drug consumption, see Padwa, *Social Poison*, 87–91, 109–38; Yvorel, *Les poisons de l'esprit*, 237–41.

196 Pick, *Faces of Degeneration*, 42–3, 222–3; Nye, *Crime, Madness and Politics*, 12, 119–24, 232.

197 Harris, *Murders and Madness*; Nye, *Crime, Madness and Politics*; Shapiro, *Breaking the Codes*; O'Brien, "Kleptomania Diagnosis."

198 Although historians of drug addiction in France have explored the issue of criminal responsibility within larger studies of the historical sociology of drug addiction in the nineteenth century, and particularly the use of opium addiction as a legal defence in the 1908 Ullmo spy case, historians of criminology more generally have not seriously engaged with medical-legal debates over morphine addiction and criminal responsibility. On the criminal responsibility of addicts and the Ullmo spy case, see Padwa, *Social Poison*, 69, 79–84; Yvorel, *Les poisons de l'esprit*, 208–13, 218–19, 232–3.

199 Harris, *Murders and Madness*, 243.

200 On alcoholism and criminal responsibility, see Harris, *Murders and Madness*, 256–67; Nye, *Crime, Madness and Politics*, 215, 235, 240–7.

201 Although alcoholism was a condition that affected all social classes, bourgeois reformers viewed it as a stereotypical vice of the working classes, particularly after 1871. Barrows, "After the Commune," 208–9.

202 Harris, *Murders and Madness*, 4–5.

203 Falret quoted in Chambard, *Les morphinomanes*, 162–3.

204 The presence or absence of free will at the time the crime was committed was also the fundamental logic of the insanity defence in Britain and the United States. Tighe, "Legal Art," 209–10; Eigen, "Lesion of the Will."

205 Dalloz and Vergé, *Code pénal annoté*, 164.

206 The 1808 Code of Criminal Procedure distinguished between two types of French criminal courts: the *tribunaux correctionnels*, which tried misdemeanor offences (*délits*) carrying a maximum penalty of five years in prison, and the *cours d'assises*, which tried felony offences. Although the *cours d'assises* utilized a trial by jury, in the *tribunaux correctionnels* a panel of three judges presided over the court and determined both verdict and sentence. After France passed the law of 1832, the power to rule on extenuating circumstances passed from judges to juries in felony cases tried in the *cours d'assises*; however, judges continued to rule on extenuating circumstances for misdemeanor offences. Donovan, *Juries*, 41, 56–9, 195n65. For more on French criminal procedure, see Donovan, "Magistrates and Juries"; Garner, "Criminal Procedure"; Esmein, Garraud, and Mittermaier, *History*.

207 For a broad comparative history of the insanity defence, see Robinson, *Wild Beasts*.

208 Goldstein, *Console and Classify*, 163–4; Watson, *Forensic Medicine*, 74.

209 Philippe Pinel (1745–1826), Jean-Étienne-Dominique Esquirol (1772–1840), and Étienne-Jean Georget (1795–1828) were key figures in the introduction of these categories of partial insanity. Goldstein, *Console and Classify*, 152–96; see also Watson, *Forensic Medicine*, 83–6.

210 Goldstein, *Console and Classify*, 166; see also Renneville, *Crime et folie*, 97–131.

211 Harris, *Murders and Madness*, 9.

212 Catherine Crawford attributes the early use of medical experts in France to its inquisitorial justice system, which required judges to investigate and compile written dossiers of evidence to establish a true account of what occurred in each case. However, rather than assessing insanity, these early medical-legal experts most frequently conducted autopsies and assessed the wounds of living victims. For comparative perspectives on the history of legal medicine under the Anglo-American accusatory and continental inquisitorial systems, see Watson, *Forensic Medicine*; Clark and Crawford, *Legal Medicine in History*, esp. 1–21, 89–116. For a detailed account of the expansion of medical expert testimony for the insanity defence, see Guignard, "L'expertise médico-légale." On the history of legal medicine in France more broadly, see Chauvaud, *Les experts du crime*; Lecuir, "La médicalisation"; Renneville, *Crime et folie*.

213 Harris, *Murders and Madness*, 2–3, 16–17. For more on positivist criminology's challenge to classical criminological theory's emphasis on free will and morality, see Wright, *Between the Guillotine and Liberty*, 111–15, 118–28.

214 Harris, *Murders and Madness*, 2–3.

215 This is the forensic psychologist C.C. Marc's definition from 1840, cited in Abelson, "Invention of Kleptomania," 135.

216 On department stores and the rise of mass consumerism in France, see Tiersten, *Marianne in the Market*; Williams, *Dream Worlds*; Miller, *Bon Marché*.

217 O'Brien, "Kleptomania Diagnosis"; Abelson, "Invention of Kleptomania."

218 Société de médecine légale de France, "Des vols aux étalages et dans les magasins: Discussion. – MM. Lunier, Motet, Gallard, Cazin, Blanche, Le Grande du Saulle, Lasègue, Brouardel." *Annales d'hygiène publique et de médecine légale* 3, no. 6 (1881): 164–86, 261–75.

219 Ibid.

220 One of these was a case from 1872, in which D…, a thirty-one-year-old woman who had been addicted to laudanum for several years, was accused of stealing the tops of two lace parasols from her employer in order to sell them for more laudanum. The medical-legal report noted that her intense opium addiction had caused "a passing alteration of her intellectual faculties and a permanent lesion of her moral sense." The court acquitted her with a "nonsuit" and her mother paid for the stolen lace parasols. Ibid., 183–5.

221 Ibid., 273.

222 Ibid., 274.

223 Brouardel does not note what Mme C…'s sentence was, and I have been unable to locate the case in the judicial records at the Archives de la Ville de Paris. Ibid., 275.

224 Garnier took over as chief physician of the Infirmerie spéciale later that same year. Paul Garnier, "Morphinisme avec attaques hystéro-épileptiques causées par l'abstinence de la dose habituelle du poison: Vol à l'étalage," *Annales d'hygiène publique et de médecine légale* 3, no. 15 (1886): 303. Henri Guimbail made a similar observation about the increasingly frequent use of morphine addiction as a legal defence in 1891. Henri Guimbail, "Crimes et délits commis par les morphinomanes," *Annales d'hygiène publique et de médecine légale* (1891): 481–501, 488–9.

225 Harris, *Murders and Madness*, 141–2.

226 Garnier, "Morphinisme," 304–5.

227 O'Brien, "Kleptomania Diagnosis," 67.

228 Garnier, "Morphinisme," 315.

229 Ibid., 308.

230 Ibid., 309–10.

231 Ibid., 313.

232 Ibid., 313–14.

233 Gaudry, *Du morphinisme chronique*, 30–1.

234 E. Marandon de Montyel, "Contribution à l'étude de la morphinomanie." *Annales médico-psychologiques* 43, no. 1 (1885): 45–64, 46–56. The case of the lawyer, known in the medical-legal literature as Paul X…, is also cited in Gaudry, *Du morphinisme chronique*, 54, and Chambard, *Les morphinomanes*, 177–8.

235 Pichon, *Le morphinisme*, 392–402.

236 Gaudry, *Du morphinisme chronique*, 72.

237 Pichon, *Le morphinisme*, 409–10. See also Chambard, *Les morphinomanes*, 178–9.

238 Pichon, *Le morphinisme*, 388.

239 Ibid., 411.

240 Neveu-Dérotrie, *De l'hystérie consécutive*, 46.

241 Gaudry, *Du morphinisme chronique*, 71.

242 "Le morphinisme devant les tribunaux," *La Semaine médicale*, 10 May 1883, 98–99; A…-V…, Gustave, no. 25117, 15 May 1883, D1U6 5994, Archives de la Ville de Paris.

243 Auguste Motet, "Morphinomanie," *Annales d'hygiène publique et de médecine légale* 3, no. 10 (1883): 22–36, 33.

244 E. Marandon de Montyel, "De la morphinomanie dans ses rapports avec la médecine légale: Affaire des époux Fiquet," *L'Encéphale* 3, no. 1 (1883): 667–706, 688.

245 Pichon, *Le morphinisme*, 271.

246 Ibid., 279.

247 This was Erlenmeyer's term, cited in Pichon, *Le morphinisme*, 279.

248 Ibid.

249 As individuals' predispositions to the influence of morphine varied widely, medical-legal experts had to assess defendants' intellectual capacity and moral responsibility on an individual basis. Dr Pichon recommended examining the strength of an addicted defendant's general mental faculties in such cases to determine the degree of moral responsibility. Although the fact of morphine addiction alone was not enough to determine complete criminal irresponsibility, Pichon believed that in some cases severe addiction merited at least some degree of irresponsibility for its impact on the moral sense. Ibid., 279–81.

250 Annette G, no. 13964, 25 November 1885, D1 U6 244, Archives de la Ville de Paris.

251 Jean-Martin Charcot, Paul Brouardel, and Auguste Motet, "Rapport médico-légal sur Annette G… (Hystérie et morphiomanie)," *Archives de neurologie* 11 (1886): 400.

252 Ibid.

253 Ibid., 404.

254 The autopsy revealed that the girl had not been sexually assaulted, so the court never reached a satisfactory conclusion about what might have motivated the kidnapping and the murder. Marandon de Montyel, "De la morphinomanie," 701.

255 Ibid., 692–3.

256 Ibid., 682; Emile Blanche, "Procès de la femme Fiquet (de Dijon) accusé d'assassinat, morphinomanie, et simulation: Rapport médico-légal," *Annales médico-psychologiques* 6, no. 10 (1883): 234–53.

257 Marandon de Montyel, "De la morphinomanie," 677–8, 682.

258 "La morphine," *Le Figaro*, 17 and 19 November 1891.

259 Ibid. It is likely that each flask contained 30 grams of a diluted morphine solution, as consuming 120 grams of pure morphine in a single evening would kill even the most experienced addict.

260 "La morphine," *Le Figaro*, 20 November 1891.

261 The French Penal Code explicitly stated that drunkenness could not be considered a legal excuse for crimes. However, in practice, juries were asked to evaluate the criminal intent of the defendant. Ruth Harris has demonstrated that juries assessed the role of alcohol on a case-by-case basis, attempting to reconcile both "a moralistic condemnation of drunkenness and a deterministic appraisal of the irresponsible behaviour alcohol caused." Harris, *Murders and Madness*, 256.

262 "La morphine," *Le Figaro*, 21 November 1891.

263 "La morphine," *Le Figaro*, 1 December 1891.

264 "La morphine," *Le Figaro*, 10 December 1891.

265 Harris, *Murders and Madness*, 267–75.

266 On the remarkable powers of paternal authority in nineteenth-century France, see Schnapper, "La correction paternelle."

267 "Une drame épouvantable," *Le Figaro*, 19 March 1892.

268 "Tour du monde: Lyon, 21 mars," *Gil Blas*, 23 March 1892.

269 *Le Figaro*, 20 March 1892. *Gil Blas* published Porteret's letter two days after the murder and, according to Chambard, the newspaper faced punitive measures for publishing the slanderous letter of an unstable murderer. "Le drame passionnel de Lyon," *Gil Blas*, 20 March 1892. See also Chambard, *Les morphinomanes*, 180–1.

270 "Le drame passionnel de Lyon."

271 Harris, *Murders and Madness*, 208–42, 285–320.

272 On the medical-legal tropes of female crime-of-passion cases, see Shapiro, *Breaking the Codes*, 136–78.

273 Harris, *Murders and Madness*, 288.

274 Ibid., 293, 296.

275 "Le drame passionnel de Lyon."

276 A. Poncet, surgeon-major at Hôtel-Dieu, and A. Lacassagne, médecin-expert des tribunaux, conducted the autopsy on 22 March. "Tour du monde," *Gil Blas*, 26 March 1892.

277 "Justice criminelle: Cour d'Assises de la Seine; Affaire Aubert. – Pour un album de timbres-poste. – Un cadavre dans un malle. – Assassinat et vol," *Gazette des tribunaux*, 26–30 October 1896, 1076–7, 1080, 1084–5, 1088.

278 Ibid., 1076.

279 Under the French inquisitorial system, judges were responsible for compiling evidence of the defendant's guilt or innocence and calling upon expert witnesses to conduct mental examinations. Watson, *Forensic Medicine*, 9–10, 19–22.

280 It is unclear why the judge denied Aubert the right to a mental examination by a medical-legal expert. The court did use a medical expert to conduct the autopsy, a chemistry expert to examine Aubert's apartment and clothes for traces of blood, and a handwriting expert to examine the handwriting on a forged letter, purportedly from Delahaef to his father. "Affaire Aubert," 1076–7, 1080, 1084–5, 1088, 1084.

281 Ibid., 1076.

282 Ibid., 1080, 1085, 1088.

283 It is possible that this was a result of the juridical shift from the punishment fitting the crime to the punishment fitting the extent to which the criminal posed a danger to society. On this shift, see Harris, *Murders and Madness*, 80; Nye, *Crime, Madness and Politics*, 232.

284 "Affaire Aubert," 1088.

285 Ibid.

286 The Penal Code prescribed capital punishment for premeditated murder (Article 302) and for murder accompanied by another crime or

misdemeanor (Article 304). The jury also granted extenuating circumstances to Aubert's mistress, who was not present at the time of the actual murder. She received a sentence of three years' imprisonment for her role as an accomplice. Aubert, no. 1356, 29 October 1896, D1 U8 102, Archives de la Ville de Paris; *Code pénal de l'empire français*, 46.

287 Bonnet explicitly mentioned Lombroso's theory of the "born criminal" as one of the most popular contemporary theories of criminological determinism. "Affaire Aubert," 1088.

288 In cases like this involving premeditated murder, juries granting extenuating circumstances would reduce the sentence from the death penalty to hard labour for life. The judges would have had the option to reduce the penalty further, to between five and twenty-five years of hard labour. Donovan, *Juries*, 59.

289 During the period from 1894 to 1908, the conviction rate for premeditated murder in the *cours d'assises* was 75.1 per cent, compared with a 67.1 per cent conviction rate for unpremeditated murder. During that same period, juries convicted 63.3 per cent of felony cases overall. James Donovan compiled this data from the *Compte général*, published annually by the Ministry of Justice. Ibid., 74–5.

290 Donovan, "Public Opinion," 578.

291 For example, Aubert met with Delahaef several times under an assumed name and then lured Delahaef to his apartment by promising to buy the stamp collection with 4,000 francs he did not possess. A few days before the murder, Aubert had the handle reattached to the axe he used as the murder weapon. He also purchased two large trunks at the Bazar de l'Hôtel de Ville and secured some sand from his landlady for the floor of his apartment, which the prosecution interpreted as evidence of a plan to conceal evidence of the murder.

292 Donovan, *Juries*, 17, 45.

293 James Donovan has written extensively on this practice; see ibid.

294 When smoked, a considerable amount of opium's potent alkaloids was lost to combustion and pipe residue.

295 Of course, as Jean-Jacques Yvorel has demonstrated, "blameworthy" pleasure-seeking morphine addicts also became an increasing focus of popular concern, particularly as morphine addiction expanded to influence all classes of society at the end of the nineteenth century. However, medical-legal arguments about criminal responsibility focused primarily on the altered physiological equilibrium of the addicted body and its influence on individual free will, not on broader debates about the spread of morphine addiction. Most defendants explored in the medical-legal literature were iatrogenic addicts, depicted as victims of an overpowering physiological dependence with therapeutic origins. Yvorel, *Poisons de l'esprit*, 197–8.

296 Dr Dupré, "L'affaire Ullmo," *Archives d'anthropologie criminelle, de médecine légale, et de psychologie normale et pathologique* (1908): 545–85, 561. See also Datta, *Heroes and Legends*, 179–225; Padwa, *Social Poison*, 79–84; Yvorel, *Les poisons de l'esprit*, 218–19.

297 Ibid., 562–6, 565, 568–9.

298 Ibid., 569.

299 Ibid., 571.

300 The report noted that *morphinomanie* was much more difficult to cure than opium eating, which, in turn, was more difficult to cure than opium smoking. Ibid., 579.

301 Ibid., 578.

302 Venita Datta argues that the Ullmo case did not become a platform for a polarized national debate in the way that the Dreyfus case did because Ullmo's guilt was never contested. Furthermore, the fact that Ullmo was Jewish did not dominate the headlines as it had with the Dreyfus case. Datta, *Heroes and Legends*, 180, 196, 211.

303 Dupré, "L'affaire Ullmo," 585.

304 The phrasing of the 1916 legislation makes the legal status of the drug user somewhat ambiguous, as an individual's criminal culpability was based on the specific conditions of the act of consumption. Although the justice system prosecuted drug traffickers more frequently, Emmanuelle Retaillaud-Bajac has demonstrated that in the 1920s and 1930s, drug users increasingly faced criminal prosecution for the consumption of psychotropic drugs, including morphine. Retaillaud-Bajac, *Les paradis perdus*, 231–71. The 1970 drug legislation that continues to shape French drug policy today still portrays morphine addicts ambiguously, both as patients to be cured and as delinquents to be disciplined. The Law of 31 December 1970 contains more explicit language condemning the illicit use of psychotropic substances than the 1916 legislation. However, it includes provisions for mandatory therapeutic treatment options in addition to possible sentences of fines and imprisonment. "No. 70-1320. —Loi du 31 décembre 1970."

305 In their 1911 monograph on criminal responsibility, Paul Dubuisson and Auguste Vigoroux argued that legal medicine should distinguish between iatrogenic addicts, whose morphine habit developed as an unintended side effect of medical treatment, and blameworthy addicts, whose morphine habit began from wilful pleasure seeking. Dubuisson and Vigoroux compared pleasure-seeking morphine addicts to alcoholics, whom they considered to be the wilful authors of their own condition. However, in each of the three cases of morphine addiction they cited as examples, the defendants were iatrogenic addicts who were found irresponsible or deserving of lenience. Dubuisson and Vigoroux, *Responsabilité pénale*, 369–81.

CHAPTER FOUR

1 *Les Feurs du Sommeil*, an oil painting by Achille Theodore Cesbron (1849–1913) depicts a field of opium poppies with the pale nude form of a woman emerging from one of the blossoms, illustrating the imagined eroticism of opium. Cécile Paul Baudry's painting *Fumeuse d'opium* (1912) depicts a nude female opium smoker reclined in a state of ecstasy. Taillac, *Les paradis artificiels*, 54–5.
2 Willy, *Lélie, fumeuse d'opium*; Mallat de Bassilan, *La Comtesse Morphine*.
3 "Fumeries d'opium," *La Dépêche de Brest*, 7 December 1906.
4 Courtois-Suffit and Giroux, *Extension du traffic*, 482–97, 492.
5 For more on the degeneration debates, see Pick, *Faces of Degeneration*; Nye, *Crime, Madness and Politics*.
6 "Académie des sciences. Séance du 1er Février. Inhalations d'éther," *Gazette médicale de Paris*, 6 February 1847, 111–15.
7 Dr Lutaud, "Peut-on violer un femme pendant l'anesthésie?," *Revue de psychiatrie* 4 (1901): 76–80, 77.
8 "Pharmacien in Trouble," *Pharmaceutical Journal* 66 (8 February 1901): 124.
9 Lutaud, "Peut-on violer," 77.
10 Vigarello, *History of Rape*, 130, 134–40.
11 Lutaud, "Peut-on violer," 78.
12 Vigarello, *History of Rape*, 141.
13 Lutaud, "Peut-on violer," 78.
14 Ibid., 79.
15 Tourdes and Metzquer, *Traité de médecine légale*, 215.
16 Baron, Étude psychologique, 110; Dolbeau, "De l'emploi du chloroforme au pointe de vue de la perpétration des crimes et délits," *Annales d'hygiène publique et de médecine légale* (1874): 168–84, 170; Vigarello, *History of Rape*, 136.
17 Baron, Étude psychologique, 109.
18 In Willy's 1911 novel, *Lélie, fumeuse d'opium*, M. Lorbin, a handsome young opportunist, lures wealthy young heiress Lélie into an opium den, using the drug to lower her inhibitions in an attempt to seduce her and seize her fortune. Willy, *Lélie, fumeuse d'opium*. The mimodrama *Ivresse d'opium*, written by Lucien Kra and René Louis around 1919, reverses the gender dynamics of the opium seduction plot. Gilda, the wife of a French engineer stationed in Cambodia, uses opium to try to seduce their native servant Divaï. When he becomes unresponsive to her seductions following a large dose of opium, she murders him in a fit of rage. Kra and Louis, *Ivresse d'opium*.
19 Cited in Vigarello, *History of Rape*, 136.
20 Béchet, *Le Docteur Morphine*.
21 Vigarello, *History of Rape*, 136.

22 Hewitt, *Institutionalizing Gender*, 9–10; Quin and Bohuon, "Muscles," 172–86; Foucault, *History of Sexuality*, 104, 121, 153.

23 Lutaud, "Peut-on violer," 79 (italics in original).

24 Ibid., 79.

25 Ibid., 80.

26 Rey, *Histoire de la douleur*, 194; Tourdes and Metzquer, *Traité de médecine légale*, 215.

27 Lacassagne, "Des phenomens psychologiques avant, pendant et après l'anesthésie provoquée," *Mémoires de l'Académie de médecine* 29 (1869): 1–72, 45, 65.

28 Ibid, 45.

29 Ibid.

30 Courty cited in ibid., 47.

31 Ibid., 64.

32 Ibid., 65.

33 Ibid.

34 Although more people became addicted to morphine as a result of medical treatment than from pleasure seeking, morphine gained a reputation as an aphrodisiac in the popular imagination, which contributed, in part, to the expansion of addiction in French society.

35 Pouchet, *Leçons de pharmacodynamie*, 594.

36 Piouffle, *Les psychoses cocaïniques*, 131.

37 André Cleyer had observed its use as an aphrodisiac in the Far East in 1642. Fonssagrives, "Anaphrodisie et aphrodisiaques (thérapeutique)," in Dechambre, *Dictionnaire encyclopédique* (1870), 109.

38 Virey, *Des médicamens aphrodisiaques*, 13–14.

39 Corbin, *Women for Hire*, 23–4. As medical research on the hereditary transmission of syphilis became more sophisticated in the 1870s and 1880s, fears of venereal contagion compounded this demographic threat. Nye, *Crime, Madness and Politics*, 158–69; Surkis, *Sexing the Citizen*, 189–211.

40 On how the illegal opiate trade eluded regulation in France leading up to the 1916 poisonous substances legislation, see Padwa, *Social Poison*, 109–27.

41 Procurer of Rennes to the Minister of Justice, handwritten letter, 17 June 1909, Correspondance Générale de la Division Criminelle, Le Cour d'Appel de Rennes, BB18 2488 (2), Archives Nationales.

42 The non-medical consumption of opium was not considered a crime until the 1916 poisonous substances legislation.

43 Padwa, *Social Poison*, 86–91, 115–37; Boekhout van Solinge, "Handling Drugs," 37–47.

44 Brunet, *Une avarie d'extrême-orient*, 24–5.

45 On the history and organization of the French police, see Berlière and Lévy, "Evolving Organization of Policing."

46 Corbin, *Women for Hire*, 77; Harsin, *Policing Prostitution*, 6, 39.
47 Report to the Procurer General of the Cour d'Appel de Rennes, Paris, 12 April 1912, Correspondance Générale de la Division Criminelle, Le Cour d'Appel de Rennes, BB18 2488 (2), Archives Nationales. In the world of prostitution, Alain Corbin distinguishes the *amant de coeur*, the kept lover of a prostitute chosen to satisfy a need for affection, from the *souteneur* (pimp). Corbin, *Women for Hire*, 155–6.
48 Report to the Procurer General of the Cour d'Appel de Rennes, Paris, 12 April 1912.
49 Ibid.
50 Cour d'Appel de Rennes (Brest), letter, 21 September 1912, BB18 2488 (2), Archives Nationales.
51 Report to the Procurer General of the Cour d'Appel de Rennes, Paris, 12 April 1912.
52 Commissaire spécial de Police, Toulon, to M. Le Commissaire Principal Chargé du Contrôle Général des Services de Recherche à Paris, letter, 11 May 1912, BB12 2488 (2) Archives Nationales.
53 Parquet du Procureur générale, Direction Criminelle, to Garde des Sceaux, Ministre de la Justice, letter, 19 March 1913, BB12 2488 (2), Archives Nationales.
54 Procurer General, Cour d'Appel de Rennes, to the Ministry of Justice, letter, 29 May 1913, BB18 2488 (2), Archives Nationales.
55 Cour d'Appel de Rennes to the Ministry of Justice, letter, 14 June 1913, BB18 2488 (2), Archives Nationales.
56 Cour d'Appel de Rennes to Ministry of Justice, 14 June 1913.
57 It is unclear from the archives whether the police ever attempted to carry out this plan.
58 "Mort d'une fumeuse d'opium," *Journal des débats politiques et littéraires*, 17 August 1908.
59 Procurer General of Rennes to the Ministry of Justice, letter, 31 May 1913, BB18 2488 (2), Archives Nationales.
60 Procurer General of Rennes to the Ministry of Justice, letter, 30 May 1913, BB18 2488 (2), Archives Nationales.
61 The Ministry of Navy to the Minister of Justice, letter, 11 December 1923, File 978.A.12 Rennes-Aix, 14-12-23, Affairs de stupéfiants et interdiction de sejour (Brest et Toulon), BB18 2488 (2), Archives Nationales.
62 Gustave le Poittevin, vice-president à la cour d'appel de Paris, to a minister [minister of justice?], letter, 25 August [year torn off], BB18 2488 (2), Archives Nationales.
63 Yvorel, *Les poisons de l'esprit*, 161.
64 Piouffle, *Les psychoses cocaïniques*, 132.
65 Courtois-Suffit and Giroux, *La cocaïne*, 10.
66 Ibid., 16.
67 Charles Bernard's report in the name of the commission of public hygiene, 15

February 1916, Folder: Opium, Dossier de Principe, Document No. 1802, Chambre des Députées, Procès verbal, BB18 2488 (2), Archives Nationales.

68 Retaillaud-Bajac, *Les paradis perdus*, 138–40.

69 The vast zone that encompasses Montmartre, the Faubourg-Montmartre, the neighborhood around l'Europe, La Madelaine, and Étoile comprises 42.7 per cent of the users and 49.2 per cent of the *"détenteurs"* in Retaillaud-Bajac's statistics. Ibid., 138.

70 Ibid., 139.

71 Ibid., 132.

72 Chambard, *Les morphinomanes*, 79.

73 Ibid., 8.

74 Guimbail, "Crimes et délits commis par les morphinomanes," *Annales d'hygiène publique et de médecine légale* (1891): 481–501, 486.

75 Chevallier, *Essai sur le cocaïnisme nasal*, 31, cited in Yvorel, *Les poisons de l'esprit*, 160.

76 Courtois-Suffit and Giroux, *La cocaïne*, 161.

77 Courtois-Suffit claimed to have seen prices of 20, 30, 60, and even 80 francs per gram for black-market cocaine. Courtois-Suffit et Giroux, *Extension du traffic*, 494.

78 Courtois-Suffit and Giroux, *La cocaïne*, 56–7.

79 Yvorel, *Les poisons de l'esprit*, 163.

80 Armengaud, *La population française*, 47, 108; Nye, *Crime, Madness and Politics*, 134.

81 Accampo, "Gendered Nature," 236.

82 Nye, *Crime, Madness and Politics*, 135; McMillan, *France and Women*, 48.

83 Nye, "Sexuality," 63.

84 Nye, *Masculinity*, 75.

85 Fonssagrives, "Anaphrodisie et aphrodisiaques," 108–9, 121.

86 Ibid., 108.

87 Fauconney, *L'impuissance et la stérilité*, 7.

88 Jouet, Étude sur le morphinisme chronique, 39; Ball, *La morphinomanie*, 24; Pichon, *Le morphinisme*, 118–19; Chambard, *Les morphinomanes*, 100–1; Pouchet, *Leçons de pharmacodynamie*, 829; Noirot, *Des troubles génitaux*, 20; Fauconney, *Les morphinomanes*, 39–40; Dupouy, *Les opiomanes*, 34–6; Gamel, *Chiqueurs, mangeurs, buveurs*, 61.

89 Courtois-Suffit and Giroux, *Extension du traffic*, 488.

90 Chambard, *Les morphinomanes*, 101.

91 Alfred Fouillée, "La Psychologie des sexes et ses fondements physiologiques," *Revue des deux mondes* 119 (September 1893): 400, quoted in Nye, *Masculinity*, 88. Scientists had been aware of the existence of male sperm since 1677, when Dutch scientist Anton van Leuwenhoek discovered that male ejaculate contained millions of tiny "animalcules." Thomas Laqueur argues that from that point forward, sperm and egg could be

used to represent man and woman as descriptors of the biology of sexual difference. Laqueur, *Making Sex*, 171.

92 Noirot, *Des troubles génitaux*, 20–1. See also Fauconney, *Les morphinomanes*, 42, 47.

93 As Emily Martin has demonstrated, the myth of the active sperm and passive egg was constructed to reflect patriarchal gender norms rather than to reflect the actual nature of the interactions between these gametes during reproduction. Martin, "Egg and the Sperm."

94 Nye, *Masculinity*; Forth, *Dreyfus Affair*.

95 Forth, *Dreyfus Affair*, 11. Rather than treating this gender instability as a "crisis," Judith Surkis seeks to displace the framework of a "crisis" of masculinity, arguing that "masculinity, and the gender and sexual order that organized it, were … contingent norms, constituted by ever-present possibilities of abnormal deviation." Surkis, *Sexing the Citizen*, 12, 71.

96 Pouchet, *Leçons de pharmacodynamie*, 595–6; Pichon, *Le morphinisme*, 119.

97 Nicolas, *Quelques recherches*, 33.

98 Ibid., 32.

99 On masturbation as both a measure of and catalyst for deviant sexuality, see Laqueur, *Solitary Sex*; Rosario, *Erotic Imagination*.

100 Nicolas, *Quelques recherches*, 33.

101 Dupouy, *Les opiomanes*, 176.

102 Nicolas, *Quelques recherches*, 33.

103 Ibid., 34.

104 Noirot, *Des troubles génitaux*.

105 Laqueur, *Making Sex*, vii–viii, 3.

106 G. Tourdes, "Anaphrodisie et aphrodisiaques (Médecine légale)" in Dechambre, *Dictionnaire encyclopédique* (1870), 122.

107 Noirot, *Des troubles génitaux*, 17–18.

108 Ibid., 20.

109 Tourdes, "Anaphrodisie et aphrodisiaques," 122.

110 Observation 9: Mme B…, quoted from Veisenburger's 1894 thesis. Noirot, *Des troubles génitaux*, 45.

111 Ibid., 25, 28. With a few exceptions, Jouet generally supports this claim as well. Jouet, *Étude sur le morphinisme chronique*, 39.

112 Observation 2 (Lutaud), cited in Noirot, *Des troubles génitaux*, 41–2.

113 Ibid., 26.

114 Nye, *Masculinity*, 114.

115 Millant, *La drogue*, 294.

116 Charles Féré quoted in Nye, *Masculinity*, 113.

117 Rosario, *Erotic Imagination*, 77; Morel, *Traité des dégénérescences*.

118 Nye, "Sexuality," 66.

119 Piouffle, *Les psychoses cocaïniques*, 132.

120 Ibid., 133.

121 Francis Amery, "Afterward: Some Observations on *Monsieur de Phocas*," in Lorrain, *Monsieur de Phocas*, 268.

122 Despite Lorrain's own openness about his sexuality, the same-sex desire in *Monsieur de Phocas* remains veiled and implied, channeled through the fetishization of eyes and the eroticism of Freneuse's ultimate murder of Ethal. Du Plessis, "Unspeakable Writing," 69, 74, 81.

123 Lorrain, *Monsieur de Phocas*, 133, 155.

124 Ibid, 135–6.

125 Ibid., 141.

126 Sibalis, "Regulation of Male Homosexuality," 83, 93–6; Rosario, *Erotic Imagination* 72–3; Nye, *Masculinity*, 106–7.

127 Thompson, "Creating Boundaries," 115–17; Choquette, "Homosexuals in the City," 155–6; Rosario, *Erotic Imagination*, 76–7.

128 Rosario, *Erotic Imagination*, 83–9.

129 "Les stupéfiants et la santé publique: La loi du 12 Juillet 1916 doit-êlle être réformé?," 19 July 1921, Correspondance Générale de la Division Criminelle, File: 978 A 12, Lyon, Ligue d'Hygiène Mentale, BB18 2488 (2), Archives Nationales.

130 Michaut, "Syphilis et pédérastie, fumeurs d'opium et climat," *Bulletin générale de thérapeutique médicale et chirurgicale* (1893): 274–279, 277. Along with "sodomite," the term "pederast" was used in nineteenth-century Paris to describe men who had sex with other men. The term "homosexuality" did not enter mainstream medical language in France until the 1890s. Peniston, *Pederasts and Others*, 2; Nye, *Masculinity*, 108.

131 Letter, 28 March 1916, Correspondance Générale de la Division Criminelle, Cour d'Aix, 978 A 12, Dossier Borie, Administrateur de la Marine à Nice, BB18 2488 (2), Archives Nationales.

132 Commissaire Central de la Ville de Nice to Procurer de la République, Nice, letter, 30 March 1916, Cour d'Aix, 978 A 12, Dossier Borie, Administrateur de la Marine à Nice, BB18 2488 (2), Archives Nationales.

133 On associations of opium with irregular sexual practices in French Indochina, see Proschan, "'Syphilis, Opiomania, and Pederasty.'"

134 Commissaire Central de la Ville de Nice to Procurer de la République, Nice, 30 March 1916.

135 Fauconney, *Les morphinomanes*, 24.

136 Tailhade, La "noire idole"; Millant, *La drogue*, 21.

137 Millant, *La drogue*, v.

138 "Document No. 2715, Chambre des Députées, Séance du 14 mai 1913," File: Opium, Dossier de Principe, BB18 2488 (2), Archives Nationales.

139 Jouet, Étude sur le morphinisme chronique, 46.

140 Chambard, *Les morphinomanes*, 24–5.

141 Moore and Cryle, "Frigidity at the Fin de Siècle," 250.

142 Although most medical statistics on morphine addiction include a

far greater number of male addicts than female ones, many doctors still supported the claim that female morphine use was more widespread. They explained the discrepancy in the statistics by claiming that women visited doctors at lower rates than men. Yvorel argues that this might have been a way for doctors to minimize the medical profession's culpability in the spread of morphine addiction that resulted from therapeutic practices. Yvorel, *Les poisons de l'esprit*, 137–8.

143 On the role of the bourgeois domestic interior as an important site for social and political debates over the moral regeneration of bourgeois private life during the Second Empire, see Nord, *Republican Moment*, 218–44. Although domestic spaces were strongly associated with bourgeois motherhood, as Mary Louise Roberts argues, throughout the nineteenth century domesticity was exposed as an ideology rather than a predetermined female destiny. Roberts, *Disruptive Acts*, 6.

144 Another possible interpretation is that the painting depicts a single woman in three different stages of intoxication. However, in either case, the eroticism of the image and its emphasis on self-induced pleasure and voyeurism highlight morphine's associations with female eroticism.

145 [Georges] Moreau de Tours, "Les Morphinées," *Le Petit Journal: Supplement Illustré*, 21 February 1891.

146 Rosario, *Erotic Imagination*, 26, 50.

147 Chambard, *Les morphinomanes*, 12–13; Goron, *Les parias de l'amour*, 129–30; Guimbail, *Les morphinomanes*; Fauconney, *Les morphinomanes*, 15; Bachmann and Coppel, *La drogue*, 134–5.

148 Chambard, *Les morphinomanes*, 12.

149 Goron, *Les parias de l'amour*, 129.

150 This expression refers to the *demimonde*, a common late nineteenth-century term for the class of women of loose sexual morals, including courtesans and mistresses who had lost their position in respectable society. The expression does not translate well into English, but *demi* ("half") and *quart du* ("a quarter") *monde* suggests that he is referring to mistresses, courtesans, prostitutes, and everyone in between.

151 Goron, *Les parias de l'amour*, 130.

152 Ibid., 130–1.

153 Ball quoted in Fauconney, *Les morphinomanes*, 15.

154 Rosario, *Erotic Imagination*, 31.

155 Surkis, *Sexing the Citizen*, 54.

156 Pedersen, "Regulating Abortion," 680–1; Schneider, *Quality and Quantity*, 39.

157 Mallat de Bassilan, *La Comtesse Morphine*, v.

158 Ibid., 54.

159 Ibid., 120–1.

160 Ibid., 134.

161 Ibid., 141.

162 Ibid., 145–6.
163 Ibid., 268.
164 Ibid., 278.
165 Ibid., 288.
166 Ibid., 67.
167 Pouchet, *Leçons de pharmacodynamie*, 830.
168 Pichon, *Le morphinisme*, 119.
169 Henri Guimbail, "L'affaire Wladimiroff, Étude médico-légale sur un cas de morphinomanie conjugale," *Annales de psychiatrie et d'hypnologie* (1891): 38–46, 40.
170 Ibid., 40–1.
171 This practice was not limited to morphine. According to Courtois-Suffit, when cocaine became popular after the turn of the century, "*cocaïonomanie à deux*" – or conjugal cocaine addiction – became "relatively frequent" as well. Courtois-Suffit, *La cocaïne*, 9.
172 Nye, *Masculinity*, 81; Surkis, *Sexing the Citizen*, 154.
173 "Gazette des Tribunaux: L'Affaire Wladimiroff," *Le Figaro*, 19 January 1891, 3; "Gazette des Tribunaux: L'Affaire Wladimiroff," *Le Figaro*, 22 January 1891, 2–3.
174 Guimbail, "L'affaire Wladimiroff," 43.
175 Ball, *La morphinomanie*, 40–1.
176 Observation 4. Mme E… (Lutaud), cited in Noirot, *Les troubles génitaux*, 42–3.
177 McMillan, *France and Women*, 51–2.
178 Guimbail, "Crimes et délits," 495.
179 Ibid., 499.
180 Courtois-Suffit et Giroux, *Extension du traffic*, 492.
181 Ibid., 492–3.
182 This was also a trope of medical literature on alcoholism at the time, which reformers viewed as another major sign and symptom of national degeneration.
183 Brouardel, *Opium, morphine, et cocaïne*, 68.
184 Piouffle, *Les psychoses cocaïnique*, 131.
185 Lutaud, *Du vaginisme*, 3, 5, 13.
186 Ibid., 15.
187 Ibid., 18–19.
188 Ibid., 20, 22.
189 While historians of medicine often point to Carl Koller's research on cocaine from 1884 as a major breakthrough in local anesthesia, doctors had been experimenting with different types of topical and local anesthetics for decades, including opiates, refrigeration, and the local application of ether, with some limited success. Rey, *Histoire de la douleur*, 211.
190 Lutaud, *Du vaginisme*, 44–9.

191 Ibid., 23, 33, 37.
192 Cazin, "Traitement du vaginisme par la cocaïne," *La revue médico-chirurgicale des maladies des femmes* (1885): 155–6, 155.
193 Ibid., 156.
194 Plott, "Rules of the Game."
195 Cazin, "Traitement du vaginisme," 156.
196 Garnier, *Anomalies sexuelles*, 136.
197 Ibid., 135.
198 Ibid., 136.
199 Franc, *De l'anesthésie locale*, 12; Jules Bautaud, "Des applications thérapeutiques de la cocaïne en gynécologie," *La Revue médico-chirurgicale des maladies des femmes* (1885): 208–10.
200 Bautaud, "Des applications thérapeutiques," 220.

CHAPTER FIVE

1 Gerdy, *Pathologie générale*, 173.
2 England had specialist anesthetists – that is, trained experts who controlled the application of anesthetic agents during surgical procedures – from the very beginning. John Snow (1813–1858) from Yorkshire, who administered anesthesia to Queen Victoria during the birth of her son Leopold in 1853, was the first professional anesthetist. France, however, did not have specialists for administering anesthesia at the time. Duncum, *Development of Inhalation Anaesthesia*, 19; Auvrard and Caubet, *Anesthésie*, 1–2.
3 Nye, *Masculinity*, 218; Nye, *Crime, Madness and Politics*, 310–29.
4 Nye, *Masculinity*, 218–19.
5 Accampo, *Blessed Motherhood*, 33.
6 Rey, *Histoire de la douleur*, 6–7; Bourke, *Story of Pain*, 7–19.
7 Rey, *Histoire de la douleur*, 59, 66–7, 104–6; Bourke, *Story of Pain*, 88–130.
8 Rey, *Histoire de la douleur*, 107–10, 113–21.
9 Ibid., 154–5. See also Peter, "Silence et cris."
10 Gelfand, *Professionalizing Modern Medicine*, 12.
11 "Lettre de M. Alphonse Sanson sur les divers moyens de rendre les malades insensibles pendant les opérations chirurgicales," *Bulletin de l'Académie de médecine* 12 (19 January 1847): 273–4; Auvrard and Caubet, *Anesthésie*, 3; Rey, *Histoire de la douleur*, 149–55; Peter, "Silence et cris," 184.
12 Velpeau, *Leçons orales de clinique*, 59.
13 Ibid., 65–6.
14 Peter, "Silence et cris," 185.
15 Ibid., 187–8.
16 Rey, *Histoire de la douleur*, 167.
17 Roux, "Physiologie. – Sur les effets d'éther," *Comptes rendus des séances de l'Académie des sciences* 24 (1 February 1847): 145–9, 148–9.

18 Velpeau, "Physiologie. – Sur les effets d'éther," and Magendie, "Remarques
    … à l'occasion de cette communication," *Comptes rendus des séances de
    l'Académie des sciences* 24 (1 February 1847): 129–44. For more on this
    debate, see Rey, *Histoire de la douleur*, 192–5.

19 Peter, "Silence et cris," 180–3.

20 Magendie, "Remarques," 143.

21 Ibid., 134.

22 Velpeau, "Physiologie," 141.

23 H. Scoutetten, "Histoire du chloroforme et de l'anesthésie en général," in
    *Extrait des Travaux de la Société des Sciences médicales de la Moselle, 1852–
    1853* (Metz: Verronnais, 1853), 4, in Baron Larrey, *Mélanges sur l'Anesthésie*,
    L 1278/ F. 63, Bibliothèque Centrale de Val-de-Grace.

24 Velpeau, "Physiologie," 141.

25 Lordat, *Extrait de la dernière leçon*.

26 Ozanam, *L'anesthésie*, 20.

27 Scoutetten, "Histoire du chloroforme," 4.

28 Lacassagne, "Des phenomens psychologiques avant, pendant et après
    l'anesthésie provoquée," *Mémoires de l'Académie de médecine* 29 (1869),
    1–72, 32.

29 Bouisson cited in ibid., 21.

30 Scoutetten, "Histoire du chloroforme," 5.

31 "M. Marshall," *La Presse*, 29 January 1847, 4.

32 Advertisements from all three dentists appeared in *La Presse* on 7 February
    1847.

33 Velpeau, "Communication relative aux effets de l'éther introduit par la
    respiration," *Comptes rendus des séances de l'Académie des sciences* 24 (25
    January 1847): 91–4, 93.

34 For more on the introduction of ether anesthesia in France, see Zimmer,
    Histoire de l'anesthésie.

35 Flourens, "Note touchant l'action de l'éther sur les centres nerveux,"
    Comptes rendus des séances de l'Académie des sciences 24 (8 March 1847):
    340–4.

36 Zimmer, *Histoire de l'anesthésie*, 237.

37 In Lyon, however, doctors were suspicious of chloroform and continued to
    employ ether for surgical operations. Ibid, 257–61, 300–2.

38 Gorré, "Observation sur un cas de mort causée par l'inhalation du
    chloroforme," *Bulletin de l'Académie de médecine* 13 (4 July 1848): 1144–60.

39 Gorré was chief surgeon at the hospital of Boulogne. Ibid., 1148.

40 Ibid., 1149.

41 Surprisingly, no one seems to have criticized Gorré and his colleague for
    not realizing that their patient was dead for two hours. Ibid., 1150.

42 Ibid., 1152–3.

43 Gorré cited the case of Hannah Greener, a fifteen-year-old girl who had
    died while under the influence of chloroform for a toenail extraction

in December 1847. Ibid., 1145–8. The following week, Dr Robert presented another case of sudden chloroform death. His patient, Daniel Schlyg, was a twenty-four-year-old Alsacian who had been shot in the thigh during the June Days. Weakened by a huge loss of blood, he died on the operating table under the influence of chloroform while undergoing amputation. *Bulletin de l'Académie de médecine* 13 (11 July 1848): 1173–4.

44 *Bulletin de l'Académie de médecine* 13 (4 July 1848): 1155–6.

45 *Bulletin de l'Académie de médecine* 13 (25 July 1848): 1209–10.

46 Only Gorré's and Robert's cases occurred in France. There were several in Britain, one in America, and one woman in Hyderabad in British India. "Sur divers cas de mort attribués au chloroforme, et sur les dangers qui peut présenter l'inhalation de cet agent; par une commission composée de MM. Roux, Velpeau, Bégin, Jules Cloquet, Amussat, Jobert, Honoré, Poiseuille, Bussy, Renaud, Gibert, Guibourt, et Malgaigne, rapporteur," *Bulletin de l'Académie de médecine* 14 (31 October 1848): 201–55, 243.

47 For example, in Maria Stock's case, the commission concluded that her death could have occurred unexpectedly for reasons unrelated to chloroform inhalations. It noted that a large quantity of air had been found in her blood during the autopsy. In the case of Daniel Schlyg, the commission argued that the severe blood loss had weakened him and most likely caused his death, and not the chloroform. Ibid., 219–20, 242–3.

48 Methods of administration varied widely, with some practitioners favoring specific apparatuses and others administering chloroform using a simple handkerchief. Dosage was incredibly difficult to measure precisely because chloroform evaporates very quickly. Also, because different patients required different doses to produce insensibility, a standard dosage could not be established. "Discussion du rapport sur divers cas de mort attribué au chloroforme, et sur les dangers que peut présenter l'inhalation de cet agent," *Bulletin de l'Académie de médecine* 14 (7 November 1848): 260–79, 266.

49 J. Guérin, *Bulletin de l'Académie de médecine* 14 (14 November 1848): 289–305, 302, 305.

50 J. Guérin, *Bulletin de l'Académie de médecine* 14 (9 January 1849): 396–411.

51 "Discussion du rapport," 279.

52 "Suite de la discussion sur le chloroforme," *Bulletin de l'Académie de médecine* 14 (12 December 1848): 355–9, 357.

53 Roux, "Suite de la discussion sur le chloroforme," *Bulletin de l'Académie de médecine* 14 (16 January 1849): 419–31, 423.

54 Ibid., 428–9.

55 Amusat, *Bulletin de l'Académie de médecine* 14 (23 January 1849): 450–1.

56 Roux, "Suite de la discussion," 423.

57 While most French practitioners sanctioned its use in complicated births that required the intervention of the obstetrician, the official teachings of French obstetrics advised against anesthesia in cases of natural childbirth. Even

after the introduction of local anesthetics in the late nineteenth century, opponents to anesthesia during natural childbirth remained entrenched in their positions into the twentieth century. Thébaud, *Quand nos grand-mères donnaient la vie*, 179. Auvrard and Caubet describe the 1890s as a period of "triumph" for obstetric anesthesia. Émile Dutertre claimed that in France natural childbirth anesthesia was still proscribed by official teachings in 1882 when he published his monograph on the subject. Dutertre, *De l'emploi du chloroforme*, 6, 14.

58 Gélis, *History of Childbirth*, 155.

59 Simpson, *Answer to the Religious Objections*.

60 Historian Jules Michelet (1798–1874) was one of the most prominent nineteenth-century thinkers who adopted this view of women defined through the cyclical processes of nature. Jordanova, *Sexual Visions*, 79–86; Accampo, *Blessed Motherhood*, 3, 6; Hewitt, *Institutionalizing Gender*, 10, 23–4. On Enlightenment associations of women and nature, see Steinbrügge, *Moral Sex*, 28–30; Lacqueur, *Making Sex*, 193–223.

61 This does not necessarily mean that opponents did not have religious objections. It is possible that they might have believed such arguments would not have held much weight with their medical colleagues. Dutertre, *De l'emploi du chloroform*, 170–6; Chaigneau, *Étude comparative*, 51.

62 Accampo, "Class and Gender," 99.

63 Accampo, *Blessed Motherhood*, 4–6. On women's exclusion from the public sphere in the aftermath of the French Revolution, see Landes, *Women and the Public Sphere*. On the importance of women's role in raising future republican citizens by serving as mother-educators within the family, see Pope, "Maternal Education"; L.L. Clark, *Schooling the Daughters*, 13–59; Popiel, *Rousseau's Daughters*; Offen, *Debating the Woman Question*, 18, 53–9.

64 Accampo, *Blessed Motherhood*, 9–10.

65 On the demographic crisis, see Pick, *Faces of Degeneration*; Nye, *Crime, Madness and Politics*; Offen, "Depopulation, Nationalism, and Feminism."

66 Rey, *Histoire de la douleur*, 188; Caton, *What a Blessing*.

67 P. Dubois, "De l'application de l'inhalation de l'éther aux accouchements," *Bulletin de l'Académie de médecine* 12 (23 February 1847): 400–11.

68 Dr Fournier-Deschamps used ether in childbirth for the first time in France on 29 January 1847. Dubois cited only this case and Simpson's research as precedents for his 8 February case. "Inspiration d'éther. Application du forceps," *Gazette des hôpitaux* 9, no. 12 (30 January 1847): 52; Blot, *De l'anesthésie*, 8–9.

69 Dubois, "De l'application de l'inhalation," 401.

70 Ergot (*seigle ergoté*) is a fungus that both doctors and midwives used to try to induce labour.

71 Dubois, "De l'application de l'inhalation," 402.

72 Ibid., 402–3.

73 Ibid., 407–8.

74 Ibid., 408–11.

75 "De l'anesthésie dans les accouchements simples," *Bulletin de la Société de chirurgie* 4 (24 May 1854): 560–70.

76 Charles James Campbell noted that this statistic refered to births since 1850. Campbell, *Mémoire sur l'anesthésie obstétricale*.

77 For more on Queen Victoria's use of chloroform, see Dutertre, *De l'emploi du chloroforme*, 12–13.

78 Campbell, *Mémoire sur l'anesthésie obstétricale*, 3–4.

79 Caesarian sections on live mothers were quite rare interventions before the nineteenth century because of their high mortality rate – as much as 66 per cent. Brockliss and Jones, *Medical World*, 560–1. In the nineteenth century, C-sections had a mortality rate of 50 per cent for both mother and child. To combat peritonitis (abdominal inflammation caused by infection), doctors had two options: first, the Porro C-Section, a radical intervention in which the uterus was removed following the C-section; and second, the uterine suture, first practiced by Dr Jean Lebas in 1769 and popularized in the 1860s. Michel Dumas cites statistics of 1,097 Porro C-Sections performed between 1876 and 1901, with only a 24.8 per cent mortality rate for the mother and 22 per cent for the child, which was significantly less than the classical C-section, with a mortality rate of 50 per cent. Dumas, "Historique de la césarienne," 39. Hélène Gorodnianskaia's statistics on C-section mortality at the Maternity Hospital in Lausanne, published in 1904, were much lower: 12.61 per cent for mothers and 9.3 per cent for infants. These figures included a combination of suturing and Porro procedures. Gorodnianskaia, *Étude statistique*, 17.

80 On the history of midwifery and of midwives' gradual subordination to male obstetricians, see Gélis, *La sage-femme*, 289–327; Stock-Morton, "Control and Limitation."

81 Pajot, "Anésthésie obstétricale," in Dechambre, *Dictionnaire encyclopédique* (1870), 494.

82 Ibid., 493–4.

83 Chaigneau, *Étude comparative*, 29; Auvrard and Caubet, *Anesthésie*, 11–14.

84 M.R. Lee, "Dix-Sept cas d'accouchements dans lequel l'emploi du chloroforme fut suivi d'effets pernicieux," *Gazette médicale de Paris* 3, no. 9 (1854): 573.

85 Houzelot, *Anesthésie obstétricale*; Campbell, *Mémoire sur l'anesthésie obstétricale*, 3–4.

86 Laborie, "De l'anesthésie dans les accouchements simples," *Bulletin de la Société de chirurgie* 4 (24 May 1854): 560–70, 562–3.

87 Lebert, *Des accouchements sans douleur*, 2–3.

88 Depaul, *Leçons de clinique obstétricale*, 431.

89 Lebert, *Des accouchements sans douleur*, 2.

90 Obstetric patient case notes from Charles James Campbell, Ms 115 (1047), fol. 184, 246, 290, 311, Bibliothèque de l'Académie Nationale de Médecine.

91 Pajot, "Anésthésie obstétricale," 492–3, 496.

92 Dr Piachaud recounted this case, which the American doctor had shared at an obstetric conference in Geneva. Auvrard and Caubet, *Anesthésie*, 14.

93 Poovey, "'Scenes,'" 145–6.

94 Pajot, "Anésthésie obstétricale," 497; Auvrard and Caubet, *Anesthésie*, 13.

95 Blot, *De l'anesthésie*, 31.

96 Blot also cited Lebreton's observations of chloroform calming nervous accidents published in *Revue Scientifique* (February 1848). Ibid., 41, 50.

97 Houzelot, *Anesthésie obstétricale*, 21–2.

98 Pajot, "Anésthésie obstétricale," 496; Blot, *De l'anesthésie*, 42; Chaigneau, Étude comparative, 9.

99 "De l'anesthésie dans les accouchements simples," *Bulletin de la Société de chirurgie* 4 (24 May 1854): 560–70, 567.

100 Houzelot, *Anesthésie obstétricale*, 17.

101 Auvrard and Caubet, *Anesthésie*, 5; Dumontpallier, cited in Chaigneau, Étude comparative, 59.

102 Bailly, "De l'anesthésie dans les accouchements naturels et d'un nouvel appareil (appareil de Legroux) pour administrer le chloroforme aux femmes en couches," *Bulletin générale de thérapeutique* (1878): 8–18, 8.

103 Franc, *De l'anesthésie locale*, 21.

104 Bailly, "De l'anesthésie," 9.

105 See also Dutertre, *De l'emploi du chloroforme*, 306.

106 Chaigneau, Étude comparative, 51–2.

107 Other proponents, including Laborie, did not give this argument much credence. Laborie, "De l'anesthésie," 561.

108 "Note Biographique: Charles James Campbell," 1875, Ms 106 (1038), fol. 1–30. Bibliothèque de l'Académie Nationale de Médecine.

109 Onimus, *Le Dr Charles James Campbell*.

110 Campbell, *Mémoire sur l'anesthésie obstétricale*, 4.

111 Calling on an *accoucheur* ("male midwife") for assistance in childbirth became a fashionable practice among women of means in the eighteenth century. These male *accoucheurs* distinguished themselves from female midwives not only by their superior medical education but also through the use of forceps and other interventionist techniques in abnormal cases. Obstetrics continued to be a prominent specialty for male practitioners throughout the nineteenth century, as the French state and the medical profession increasingly sought to regulate the activities of female midwives through education and licensing requirements. Weisz, *Divide and Conquer*, 4; Brockliss and Jones, *Medical World*, 263–6. On the regulation of female midwives in the nineteenth century, see Stock-Morton, "Control and Limitation."

112 Bailly, "De l'anesthésie," 12–13.

113 Later in the century, poor women began to have more options for

childbirth. The insalubrious reputations and high death rates in maternity hospitals eventually led the French government to act. In 1869, it began sponsoring public assistance programs to pay licensed midwives for home deliveries for women who could not otherwise afford it. Rachel Fuchs notes that between 1869 and 1900, 25,958 poor women benefited from this type of assistance. Fuchs, *Poor and Pregnant*, 32; Stewart, *For Health and Beauty*, 128. On the Paris Maternité, see Beauvalet-Boutouyrie, *Naître à l'hôpital*.

114 Although Mary Lynn Stewart argues that women in the Maternity Hospital around 1900 rarely received anesthetic during childbirth, many of the "experiments" I have examined from studies on obstetric anesthesia in the nineteenth century were conducted in maternity hospitals, for example, Dr Jeannel's research at the Montpellier Maternité de l'Hôtel-Dieu Saint-Éloi. Stewart, *For Health and Beauty*, 128–9.

115 The Paris Maternité served as a teaching institution for the instruction of midwives and obstetrical students. Beauvalet-Boutouyrie, *Naître à l'hôpital*, 157–83. However, it also served as an important site for clinical research, as demonstrated by the numerous case studies from Maternité patients published in the medical press.

116 Elinor Accampo notes that although antisepsis and asepsis reduced puerperal fever deaths beginning in the 1880s, these deaths remained relatively high until 1934, when *Streptococcus* was identified. Accampo cites maternal mortality rates between 0.25 per cent and 6.6 per cent but notes that the rate could be as high as 9 per cent in lying-in hospitals. Accampo, *Blessed Motherhood*, 29; Thébaud, *Quand nos grand-mères*, 178.

117 Loudon, *Death in Childbirth*, 430–1.

118 Smith, *Ladies of the Leisure Class*, 82; Accampo, *Blessed Motherhood*, 29; Stewart, *For Health and Beauty*, 95–111.

119 Bailly, "De l'anesthésie," 8.

120 Campbell, *Mémoire sur l'anesthésie obstétricale*, 4–5.

121 Ibid., 5.

122 Ibid., 7; Obstetric patient case notes from Campbell, Ms 115 (1047); Ms 116 (1048), Bibliothèque de l'Académie Nationale de Médecine.

123 Campbell, *Mémoire sur l'anesthésie obstétricale*, 8–10.

124 Ibid., 11–12.

125 Blot, *De l'anesthésie*, 5.

126 Dastre, Étude critique, 15–16.

127 Houzelot, *Anesthésie obstétricale*, 23–4.

128 Ibid., 25.

129 Larrey, *De l'éthérisation*, 21.

130 For more on anesthesia apparatuses, see Zimmer, *Histoire de l'anesthésie*.

131 Sédillot, *De l'insensibilité produite par le chloroforme* (1848), cited in Larrey, *De l'éthérisation*, 19.

132 Bailly, "De l'anesthésie," 12–13.

133 Lebert, *Des accouchements sans douleur*, 9; Laborie, "De l'anesthésie."

134 Chaigneau, Étude comparative, 69–72.

135 In practically all of Houzelot's observations, he notes that once the woman experienced the relief of chloroform, she asked for it with subsequent contractions. Houzelot, *Anesthésie obstétricale*.

136 Chaigneau, Étude comparative, 69.

137 Le Roux, *Le chemin du crime*, 214. While the woman's arguments about Adam echoed those of James Young Simpson and other proponents of childbirth anesthesia, Le Roux's conclusions and the woman's quote seem to have received a lot of attention. Several medical journals published a short excerpt of the conclusions in 1888 and 1889 under the title "L'anesthésie en obstétrique et la côte d'Adam," including *La France médicale* 2 (1888): 1359; *Lyon médicale* 59 (1888): 107; *Revue de l'hypnotisme et de la psychologie physiologique* (1888): 126–27; *Gazette de gynécologie* 3 (1888): 367; *Répertoire de pharmacie* 16 (1888): 399–400; and *Revue générale de clinique et de thérapeutique: Journal des praticiens* (1889): 148.

138 G. Lebert, "Des accouchements sans douleur ou de l'anodynie obstétricale par le Chloroforme et spécialement par la bromure d'éthyle," *Concours médical* (1881): 218–20, 220.

139 Ethyl bromide (*bromure d'éthyl* or *éther bromhydrique*) is produced by combining potassium bromide, sulfuric acid, and alcohol. British surgeon Thomas Nunneley first discovered ethyl bromide's anesthetic properties in 1849 while conducting research on animals. Fraenkel, *Contribution a l'étude*, 32–3; Zimmer, *Histoire de l'anesthésie*, 374–6. See also *Codex medicamentarius* (1884), 208–9.

140 Lebert, "Des accouchements sans douleur," 218.

141 Ibid., 219.

142 Ibid., 220.

143 Early experiments on ethyl bromide were conducted around 1850 but the substance was abandoned and not taken up again until the 1880s. Auvrard and Caubet, *Anesthésie*, 9–10; Lebert, *Des accouchements sans douleur*, 2–3.

144 It is unclear how many women it might have reached. The pamphlet cost 1 fr. 50 c., so it may not have been affordable for poorer women.

145 Lebert, *Des accouchements sans douleur*, 1.

146 Offen, "Depopulation, Nationalism, and Feminism." Coitus interruptus was the most common method of birth control employed in the nineteenth century. Couples could also use other traditional methods – abstinence, birth spacing, non-vaginal intercourse – or, depending on their income, mechanical methods, including douching, pessaries, and condoms. McLaren, *Sexuality and Social Order*, 12–25; McLaren, *History of Contraception*; Offen, *Debating the Woman Question*, 86–93.

147 Offen, *Debating the Woman Question*, 187–200; Roberts, *Disruptive Acts*, 26–7.

148 Neo-Mathusianism supported birth control as a means of regenerating France by increasing the quality of its population through planned pregnancies. Robin founded the neo-Malthusian League of Human Regeneration in 1896, which published a journal, *Régénération*, and distributed a pamphlet titled "Means of Avoiding Large Families," which contained explicit instructions for avoiding pregnancy. Robin received over five hundred requests for copies of the pamphlet within the first month after its publication. Accampo, *Blessed Motherhood*, 4–5, 41–5; Offen, *Debating the Woman Question*, 255–9.

149 Accampo, *Blessed Motherhood*, 52–8; Fuchs, *Poor and Pregnant*, 96–8.

150 Accampo, *Blessed Motherhood*, 28–34, 49.

151 Ibid., 85–92.

152 Offen, "Depopulation, Nationalism, and Feminism," 654–6; Jensen, "Paradigms and Political Discourse."

153 Lebert, *Des accouchements sans douleur*, 28.

154 Pinard, *De l'action comparée*; Chaigneau, *Étude comparative*.

155 Koller's findings were reported to the French medical community in an article in *Semaine médicale* on 23 October 1884. Guinier, *De l'anesthésie locale*, 14; Doléris, *De l'analgésie*; Alphonse Herrgott, "De l'emploi de la cocaïne en obstétrique," *Annales de gynécologie et d'obstétrique* (February 1885): 81–97; Jeannel, *De la suppression de la douleur*; Franc, *De l'anesthésie locale*. While doctors including Doléris, Chartier, Aubert, and Rouville experimented with spinal anesthesia using cocaine and stovaine during childbirth between 1900 and 1908, French doctors did not reach a consensus on the safety of this practice. Keim, *Les médications nouvelles*, 77–82; Rouville, *Consultations de gynécologie*, 5–10.

156 Jeannel, *Supression de la douleur*, 13–14.

157 Dr Rabey to Dr Doléris, 16 February 1886, cited in Guinier, *De l'anesthésie locale*, 57.

158 Franc, *De l'anesthésie locale*, 16–17; Herrgott, "Cocaïne en obstétrique," 92–7.

159 Herrgott, "Cocaïne en obstétrique," 94.

160 Purrey, *Conseils aux mères de famille*, 29.

161 Stewart, *For Health and Beauty*, 128–9.

162 Auvrard and Caubet, *Anesthésie*, 2.

163 Quoted in Offen, *Debating the Woman Question*, 394.

164 On the history of conscription in France, see Stoker, Schneid, and Blanton, *Conscription*, 1–23; Flynn, *Conscription and Democracy*, 14–21, 27–30.

165 Bell, *First Total War*, 78, 80–1, 210. On the image of the citizen-soldier as popularized by Enlightenment thinkers leading up to the Revolution, see Hippler, *Citizens*, 37–45.

166 The term of service varied from five to eight years between 1818 and 1889 and was reduced to three years after 1889. Weber, *Peasants into Frenchmen*, 292–4.

167 Forth, *Dreyfus Affair*, 43; Nye, *Masculinity*, 79.

168 Rey, *Histoire de la douleur*, 161–3.

169　Larrey served as First Surgeon to Napoleon's Imperial Guard. Delorme, *Traité de chirurgie*, 196.

170　Ferrandis, "Histoire de l'anesthésie." For more on the history of military anesthesia, see Micaelli-Queyriaux, "Evolution de l'anesthésie militaire"; Brisou, "Débuts de l'anésthésie générale."

171　Haller, *Battlefield Medicine*, 156.

172　French military surgeons also began to use chloroform during conflicts in the Kabylie region of Algeria in 1854, 1856, and 1857; however, the medical literature tends to focus more on Crimea. Delorme, *Traité de chirurgie*, 307; Ferrandis, "Histoire de l'anesthésie militarie," 254; Zimmer, *Histoire de l'anesthésie*, 405–11; Goldfrank, *Origins*.

173　Marroin, *Histoire médicale*, 72.

174　Scrive, *Relation médico-chirurgicale*, 120.

175　Lucien Baudens, "Une mission médicale à l'Armée d'Orient," *Revue des deux mondes* 8 (1857): 587–616, 613. Of the 51,620 total French wounded, 39,870 soldiers survived their wounds. Clodfelter, *Warfare and Armed Conflicts*, 180.

176　Scrive, *Relation médico-chirurgicale*, 120.

177　Ibid., 465–6; Delorme, *Traité de chirurgie*, 297.

178　Quesnoy, *Souvenirs historiques*, 203–4.

179　Scrive, *Relation médico-chirurgicale*, 468.

180　Marroin, *Histoire médicale*, 73.

181　Scrive, *Relation médico-chirurgicale*, 468.

182　Ibid., 122.

183　Ibid., 121.

184　Ibid., 120–1, 466.

185　Legouest, *De chirurgie d'armée*, 774–5.

186　Ibid., 775.

187　Delorme, *Traité de chirurgie*, 356.

188　Just Lucas-Championnière studied antiseptic methods in Glasgow under Joseph Lister in 1868 and introduced them into French surgical practice in 1869. Duncum, *Development of Inhalation Anaesthesia*, 32.

189　Delorme, *Traité de chirurgie*, 355. See also Moison, *Le service pharmaceutique*, 100–5; Laventure, *Le choix de l'anesthésie*, 25.

190　For more on the history of the war, see Taithe, *Defeated Flesh*; Wawro, *Franco-Prussian War*; Howard, *Franco-Prussian War*.

191　Sabatier, *Rapport sur la campagne de l'ambulance*, 117.

192　Delorme, *Traité de chirurgie*, 230.

193　Championnière cited in Moison, *Le service pharmaceutique*, 111.

194　Grellois, *Histoire médicale du siège de Metz*, 32, cited in Moison, *Le service pharmaceutique*, 108.

195　In March of 1871, the city of London made a large gift of medicines to the Pharmacie Centrale des Hôpitaux de Paris; however, the medicines did not arrive until June, after the fall of the Paris Commune. Unsigned letter, n.d., 542 FOSS 94, Archives de l'Assistances Publique-Hôpitaux de Paris.

196 Sabatier, *Rapport sur la campagne de l'ambulance*, 116.

197 Ibid., 116–17.

198 Ibid., 117.

199 Ibid., 114–15; Chenu, *Aperçu historique*, ii–v.

200 National Aid Society, *Report of the Operations*, 11–13, 102.

201 Sabatier, *Rapport sur la campagne de l'ambulance*, 114, 116.

202 Chassagne and Emery-Desbrousses, *Guide médical pratique*, 182.

203 Ibid., 183.

204 Demmler, *La chirurgie du champ de bataille*, 121.

205 *Formulaire pharmaceutique à l'usage des hôpitaux militaires*, 70–6, 134–6, 142–4, 147.

206 Service de Santé, *Formulaire pharmaceutique*, 24–40.

207 Laventure, *Choix de l'anesthésie*, 33, 38.

208 M. Harrison, *Medical War*, 10; Van Bergen, *Before My Helpless Sight*, 285.

209 "Demandes d'exportation: produits chimiques et pharmaceutiques," 1914–19, F/12/7893, Archives Nationales.

210 Courington and Calverley, "Anesthesia," 644.

211 Van Bergen, *Before My Helpless Sight*, 287; Haller, *Battlefield Medicine*, 154.

212 Van Bergen, *Before My Helpless Sight*, 293, 299–300.

213 R. Romme, "La narcose et l'auto-narcose par le mélange de Schleich," *La Presse médicale*, 4 April 1906, 212–13.

214 Association français de chirurgie, *Dix-Neuvième Congrès*, 858.

215 Schleich, *Those Were Good Days*, 225.

216 British stretcher-bearers administered water and blue morphine tablets to the wounded as they dressed their wounds on the battlefield – but they may have been conservative with this practice so their wounded did not become unconscious dead weights when transported. Mayhew, *Wounded*, 24, 26, 29.

217 Any nurses present would have been male, as the French Army banned female nurses from the front lines, restricting them to hospitals farther back until 1918. Darrow, "French Volunteer Nursing," 88.

218 Van Bergen, *Before My Helpless Sight*, 288.

219 Ibid., 287; Micaelli-Queyriaux, "Evolution de l'anesthésie militaire," 68.

220 Jacques Carles and André Charrier, "L'anesthésie générale au chloride d'éthyle et la chirurgie de guerre," *Le progrès médical*, no. 39 (October 1915): 478–80.

221 Carles and Charrier also noted that ethyl chloride did not provoke nausea as often as chloroform, so patients could eat a meal right after a procedure. However, ethyl chloride, like ether, was highly flammable, an added danger for surgeons operating in battlefield conditions.

222 Demmler, *Chirurgie du champ de bataille*, 119.

223 Haller, *Battlefield Medicine*, 149; Courington and Calverley, "Anesthesia," 644.

224 H. Rouvillois, "The H.O.E. in the French Army (Primary and Secondary

Evacuation Hospitals)," trans. J.R. Kean, *The Military Surgeon* 56, no. 5 (May 1925): 529–57.

225 Henri Vignes, "A propos de l'anesthésie en chirurgie de guerre. Communication fait a la *Société de Pathologie Comparée*. Séance du 14 novembre 1916," pamphlet, HS 510, Bibliothèque Centrale du Service de Santé des Armées, Val-de-Grâce.

226 Courington and Calverley, "Anesthesia," 644; Haller, *Battlefield Medicine*, 149.

227 Henry Reynès (de Marseille), "IV. Neuf mois de chirurgie de l'avant, à Verdun," *Bulletin de l'Académie de médecine* 74 (27 July 1915): 111–13, 112–13.

228 Ibid., 112.

229 Dr Victor Pauchet, "Matériel chirurgical de l'ambulance de corps d'armée," *Gazette médicale de Paris*, 21 April 1915, 28–9.

230 Ibid., 28–9.

231 James Corning of New York first discovered spinal anesthesia in 1885 while experimenting on dogs, yet spinal anesthesia remained virtually unknown in medical practice until 1898, when German doctor Auguste Bier first used it to anesthetize a human for surgery. Laventure, *Choix de l'anesthésie*, 41–2; Paul Reclus, "De la méthode de Bier," *Bulletin de l'Académie de médecine* 45 (19 March 1901): 345–51.

232 Laventure, *Choix de l'anesthésie*, 43.

233 Demmler, *La chirurgie du champ de bataille*, 120–1; Picard, *Contribution à l'étude*, 8–9.

234 La Motte noted that the patient experienced no pain or sensation from the waist down but jabbered away in a state of animated delirium. Ellen N. La Motte, "At the Telephone," in Higonnet, *Nurses at the Front*, 65–7.

235 Demmler, *La chirurgie du champ de bataille*, 120–1.

236 *Maître-infirmiers* (master-nurses) were recruited from among re-enlisted soldiers and corporals. They received three months of theoretical training at a military hospital and were required to pass an exam in front of a committee. Given the shortages of medical personnel during the war, some of the individuals charged with administering anesthesia during surgery may have had even less training. Ministère de la Guerre, *Manuel technique*, 1–2, 75–6.

237 Picard, *Anesthésie en chirurgie d'armée*, 27.

238 Colombel, *Journal d'une infirmière*, 99.

239 Ibid., 100–1.

240 Medical manuals instructed military surgeons to avoid running out of supplies by not wasting them. Demmler, *Chirurgie du champ de bataille*, 7.

241 Duhamel, *La vie des martyrs*, 66.

242 Ibid., 67–8.

243 Ibid., 66.

244 Ibid., 68.

245 Ibid., 46–7. In some cases, medical personnel hesitated to administer anesthetics for fear that opiates could slow the patient's circulation or that chloroform could cause respiratory issues and intense vomiting. Still, Christine Hallett notes, they expressed far less reluctance to administer anesthetics to ease the suffering of dying patients. Hallett, *Containing Trauma*, 66, 104–6.

246 Ellen N. La Motte, "Alone," in Higonnet, *Nurses at the Front*, 15.

247 Borden, *Forbidden Zone*, 147–8.

248 Savariaud, "L'anesthésie prolongée au chlorure d'éthyle dans la pratique des grandes pansements," *La Presse médicale* no. 6 (31 January 1916): 45.

249 Edmond Delorme, "II. Des raideurs articulaires et des ankyloses consécutives aux blessures de guerre. Des rôles respectifs de la mécanothérapie et de la chirurgie orthopédique," *Bulletin de l'Académie de médecine*, 30 November 1915, 611–49, 612–13, 629. However, Delorme noted that for ankylosis, doctors had to resort to orthopedic surgery.

250 Ibid., 631.

251 Ibid., 631, 645.

252 Ibid., 635.

253 Ibid., 649.

254 On efforts to rehabilitate wounded and dismembered soldiers after the war, see Koven, "Remembering and Dismemberment"; Panchasi, "Reconstructions."

CONCLUSION

1 "No. 10090. – Loi … du 12 Juillet 1916." For a detailed social history of drugs and drug users in the interwar period following the passage of this legislation, see Retaillaud-Bajac, *Les paradis perdus*.

2 Véronal was the first of several barbiturate derivatives developed between 1903 and 1911. Another popular barbiturate was phenobarbital, sold commercially in France as "Gardénal" and in Germany as "Luminal" beginning in 1912. These addictive substances were sold in France without restriction until 1930. Retaillaud-Bajac, *Les paradis perdus*, 78.

3 Based on reported medical statistics on addicted patients from the interwar period, Emmanuelle Retaillaud-Bajac determined that medical prescriptions remained a major cause in the spread of morphine and other drug addictions even after the passage of the 1916 poisonous substances law. To take one example, between 1922 and 1928 Dr Ghelerter reported that twenty-nine of fifty morphine and heroin addicts he observed at Henri-Rousselle Hospital had become addicted as a result of medical treatment that, in the majority of cases, had been prescribed after the 1916 law. Ibid., 80–9.

4 Boekhout van Solinge, "Handling Drugs," 65–103.

5 In 2018, the US Substance Abuse and Mental Health Services Administration reported that 9.3 million adults had misused prescription pain relievers in the previous year. Substance Abuse and Mental Health Services Administration, "2018 Key Substance Abuse." On the marketing of OxyContin specifically, see Van Zee, "Promotion and Marketing."

6 Researchers have argued that France has not experienced an opioid crisis comparable to the one in the United States for several reasons: France restricts opioid prescriptions to a twenty-eight-day supply and prohibits direct-to-consumer marketing of pharmaceuticals. France also widely distributes naloxone to addicts to help them avoid overdosing, and Paris has introduced a safe drug consumption room where addicts can get clean needles and free optional counseling from psychiatrists and other health care providers. Bellefonds, "How France Is Confronting"; Hider-Mlynarz, Cavalié, and Maison, "Trends in Analgesic Consumption"; Authier, "Dossier Antalgiques."

7 Agence nationale de sécurité du médicament et des produits de santé, *Situation Report.*

8 Authier, "Dossier Antalgiques," 111.

9 On 9 January 2014, the Agence national de sécurité des médicaments (ANSM) approved the therapeutic prescription of Sativex, a cannabis-based throat spray designed to treat contractures in multiple sclerosis patients. Sativex is the first cannabis-based medication to be approved for use in France since cannabis was removed from the French pharmacopoeia in 1953. However, price disputes with the British pharmaceutical company that makes the drug have prevented Sativex from being sold in French pharmacies. Official approval of the use of medical cannabis has been much slower to come in France than in the United States. An experimental trial of medical cannabis for three thousand pain patients initially scheduled to begin in 2019 was delayed for two years. The trial finally commenced in March 2021 and is scheduled to be completed in March 2023. Advocates are hopeful that the two-year experimental trial might lead to the legalization of medical cannabis in France. Hecketsweiler and Clavreul, "Le Sativex"; Guba, *Taming Cannabis*, 218; Mufson, "France to Launch"; Vinogradoff, "'Une aberration'"; Fullalove, "Medical Cannabis Trials."

10 The ANSM published a report on benzodiazepine consumption in France, which found that 11.5 million people had consumed benzodiazepines at least once in 2012. Agence nationale de sécurité du médicament et des produits de santé, État des lieux de la consommation; Mascret, "Les Français Consomment"; "France's Drug Addiction"; "Un Français sur trois."

11 "France Clinical Trial"; Whitman, "French Clinical Trial Disaster"; Bisserbe, "French Drug Trial."

BIBLIOGRAPHY

ARCHIVES

Archives de l'Assistance Publique-Hôpitaux de Paris
Archives Nationales
Archives Nationales d'Outre Mer
Archives de la Préfecture de Police de Paris
Archives de la Ville de Paris
Bibliothèque de l'Académie Nationale de Médecine
Bibliothèque Centrale du Service de Santé des Armées, Val-de-Grâce
Bibliothèque Charcot
Bibliothèque Interuniversitaire de Santé
Bibliothèque Médicale Henry-Ey, Centre Hospitalier Sainte-Anne
Bibliothèque Nationale de France

HISTORICAL PERIODICALS

Annales de chimie et de physique
Annales de gynécologie et d'obstétrique
Annales d'hygiène publique et de médecine légale
Annales médico-psychologiques
Annales de psychiatrie et d'hypnologie
Archives d'anthropologie criminelle
Archives générales de médecine
Archives de neurologie
Bulletin de l'Académie de médecine
Bulletin commercial: Annexe de l'Union pharmaceutique
Bulletin général de thérapeutique médicale et chirurgicale
Bulletins et mémoires de la Société médicale des hôpitaux de Paris
Bulletin de la Société de chirurgie
Bulletin de la Société de thérapeutique
Comptes rendus des séances de l'Académie des sciences
Comptes rendus des séances de la Société de biologie
Concours médical
La Dépêche de Brest

L'Encéphale
Le Figaro
La France médicale
Gazette des hôpitaux
Gazette médicale de Paris
Gazette des tribunaux
Gil Blas
Journal de chimie médicale, de pharmacie et de toxicologie
Journal des débats politiques et littéraires
Journal de médecine et de chirurgies pratiques
Journal des maladies mentales
Lyon médicale
McClure's Magazine
Mémoires de l'Académie de médecine
Mémoires de l'Institut des sciences, lettres et arts
The Military Surgeon
Moniteur Algérien
New York Times
Pharmaceutical Journal
Le Petit Journal
Le Progrès médical
La Presse
La Presse médicale
Répertoire de pharmacie
Revue des deux mondes
Revue de l'hypnotisme et de la psychologie physiologique
Revue générale de clinique et de thérapeutique: Journal des praticiens
La Revue médico-chirurgicale des maladies des femmes
Revue de psychiatrie
Revue scientifique
La Semaine médicale
Union médicale
Union pharmaceutique

PUBLISHED SOURCES

Aaslestad, Katherine, and Johan Joor, eds. *Revisiting Napoleon's Continental System: Local, Regional and European Experience*. Basingstoke: Palgrave Macmillan, 2015.
Abelson, Elaine S. "The Invention of Kleptomania." *Signs* 15, no. 1 (1989): 123–43.
Abrams, M.H. *The Mirror and the Lamp: Romantic Theory and the Critical Tradition*. New York: Oxford University Press, 1953.
Accampo, Elinor. *Blessed Motherhood, Bitter Fruit: Nelly Roussel and the*

Politics of Female Pain in Third Republic France. Baltimore: Johns Hopkins University Press, 2006.

– "Class and Gender." In *Revolutionary France: 1788–1880*, edited by Malcolm Crook, 93–122. Oxford: Oxford University Press, 2002.

– "The Gendered Nature of Contraception in France: Neo-Malthusianism, 1900–1920." *Journal of Interdisciplinary History* 34, no. 2 (2003): 235–62.

Ackerknecht, Erwin H. "Anticontagionism between 1821 and 1867." *Bulletin of the History of Medicine* 22, no. 5 (1948): 570–5.

– "Health and Hygiene in France, 1815–1848." *Bulletin of the History of Medicine* 22, no. 2 (1948): 117–55.

– *Medicine at the Paris Hospital, 1794–1848*. Baltimore: Johns Hopkins University Press, 1967.

Ackerman, Evelyn Bernette. *Health Care in the Parisian Countryside, 1800–1914*. New Brunswick, NJ: Rutgers University Press, 1990.

Agence nationale de sécurité du médicament et des produits de santé. *Analyse des ventes de médicaments en France en 2013*. Edited by Philippe Cavalié and Alia Djeraba. Saint-Denis, June 2014.

– *État des lieux de la consommation des benzodiazépines en France*. Edited by Nathalie Richard. Saint-Denis, December 2013. https://archiveansm. integra.fr/var/ansm_site/storage/original/application/3e06749ae5a50cb-7ae8ofb655dee103a.pdf.

– *Situation Report: Use and Abuse of Opioid Analgesics*, By Emilie Monzon. Coordinated by Nathalie Richard. Saint-Denis, February 2019. https:// archiveansm.integra.fr/var/ansm_site/storage/original/application/ c303ea105c0f450eacb436c987ad9e51.pdf.

Altman, Lawrence K. *Who Goes First? The Story of Self-Experimentation in Medicine*. Berkeley: University of California Press, 1998.

Appignanesi, Lisa. *Sad, Mad, and Bad: Women and the Mind-Doctors from 1800*. Toronto: McArthur, 2007.

Armengaud, André. *La population française au XIXe siècle*. Paris: Presses Universitaires de France, 1971.

Artières, Philippe, ed. *Journal d'un morphinomane: 1880–1894*. Paris: Editions Allia, 1997.

Arveiller, Jacques. "Cannabis et formation du médecin: Moreau de Tours et ses internes." *Pratiques en santé médicale* 63, no. 2 (2017): 21–8.

– "Le Cannabis en France au XIXe siècle: Une histoire médicale." *L'Évolution psychiatrique* 78, no. 3 (2013): 451–484.

Association français de chirurgie. *Dix-Neuvième Congrès de Chirurgie, Paris 1906: Procès-verbal, mémoires et discussions*. Paris: Félix Alcan, 1906.

Aubergier, Hector. *Des préparations d'opium indigène de H. Aubergier approuvées par l'Académie Impériale de Médecine*. Clermont: Hubler et Dubus, 1855.

– *Mémoire sur l'opium indigène*. Paris: J.-B. Baillière, 1853.

Aubert-Roche, Louis-Rémy. *De la peste ou typhus d'Orient ... Suivis d'un essai sur le hachisch.* Paris: J. Rouvier, 1840.

Auslander, Leora. *Taste and Power: Furnishing Modern France.* Berkeley: University of California Press, 1996.

Authier, Nicolas. "Dossier Antalgiques." *La Lettre du pharmacologue* 31 no. 4 (2017): 110–12.

Auvrard, Alfred, and Edmond Caubet. *Anesthésie chirurgicale et obstétricale.* Paris: Rueff, 1892.

Bachmann, Christian, and Anne Coppel. *La drogue dans le monde: Hier et aujourd'hui.* Paris: A. Michel, 1991.

Baker, Keith. "Scientism at the End of the Old Regime: Reflections on a Theme of Professor Charles Gillispie." *Minerva* 25, no. 1 (1987): 21–34.

Ball, Benjamin. *La morphinomanie.* Paris: Asselin et Houzeau, 1885.

Balzac, Honoré de. *Lettres à Madame Hanska.* Vol. 3. Paris: Editions du Delta, 1969.

Barnes, David S. *The Great Stink of Paris and the Nineteenth-Century Struggle against Filth and Germs.* Baltimore: Johns Hopkins University Press, 2006.

– *The Making of a Social Disease: Tuberculosis in Nineteenth-Century France.* Berkeley: University of California Press, 1995.

Baron, Baptiste. *Étude psychologique de l'anesthésie par l'éther avec quelques considérations médico-légales.* Lyon: A.H. Storck, 1896.

Barret, Émile. "De la morphimétrie." In *Étude sur les préparations galéniques de l'opium inscrites au Codex de 1866,* 19–24. Paris: Imprimerie Administrative et des Chemins de Fer de Paul Dupont, 1866.

Barrows, Susanna. "After the Commune: Alcoholism, Temperance, and Literature in the Early Third Republic." In *Consciousness and Class Experience in Nineteenth-Century Europe,* 205–18. New York: Holmes and Meier, 1979.

– "Alcohol, France and Algeria: A Case Study in the International Liquor Trade." *Contemporary Drug Problems* 11 (1982): 525–43.

– *Distorting Mirrors: Visions of the Crowd in Late Nineteenth-Century France.* New Haven: Yale University Press, 1981.

Battandier, J. *Algérie: Plantes médicinales.* Alger-Mustapha: Giralt, 1900.

Baudelaire, Charles. *Artificial Paradises.* Translated by Stacy Diamond. New York: Carol, 1996.

– *Oeuvres complètes de Charles Baudelaire.* Vol. 4, *Petits poèmes en prose; Les Paradis artificiels.* Paris: Michel Lévy frères, 1869.

Beauvalet-Boutouyrie, Scarlett. *Naître à l'hôpital au XIXᵉ siècle.* Paris: Belin, 1999.

Béchet, Louis. *Le Docteur Morphine.* Marseille: Imprimerie Méridionale, 1906.

Belhoste, Bruno. *Paris Savant: Capital of Science in the Age of Enlightenment.* Oxford: Oxford University Press, 2019.

Bell, David. *The First Total War: Napoleon's Europe and the Birth of Warfare as We Know It.* New York: Mariner Books, 2008.

Bellefonds, Colleen de. "How France Is Confronting Opioid Use." *US News and*

World Report, 5 July 2018. https://www.usnews.com/news/best-countries/
articles/2018-07-05/rise-in-opioid-deaths-in-france-stirs-new-alarm.

Belon, Pierre. *Les observations de plusieurs singularitez et choses memorables, trouvees en Grèce, Asie, Judée, Egypte, Arabie & autres pays estranges.* Paris: G. Cavellat, 1588.

Bénard, J.-P. *Résumé des expériences faites à Amiens en 1854, 1855, 1856, sur l'extraction de l'opium-oeillette.* Amiens: E. Yvert, 1857.

Ben-David, Joseph. "The Rise and Decline of France as a Scientific Centre." *Minerva* 8, no. 2 (1970): 160–79.

Benjamin, Walter. *On Hashish.* Translated by Howard Eiland. Cambridge, MA: Belknap Press of Harvard University Press, 2006.

Berg, Maxine, and Helen Clifford, eds. *Consumers and Luxury: Consumer Culture in Europe, 1650–1850.* Manchester: Manchester University Press, 1999.

Bergmann, Norman A. "Humphry Davy's Contribution to the Introduction of Anaesthesia: A New Perspective." *Perspectives in Biology and Medicine* 34 (1991): 534–41.

Berlanstein, Lenard R. *The Working People of Paris, 1871–1914.* Baltimore: Johns Hopkins University Press, 1984.

Berlière, Jean-Marc, and René Lévy. "The Evolving Organization of Policing: From the Ancien Régime to De Gaulle and the *Police Nationale*." In *Policing in France*, edited by Jacques de Maillard and Wesley G. Skogan, 21–38. New York: Routledge, 2020.

Berman, Alex. "The Persistence of Theriac in France." *Pharmacy in History* 12, no. 1 (1970): 5–12.

– "Drug Control in Nineteenth-Century France: Antecedents and Directions." In *Safeguarding the Public: Historical Aspects of Medicinal Drug Control*, edited by John B. Blake, 3–14. Baltimore: Johns Hopkins University Press, 1970.

Bernard, Claude. *Introduction à l'étude de la médecine expérimentale.* Paris: J.-B. Baillière et fils, 1865.

Berridge, Virginia, and Griffith Edwards. *Opium and the People: Opiate Use in Nineteenth-Century England.* New York: St Martin's Press, 1981.

Berthé, P. *Examen critique des divers procédés qui ont été proposés pour doser la morphine de l'opium, Considérations sur la possibilité du titrage et sur l'utilité pour la médecine de la culture du pavot en France.* Paris: Dubuisson, 1858.

– *Du titrage de l'opium: Lettre à M. Favrot, Rédacteur de la partie pharmaceutique de la France médicale.* Paris: Dubuisson, 1859.

– *Lettre à M. Le Professor Chevallier sur le titrage de l'opium.* Paris: Dubuisson, 1859.

– *Note sur le titrage de l'opium present à l'Académie impériale de médecine.* Paris: Henri Elon, 1859.

Binder, E. *Des indications de l'opium dans les différentes formes d'aliénation mentale.* Strasbourg: Berger-Levrault, 1856.

Bisserbe, Noemie. "French Drug Trial Leaves One Person Brain Dead, Four with

Serious Disorders." *Wall Street Journal*, 15 January 2016. http://www.wsj.com/articles/french-prosecutors-investigate-drug-trial-injuries-1452861924.

Black, Sara E. "Doctors on Drugs: Medical Professionals and the Proliferation of Morphine Addiction in Nineteenth-Century France." *Social History of Medicine* 30, no. 1 (2017): 114–36.

– "Morphine on Trial: Legal Medicine and Criminal Responsibility in the *Fin de Siècle*." *French Historical Studies* 42, no. 4 (2019): 623–53.

Blot, Hippolyte. *De l'anesthésie appliquée à l'art des accouchements*. Paris: Victor Masson, 1857.

Boekhout van Solinge, Tim. "Handling Drugs à la Française." In *Dealing with Drugs in Europe: An Investigation of European Drug Control Experiences; France, the Netherlands, and Sweden*, 65–103. The Hague: BJu Legal Publishers, 2004.

Booth, Martin. *Opium: A History*. New York: St. Martin's Press, 1998.

Borden, Mary. *The Forbidden Zone*. Garden City, NY: Doubleday, 1930.

Bosc, Ernest. *Traité théorique et pratique du haschich*. 2nd ed. Nice: Bureau de "La Curiosité," 1904.

Bouchardat, Apollinaire. *Nouveau formulaire magistral*. 14th ed. Paris: Germer Baillière, 1867.

Bourke, Joanna. *The Story of Pain: From Prayer to Painkillers*. New York: Oxford University Press, 2014.

Bourneville, Désiré Magloire, and Paul Regnard. *Iconographie photographique de la Salpêtrière*. Paris: Progrès médical, A. Delahaye, 1877–79.

Brennan, Thomas. *Burgundy to Champagne: The Wine Trade in Early Modern France*. Baltimore: Johns Hopkins University Press, 1997.

– *Public Drinking and Popular Culture in Eighteenth-Century Paris*. Princeton, NJ: Princeton University Press, 1988.

– "Towards the Cultural History of Alcohol in France." *Journal of Social History* 23, no. 1 (1989): 71–92.

Brisou, B. "Débuts de l'anésthésie générale dans la marine de guerre." *Médecine et armées* 25, no. 7 (1997): 543–50.

Brockliss, Laurence, and Colin Jones. *The Medical World of Early Modern France*. Oxford: Oxford University Press, 1997.

Brouardel, Paul. *Opium, morphine et cocaïne: Intoxication aiguë par l'opium, mangeurs et fumeurs d'opium, morphinomanes et cocaïnomanes*. Paris: J.-B. Baillière et fils, 1906.

Brunet, Felix. *Une avarie d'extrême-orient: La fumerie d'opium, nécessité de l'éviter et possibilité de la guérir*. Paris: J. Gainche, 1903.

Calvet, Léopold. *Essai sur le morphinisme aigu et chronique*. Paris: V. Goupy, 1876.

Campbell, Charles James. *Mémoire sur l'anesthésie obstétricale*. Paris: G. Masson, 1874.

Canguilhem, Georges. *The Normal and the Pathological*. New York: Zone Books, 1989.

Carroy, Jacqueline. "Observation, expérimentation et clinique de soi: Haschich, folie, rêve et hystérie au XIXe siècle." In *L'envers de la raison alentour Canguilhem*, edited by Pierre F. Daled, 53–71. Paris: Vrin, 2009.

Caton, Donald. *What a Blessing She Had Chloroform: The Medical and Social Response to the Pain of Childbirth from 1800 to the Present*. New Haven: Yale University Press, 1999.

Cavaillès. *Guide pratique pour l'usage des pharmacies portatives*. Paris: Pharmacie Rogé, 1868.

Chaigneau, Jules. *Étude comparative des divers agents anesthésiques employés dans les accouchements naturels*. Paris: Steinheil, 1890.

Chast, François. "Les origines de la législation sur les stupéfiants en France." *Histoire des sciences médicales* 43 no. 3 (2009): 293–305.

Chamayou, Grégoire. *Les corps vils: Expérimenter sur les êtres humains aux XVIIIe et XIXe siècles*. Paris: La Découverte, 2014.

Chambard, Ernest. *Les morphinomanes: Étude clinique, médico-légale et thérapeutique*. Paris: Rueff, 1893.

Chambrin, Émile. *Contribution à l'étude des accidents nerveux consécutifs à l'intoxication par l'éther*. Paris: Jouve et Boyer, 1899.

Charcot, J.M. *Leçons du mardi à la Salpêtrière*. Paris: Bureaux du Progrès medical/A. Delahaye et Emile Lecrosnier, 1887.

Chassagne, Amédée, and Emery-Desbrousses. *Guide médical pratique de l'officier*. Paris: Librarie Ch. Delagrave, 1876.

Chauvaud, Frédéric. *Les experts du crime: La médecine légale en France au XIXe siècle*. Paris: Aubier, 2000.

Chauveau, Sophie. "Les origines de l'industrialisation de la pharmacie avant la Première Guerre mondiale." *Histoire, économie et société* 14, no. 4 (1995): 627–42.

Chenu, Jean Charles. *Aperçu historique, statistique et clinique sur le service des ambulances et des hôpitaux de la Société francaise de secours aux blessés des armées de terre et de mer: pendant la guerre de 1870–1871*. Paris: Dumaine, 1874.

Chevallier, Alphonse. *Notice historique sur l'opium indigène*. Paris: W. Remiquet, 1852.

Choquette, Leslie. "Homosexuals in the City: Representations of Lesbian and Gay Space in Nineteenth-Century Paris." *Journal of Homosexuality* 41, no. 3–4 (2002): 149–67.

Clark, Linda L. *Schooling the Daughters of Marianne: Textbooks and the Socialization of Girls in Modern French Primary Schools*. Albany: State University of New York Press, 1984.

Clark, Michael, and Catherine Crawford, eds. *Legal Medicine in History*. Cambridge: Cambridge University Press, 1994.

Clodfelter, Micheal. *Warfare and Armed Conflicts: A Statistical Encyclopedia of Casualty and Other Figures, 1492–2015*. 4th ed. Jefferson, NC: McFarland, 2017.

Code des médicamens ou pharmacopée française publiée ... par la Faculté de médecine de Paris l'an 1818. Paris: Hacquart, 1819.

Code pénal de l'empire français. Paris, 1810.

Codex: Pharmacopée française. Paris: Béchet, 1837.

Codex medicamentarius: Pharmacopée française rédigée par ordre du gouvernement. Paris: J.-B. Baillière et fils, 1866.

Codex medicamentarius: Pharmacopée française rédigée par ordre du gouvernement. Paris: G. Masson, 1884.

Codex medicamentarius gallicus: Pharmacopée française rédigée par ordre du gouvernement. Paris: Masson, 1908.

Cohen, Deborah. *Household Gods: A History of the British and Their Possessions*. New Haven: Yale University Press, 2006.

Cole, Joshua. *The Power of Large Numbers: Population, Politics, and Gender in Nineteenth-Century France*. Ithaca: Cornell University Press, 2000.

Coleman, William. *Death Is a Social Disease: Public Health and Political Economy in Early Industrial France*. Madison: University of Wisconsin Press, 1982.

Colombel, Emmanuel. *Journal d'une infirmière d'Arras: Août–septembre–octobre 1914*. Paris: Bloud et Gay, 1916.

Cooter, Roger. "Anticontagionism and History's Medical Record." In *The Problem of Medical Knowledge: Examining the Social Construction of Medicine*, edited by Peter Wright, 87–108. Edinburgh: Edinburgh University Press, 1984.

Corbin, Alain. *Women for Hire: Prostitution and Sexuality in France after 1850*. Translated by Alan Sheridan. Cambridge, MA: Harvard University Press, 1990.

Courington, Frederick W., and Roderick K. Calverley. "Anesthesia on the Western Front: The Anglo-American Experience of World War I." *Anesthesiology* 65, no. 6 (1986): 642–53.

Courtive, Edmond de. *Haschish: Étude historique, chimique, et physiologique*. Paris: Édouard Bautruche, 1848.

Courtois-Suffit, Maurice, and René Giroux. *La cocaïne: Ètude d'hygiène sociale et de médecine légale*. Paris: Masson, 1918.

– *Extension du traffic de la cocaïne et de la cocaïnomanie*. Extract from *Revue de médecine*. Paris: Félix Alcan, n.d. 14196 (71). Bibliothèque Interuniversitaire de Santé.

Courtwright, David T. *Dark Paradise: Opiate Addiction in America before 1940*. Cambridge, MA: Harvard University Press, 1982.

– *Forces of Habit: Drugs and the Making of the Modern World*. Cambridge, MA: Harvard University Press, 2001.

Crosland, Maurice. *Science under Control: The French Academy of Sciences, 1795–1914*. Cambridge: Cambridge University Press, 2002.

Daftary, Farhad. *The Assassin Legends: Myths of the Isma'ilis*. London: I.B. Tauris, 1995.

Dalbanne, N. *Essai sur quelques accidents produits par la morphine*. Paris: A. Parent, 1877.

Dalloz, Édouard, and Charles-Henri Vergé. *Code pénal annoté et expliqué d'après la jurisprudence et la doctrine*. Paris: Bureau de la Jurisprudence générale, 1881.

Darrow, Margaret H. "French Volunteer Nursing and the Myth of War Experience in World War I." *American Historical Review* 101, no. 1 (1996): 80–106.

Daston, Lorraine, and Peter Galison. *Objectivity*. New York: Zone Books, 2007.

Dastre, Albert. *Étude critique des travaux récents sur les anesthésiques*. Paris: G. Masson, 1881.

Datta, Venita. *Heroes and Legends of Fin-de-Siècle France: Gender, Politics, and National Identity*. Cambridge: Cambridge University Press, 2011.

Davenport-Hines, Richard. *The Pursuit of Oblivion: A Global History of Narcotics*. New York: W.W. Norton, 2002.

Davis, Diana K. "Restoring Roman Nature: French Identity and North African Environmental History." In *Environmental Imaginaries of the Middle East and North Africa*, edited by Diana K. Davis and Edmund Burke III, 60–86. Athens: Ohio University Press, 2011.

– *Resurrecting the Granary of Rome: Environmental History and French Colonial Expansion in North Africa*. Athens: Ohio University Press, 2007.

Davy, Humphry. *Researches, Chemical and Philosophical – Chiefly Concerning Nitrous Oxide, or Diphlogisticated Nitrous Air, and Its Respiration*. London: J. Johnson, 1800.

Dechambre, Amédée. *Dictionnaire encyclopédique des sciences médicales*. 100 vols. Paris: G. Masson/P. Asselin, 1864–89.

– *Dictionnaire usuel des sciences médicales*. Paris: G. Masson, 1885.

Decharme, J. Constantin. *Mémoire sur l'opium indigène*. Amiens: Duval et Herment, 1855.

Degoix, Casimir. *Maladies et médicaments à la mode*. Paris: J.-B. Baillière et fils, 1891.

Dehaut, Félix. *Manuel de médecine, d'hygiène, de chirurgie et de pharmacie domestiques*. 20th ed. Paris: The author, 1893.

Delorme, Edmond. *Traité de chirurgie de guerre*. Vol. 1. Paris: Félix Alcan, 1888.

Déloye, Yves. *École et citoyenneté: L'individualisme républicain de Jules Ferry à Vichy; Controverses*. Paris: Presses de la Fondation nationale des sciences politiques, 1994.

Demmler, Anathese. *La chirurgie du champ de bataille*. Paris: Masson, 1907.

Depaul, J.A.H. *Leçons de clinique obstétricale professées à l'Hôpital des cliniques*. Paris: Adrien Delahaye, 1872.

Deschamps, Georges. *Étude comparative des codex français*. Paris: Henri Jouve, 1891.

Descours-Gatin, Chantal. *Quand l'opium finançait la colonisation en Indochine: L'élaboration de la régie générale de l'opium, 1860 à 1914*. Paris: L'Harmattan, 1992.

Didi-Huberman, Georges. *Invention of Hysteria: Charcot and the Photographic Iconography of the Salpêtrière*. Cambridge, MA: MIT Press, 2003.

Dion, Roger. *Histoire de la vigne et du vin en France: Des origines au XIXe siècle.* Paris: CNRS, 2010.

Direction Générale des Douanes. *Tableau général du commerce.* Paris: Imprimerie Nationale, 1840–1920.

Doléris. *De l'analgésie des voies génitales obtenue par l'application locale de cocaïne pendant le travail de l'accouchement.* Paris: A Delahaye and E. Lecroisier, 1885.

Donovan, James M. *Juries and the Transformation of Criminal Justice in France in the Nineteenth and Twentieth Centuries.* Chapel Hill: University of North Carolina Press, 2010.

– "Magistrates and Juries in France, 1791–1952." *French Historical Studies* 22, no. 3 (1999): 379–420.

– "Public Opinion and the French Capital Punishment Debate of 1908." *Law and History Review* 32, no. 3 (2014): 575–609.

Dorvault, François. *Catalogue pharmaceutique ou prix courant général de la Pharmacie Centrale de France et de la Maison générale de Droguerie Ménier réunies.* Paris: n.p., 1877.

Dowbiggin, Ian. *Inheriting Madness: Professionalization and Psychiatric Knowledge in Nineteenth-Century France.* Berkeley: University of California Press, 1991.

Dubuisson, Paul, and Auguste Vigouroux. *Responsabilité pénale et folie: Etude médico-légale.* Paris, Félix Alcan, 1911.

Duhamel, Georges. *La vie des martyrs, 1914–1916.* 7th ed. Paris: Mercure de France, 1917.

Dumas, Michel. "Historique de la césarienne." Medical thesis, Université de Limoges, 1975.

Duncum, Barbara M. *The Development of Inhalation Anaesthesia; with Special Reference to the Years 1846–1900.* London: Oxford University Press, 1947.

Du Plessis, Michael. "Unspeakable Writing: Jean Lorrain's Monsieur De Phocas." *French Forum* 27, no. 2 (2002): 65–98.

Dupouy, Roger. *Les opiomanes, mangeurs, buveurs et fumeurs d'opium: Étude clinique et médico-littéraire.* Paris: Alcan, 1912.

Durkheim, Émile. *On Morality and Society.* Edited by Robert N. Bellah. Chicago: University of Chicago Press, 1973.

Dutertre, Émile. *De l'emploi du chloroform dans les accouchements naturels (physiologie).* Paris: J.-B. Baillière et fils, 1882.

Eigen, Joel Peter. "Lesion of the Will: Medical Resolve and Criminal Responsibility in Victorian Insanity Trials." *Law and Society Review* 33, no. 2 (1999): 425–59.

Ellis, Jack D. *The Physician-Legislators of France: Medicine and Politics in the Early Third Republic, 1870–1914.* New York: Cambridge University Press, 1990.

"El-Thebib: Le médecin." *L'Algérie à l'Exposition Universelle de 1900,* no. 10 (15 September 1900).

Esmein, A., R. Garraud, and C.J.A. Mittermaier. *A History of Continental Criminal Procedure, with Special Reference to France*. Boston: Little, Brown, 1913.

Fauchier, Louis. *Contribution à l'étude du rêve morphinique et de la morphinomanie*. Montpellier: Firmin et Montane, 1910.

Fauconney, Jean. [Docteur Caufeynon, pseud.]. *L'impuissance et la stérilité chez l'homme et la femme: Causes morales et physiques, vices de conformation, vaginisme, frigidité, erreurs de coït*. Paris: Nouvelle librairie médicale, 1903.

– *Les morphinomanes et les fumeurs d'opium: Les causes et les effets de la morphinomanie, suplices et voluptés, opiophages et fumeurs d'opium*. Paris: Charles Offenstadt, 1903.

Faure, Olivier. *Histoire sociale de la médecine: XVIIIᵉ–XXᵉ siècles*. Paris: Anthropos, 1994.

– *Les français et leur médecine au XIXᵉ siècle*. Paris: Belin, 1993.

– "La médecine gratuite au XIXᵉ siècle: De la charité à l'assistance." *Histoire, économie et société* 3, no. 4 (1984): 593–608.

– "Officines, pharmaciens et médicaments en France au XIXᵉ siècle." *Bulletin de la société d'histoire moderne*, no. 44 (1989): 31–9.

– "Les officines pharmaceutiques françaises: De la réalité au mythe (fin XIXᵉ–début XXᵉ siècle)." *Revue d'histoire moderne et contemporaine* 43, no. 4 (1996): 672–85.

– "Une pharmacie lyonnaise et ses clients, à la veille de la Première Guerre mondiale." *Revue d'histoire de la pharmacie* 80, no. 294 (1992): 307–14.

Ferrandis, J.-J. "Histoire de l'anesthésie militaire française." *Médecine et armées* 27, no. 4 (1999): 253–8.

Flynn, George Q. *Conscription and Democracy: The Draft in France, Great Britain, and the United States*. Westport, CT: Praeger, 2001.

Formulaire pharmaceutique à l'usage des hôpitaux militaires français. Paris: Victor Rozier, 1857.

Formulaire des pharmaciens français: Formulaire de la Société des pharmaciens du Loiret adopté par l'Association générale des pharmaciens de France. 8th ed. Orléans: Auguste Gout, 1904.

Forth, Christopher E. *The Dreyfus Affair and the Crisis of French Manhood*. Baltimore: Johns Hopkins University Press, 2004.

Foster, Claire. *The Ethics of Medical Research on Humans*. New York: Cambridge University Press, 2001.

Foucault, Michel. *The History of Sexuality*. Translated by Robert Hurley. New York: Vintage Books, 1990.

– *Madness and Civilization: A History of Insanity in the Age of Reason*. Translated by Richard Howard. New York: Vintage Books, 1988.

– *Technologies of the Self: A Seminar with Michel Foucault*. Edited by Luther H. Martin, Huck Gutman, and Patrick H. Hutton. Amherst: University of Massachusetts Press, 1988.

Fox, Robert. *The Savant and the State: Science and Cultural Politics in Nineteenth-Century France*. Baltimore: Johns Hopkins University Press, 2012.

Fraenkel, Marcus. *Contribution a l'étude du bromure d'éthyle comme anesthésique général*. Paris: Henri Jouve, 1894.

Franc, Charles. *De l'anesthésie locale par le chlorhydrate de cocaïne en obstétrique et en gynécologie*. Paris: A. Coccoz, 1890.

"France's Drug Addiction: 1 in 3 on Psychotropic Medication." *France 24*, 20 May 2014. http://www.france24.com/en/20140520-france-drug-addiction-1-3-psychotropic-medication.

"France Clinical Trial: 90 Given Drug, One Man Brain-Dead." *BBC News*, 15 January 2016. http://www.bbc.com/news/world-europe-35320895.

Fuchs, Rachel G. *Poor and Pregnant in Paris: Strategies for Survival in the Nineteenth Century*. New Brunswick, NJ: Rutgers University Press, 1992.

Fullalove, Ellie. "Medical Cannabis Trials in France Show Promise." *The Connection*, 28 September 2021. https://www.connexionfrance.com/French-news/Health/Medical-cannabis-trials-in-France-show-promise-but-how-the-country-will-make-legal-cannabis-farms-financially-viable-remains-uncertain.

Gamel, Raymond. *Chiqueurs, mangeurs, buveurs et fumeurs d'opium: Étude médico-sociale sur l'abus de l'opium en France et dans les colonies françaises*. Montpellier: Coulet et fils, 1912.

Garner, James W. "Criminal Procedure in France." *Yale Law Journal* 25, no. 4 (1916): 255–84.

Garnier, Pierre. *Anomalies sexuelles: Apparentes et cachées, avec 230 observations*. Paris: Garnier frères, 1889.

Gaudry, Claudius. *Contribution à l'étude du morphinisme chronique et de la responsabilité pénale chez les morphinomanes*. Coulommiers: Brodard et Gallois, 1886.

Gautier, Théophile, *Baudelaire*. Edited by Claude-Marie Senninger with Lois Cassandra Hamrick. Paris: Klincksieck, 1986.

Gelfand, Toby. *Professionalizing Modern Medicine: Paris Surgeons and Medical Science and Institutions in the 18th Century*. Westport, CT: Greenwood Press, 1980.

Gélis, Jacques. *History of Childbirth: Fertility, Pregnancy, and Birth in Early Modern Europe*. Translated by Rosemary Morris. Boston: Northeastern University Press, 1991.

– *La sage-femme ou le médecin: Une nouvelle conception de la vie*. Paris: Fayard, 1988.

Gerdy, Pierre-Nicolas. *Pathologie générale médico-chirurgicale: Avec recherches particulières sur la nature, la symptomatologie, les terminaisons générales des maladies sur leurs influences et leur causes sur le diagnostic etc*. Paris: Victor Masson, 1851.

Gillispie, Charles. *Science and Polity in France: The Revolutionary and*

Napoleonic Years. Princeton, NJ: Princeton University Press, 2004.

Giraud, Jules. *Testament d'un haschischéen*. Paris: H. & H. Durville, n.d.

Goetz, Christopher G., Michel Bonduelle, and Toby Gelfand. *Charcot: Constructing Neurology*. New York: Oxford University Press, 1995.

Goldfrank, David M. *The Origins of the Crimean War*. New York: Routledge, 1993.

Goldstein, Jan. *Console and Classify: The French Psychiatric Profession in the Nineteenth Century*. Chicago: University of Chicago Press, 2001.

– "Neutralizing Freud: The Lycée Philosophy Class and the Problem of the Reception of Psychoanalysis in France." *Critical Inquiry* 40, no. 1 (2013): 40–82.

– *The Post-Revolutionary Self: Politics and Psyche in France, 1750–1850*. Cambridge, MA: Harvard University Press, 2005.

Golinski, Jan. "Humphry Davy: The Experimental Self." *Eighteenth-Century Studies* 45, no. 1 (2011): 15–28.

Gootenberg, Paul. *Andean Cocaine: The Making of a Global Drug*. Chapel Hill: University of North Carolina Press, 2008.

Gorodnianskaia, Hélène. *Étude statistique sur l'opération césarienne*. Lausanne: Charles Guex, 1904.

Goron, Marie-François. *Les parias de l'amour*. Paris: Ernest Flammarion, 1899.

Gounot, Roger. *Charles Maurin, 1856–1914: Essai sur le peintre et catalogue de l'exposition de 1978*. Puy-en-Velay: Les Arts Graphiques, 1978.

Gower, Barry. *Scientific Method: A Historical and Philosophical Introduction*. London: Routledge, 1996.

Griolet, Gaston, Charles-Paul-Laurent Vergé, and Henry Bourdeaux. *Code d'instruction criminelle et code pénal annotés d'après la doctrine et la jurisprudence*. Paris: Bureau de la Jurisprudence Générale Dalloz, 1909.

Guba, David A. "Antoine Isaac Silvestre de Sacy and the Myth of the Hachichins: Orientalizing Hashish in Nineteenth-Century France." *Social History of Alcohol and Drugs* 30, no. 1 (2016): 50–74.

– *Taming Cannabis: Drugs and Empire in Nineteenth-Century France*. Montreal and Kingston: McGill-Queen's University Press, 2020.

Guibourt, Nicolas-Jean-Baptiste-Gaston. *Mémoire sur le dosage de l'opium et sur la quantité de morphine que l'opium doit contenir; Observations sur le laudanum liquide de Sydenham*. Paris: E. Thunot, 1862.

Guignard, Laurence. "L'expertise médico-légale de la folie aux Assises 1821–1865." *Le Mouvement social*, no. 197 (2001): 57–81.

Guimbail, Henri. *Les morphinomanes: Comment on devient morphinomane, les prédestinés, éphémère volupté et supplices durables, désordres physiques et troubles de l'intelligence, médecine légale, traitement*. Paris: J.-B. Baillière et fils, 1891.

Guinier, Pierre. *De l'anesthésie locale par le chlorhydrate de cocaïne en gynécologie et en obstétrique*. Montpellier: G. Firmin, 1887.

Guy, Kolleen M. *When Champagne Became French: Wine and the Making of a National Identity*. Baltimore: Johns Hopkins University Press, 2003.

Hahn, Roger. *Anatomy of a Scientific Institution: Paris Academy of Sciences, 1666–1803*. Berkeley: University of California Press, 1971.

Haine, W. Scott. *The World of the Paris Café: Sociability among the French Working Class, 1789–1914*. Baltimore: Johns Hopkins University Press, 1998.

Haller, John S. *Battlefield Medicine: A History of the Military Ambulance from the Napoleonic Wars through World War I*. Carbondale: Southern Illinois University Press, 2011.

Hallett, Christine E. *Containing Trauma: Nursing Work in the First World War*. Manchester: Manchester University Press, 2009.

Harris, Ruth. *Murders and Madness: Medicine, Law, and Society in the Fin-de-Siècle*. Oxford: Clarendon Press, 1989.

Harrison, Carol E. *The Bourgeois Citizen in Nineteenth-Century France: Gender, Sociability, and the Uses of Emulation*. Oxford: Oxford University Press, 1999.

Harrison, Mark. *The Medical War: British Military Medicine in the First World War*. Oxford: Oxford University Press, 2010.

Harsin, Jill. "Gender, Class, and Madness in Nineteenth-Century France." *French Historical Studies* 17, no. 4 (1992): 1048–70.

– *Policing Prostitution in Nineteenth-Century Paris*. Princeton, NJ: Princeton University Press, 1985.

Hayter, Alethea. *Opium and the Romantic Imagination*. Berkeley: University of California Press, 1968.

Heath, Elizabeth. *Wine, Sugar, and the Making of Modern France: Global Economic Crisis and the Racialization of French Citizenship, 1870–1910*. Cambridge: Cambridge University Press, 2014.

Hecketsweiler, Chloé, and Laetitia Clavreul. "Le Sativex, médicament à base de cannabis, autorisé en France." *Le Monde*, 9 January 2014. http://www.lemonde.fr/sante/article/2014/01/09/le-sativex-medicament-a-base-de-cannabis-autorise-en-france_4344958_1651302.html.

Herzig, Rebecca. *Suffering for Science: Reason and Sacrifice in Modern America*. New Brunswick, NJ: Rutgers University Press, 2005.

Hewitt, Jessie. *Institutionalizing Gender: Madness, the Family, and Psychiatric Power in Nineteenth-Century France*. Ithaca: Cornell University Press, 2020.

Hickman, Timothy Alton. *The Secret Leprosy of Modern Days: Narcotic Addiction and Cultural Crisis in the United States, 1870–1920*. Amherst: University of Massachusetts Press, 2007.

Hider-Mlynarz, Karima, Philippe Cavalié, and Patrick Maison. "Trends in Analgesic Consumption in France over the Last 10 Years and Comparison of Patterns across Europe." *British Journal of Clinical Pharmacology* 84, no. 6 (2018): 1324–34.

Higonnet, Margaret R., ed. *Nurses at the Front: Writing the Wounds of the Great War*. Boston: Northeastern University Press, 2001.

Hildreth, Martha L. *Doctors, Bureaucrats, and Public Health in France, 1888–1902*. New York: Garland, 1987.

– "Medical Rivalries and Medical Politics in France: The Physicians' Union Movement and the Medical Assistance Law of 1893." *Journal of the History of Medicine and Allied Sciences* 42, no. 1 (1987): 5–29.

Hilton, Frank. *Baudelaire in Chains: Portrait of the Artist as a Drug Addict.* London: P. Owen, 2004.

Hippler, Thomas. *Citizens, Soldiers and National Armies: Military Service in France and Germany, 1789–1830.* London: Routledge, 2014.

Hodder, Ian. *Entangled: An Archaeology of the Relationships between Humans and Things.* Malden, MA: Wiley-Blackwell, 2012.

– "The Entanglements of Humans and Things: A Long-Term View." *New Literary History* 45, no. 1 (2014): 19–36.

Houzelot, Paul-Crescent-Xavier. *Anesthésie obstétricale: De l'emploi du chloroforme dans l'accouchement naturel simple.* Meaux: A. Carro, 1854.

Howard, Michael. *The Franco-Prussian War: The German Invasion of France, 1870–1871.* 2nd ed. New York: Routledge, 2001.

Hustvedt, Asti. *Medical Muses: Hysteria in Nineteenth-Century Paris.* New York: W.W. Norton, 2011.

Isnard, Hildebert. "Vigne et colonisation en Algérie." *Annales de géographie* 58, no. 311 (1949): 212–19.

Jeannel, Sidoine. *De la suppression de la douleur dans les accouchements par des applications locales de chlorhydrate de cocaïne.* Montpellier: Boehm et fils, 1886.

Jennings, Jeremy. *Revolution and the Republic: A History of Political Thought in France since the Eighteenth Century.* Oxford: Oxford University Press, 2011.

Jensen, Jane. "Paradigms and Political Discourse: Labour and Social Policy in the USA and France before 1914." *Canadian Journal of Political Science* 22, no. 2 (1989): 235–58.

Jonas, Hans. "Philosophical Reflections on Experimenting with Human Subjects." In *Experimentation with Human Subjects*, edited by Paul A. Freund, 1–31. New York: George Braziller, 1970.

Jordanova, Ludmilla. *Sexual Visions: Images of Gender in Science and Medicine between the Eighteenth and Twentieth Centuries.* Milwaukee: University of Wisconsin Press, 1993.

Jourdan, A.-J.-L. *Code pharmaceutique.* Paris: Guillaume, 1821.

Julien, Pierre. "Un empire industriel issu d'une droguerie pharmaceutique." *Revue d'histoire de la pharmacie* 70, no. 254 (1982): 180–2.

Jouet, Daniel. *Étude de morphinisme chronique.* Paris: Alphonse Derenne, 1883.

Keim, Gustave. *Les médications nouvelles en obstétrique.* Paris: J.-B. Baillière et fils, 1908.

Keller, Richard. *Colonial Madness: Psychiatry in French North Africa.* Chicago: University of Chicago Press, 2007.

Kopper, Joachim. "La signification de Kant pour la philosophie française." *Archives de philosophie* 44 no. 1 (1981): 63–88.

Koven, Seth. "Remembering and Dismemberment: Crippled Children,

Wounded Soldiers, and the Great War in Great Britain." *American Historical Review* 99, no. 4 (1994): 1167–202.

Kra, Lucien, and René Louis. *Ivresse d'opium*. Paris: A. de Smith, 1919.

Kudlick, Catherine J. *Cholera in Post-Revolutionary Paris: A Cultural History*. Berkeley: University of California Press, 1996.

La Berge, Ann F. *Mission and Method: The Early Nineteenth-Century French Public Health Movement*. Cambridge: Cambridge University Press, 1992.

Lacoste-Veysseyre, Claudine, ed. *Théophile Gautier: Correspondance générale, 1843–1845*. Vol. 2. Geneva: Librarie Droz, 1986.

Landes, Joan B. *Women and the Public Sphere in the Age of the French Revolution*. Ithaca: Cornell University Press, 1988.

Laqueur, Thomas. *Making Sex: Body and Gender from the Greeks to Freud*. Cambridge, MA: Harvard University Press, 1990.

– *Solitary Sex: A Cultural History of Masturbation*. New York: Zone Books, 2003.

Larrey, Hippolyte Baron. *De l'éthérisation sous le rapport de la responsabilité médicale*. Paris: J.-B. Baillière et fils, 1857.

Latour, Bruno. *The Pasteurization of France*. Cambridge, MA: Harvard University Press, 1988.

Laventure, Fernand. *Du choix de l'anesthésie en campagne*. Nancy: Berger-Levrault, 1913.

Lebert, Gustave. *Des accouchements sans douleur par l'emploi du bromure d'éthyle: Conseils aux femmes sur le point de devenir mères*. Paris: O. Doin, 1882.

Lecuir, Jean. "La médicalisation de la société française dans la deuxième moitié du XVIIIe siècle en France: Aux origines des premiers traités de médecine légale." *Annales de Bretagne et des pays de l'ouest* 86, no. 2 (1979): 231.

Ledermann, François. "Pharmacie, médicaments et psychiatrie vers 1850: Le cas de Jacques-Joseph Moreau de Tours." *Revue d'histoire de la pharmacie* 76, no. 276 (1988): 67–76.

Lefèvre, René. *Contribution à l'étude de la morphinomanie*. Paris: H. Jouve, 1905.

Legouest, Léon. *De chirurgie d'armée*. Paris: J.-B. Baillière et fils, 1863.

Léonard, Jacques. "Femmes, religion et médecine: Les religieuses qui soignent, en France au XIXe siècle." *Annales* 32, no. 5 (1977): 887–907.

– *La France médicale au XIXe siècle*. Mesnil-sur-l'Estrée: Gallimard/Julliard, 1978.

– *La vie quotidienne du médecin de province au XIXe siècle*. Paris: Hachette, 1977.

Le Roux, Hugues. *Le chemin du crime*. Paris: V. Havard, 1889.

Lesch, John E. *The First Miracle Drugs: How the Sulfa Drugs Transformed Medicine*. Oxford: Oxford University Press, 2006.

– *Science and Medicine in France: The Emergence of Experimental Physiology, 1790–1855*. Cambridge, MA: Harvard University Press, 1984.

Lescure, François. *La médecine du peuple indispensable pour conserver la santé, se préserver et guérir des maladies et pour vivre longtemps, mise à la portée de tout le monde et de toutes les bourses*. Auch: G. Foix, 1884.

Lewis, Bernard. *The Assassins.* New York: Basic Books, 2002.

Lordat, *Extrait de la dernière leçon du cours de physiologie fait à la Faculté de médecine de Montpellier (1846–47), sur la doctrine de l'alliance des deux puissances du dynamisme humain; Leçon dont l'objet principale a été la théorie de l'éthérisation.* Montpellier: J. Martel Aine, 1847.

Lorrain, Jean. *Monsieur de Phocas.* Translated by Francis Amery. Sawtry, UK: Dedalus, 1994.

Loudon, Irvine. *Death in Childbirth: An International Study of Maternal Care and Maternal Mortality, 1800–1950.* Oxford: Oxford University Press, 1992.

Luauté, Jean-Pierre. "Contexte historique et motivations des premiers auto-expérimentateurs médicaux." *Annales médico-psychologiques* 175, no. 7 (2017): 639–44.

Lutaud, Auguste. *Du vaginisme.* Paris: G. Masson, 1874.

Mallat de Bassilan, Marcel-Jacques-Saint-Ange. *La Comtesse Morphine.* Paris: Frinzine, Klein et Cie, 1885.

Mandelbaum, Maurice. *History, Man, and Reason: A Study in Nineteenth-Century Thought.* Baltimore: Johns Hopkins University Press, 1971.

Manuel des soeurs de pharmacie: Exposé médical pharmaceutique et vocabulaire. Poitiers: H. Oudin frères, 1877.

Marroin, Auguste. *Histoire médicale de la flotte française dans la mer Nord pendant la guerre de Crimée.* Paris: J.-B. Baillière et fils, 1861.

Martin, Emily. "The Egg and the Sperm: How Science Has Constructed a Romance Based on Stereotypical Male-Female Roles." *Signs* 16, no. 3 (1991): 485–501.

Mascret, Damien. "Les Français consomment encore trop de psychotropes." *Le Figaro*, 16 January 2012. http://sante.lefigaro.fr/actualite/2012/01/16/16937-francais-consomment-encore-trop-psychotropes.

Matlock, Jann. "Doubling Out of the Crazy House: Gender, Autobiography, and the Insane Asylum System in Nineteenth-Century France." *Representations*, no. 34 (1991): 166–95.

Mayhew, Emily. *Wounded: A New History of the Western Front in World War I.* New York: Oxford University Press, 2014.

Maza, Sarah. *The Myth of the French Bourgeoisie: An Essay on the Social Imaginary, 1750–1850.* Cambridge, MA: Harvard University Press, 2003.

McLaren, Angus. *A History of Contraception: From Antiquity to the Present Day.* Oxford: Blackwell, 1990.

– *Sexuality and Social Order: The Debate over the Fertility of Women and Workers in France, 1770–1920.* New York: Holmes and Meier, 1983.

McMillan, James F. *France and Women, 1789–1914: Gender, Society and Politics.* New York: Routledge, 2002.

Ménier et Cie. Maison Centrale de Droguerie. *Prix courant général.* Paris: Schneider et Langrand, 1845.

– *Prix courant général.* Paris: Plon Frères, 1854.

Micaelli-Queyriaux, Pascale. "Evolution de l'anesthésie militaire et de ses techniques à travers les conflits (de la guerre de Crimée à la guerre d'Algérie)." Medical thesis, Université Claude Bernard-Lyon 1, 2001.

Micale, Mark S. *Hysterical Men: The Hidden History of Male Nervous Illness.* Cambridge, MA: Harvard University Press, 2008.

Michéa, Claude-François. *De l'emploi des opiacés dans le traitement de l'aliénation mentale.* Paris: F. Malteste, 1849.

Mickel, Emanuel J., Jr. *The Artificial Paradises in French Literature: The Influence of Opium and Hashish on the Literature of French Romanticism and* Les fleurs du mal. Chapel Hill: University of North Carolina Press, 1969.

Millant, Richard. *La culture du pavot et le commerce de l'opium en Turquie.* Paris: Augustin Challamel, 1913.

– *La drogue: Fumeurs et mangeurs d'opium.* Paris: Roger, 1910.

Miller, Michael B. *The Bon Marché: Bourgeois Culture and the Department Store, 1869–1920.* Princeton, NJ: Princeton University Press, 1981.

Ministère de la Guerre. *Catalogue explicatif et raisonné de l'exposition permanent des produits de l'Algérie suivi du catalogue méthodique des produits algériens à l'Exposition universelle de Paris en 1855.* Paris: Firmin Didot Frères, 1855.

– *Manuel technique du maître-infirmier.* Paris: Imprimerie Nationale, 1909.

Moison, Claude. *Le service pharmaceutique pendant la guerre Franco-Allemande de 1870–1871.* Cahors: Coueslant, 1955.

Mollet, Marc, and Dominique Pradeau. "La pharmacie centrale des hôpitaux: De 1795 à 1812." In *Cinq siècles de pharmacie hospitalière: 1495–1995,* edited by François Chast and Pierre Julien, 38–42. Paris: Editions Hervas, 1995.

Moore, Alison, and Peter Cryle. "Frigidity at the *Fin de Siècle* in France: A Slippery and Capacious Concept." *Journal of the History of Sexuality* 19, no. 2 (2010): 243–61.

Moreau [de Tours], Jacques-Joseph. *Du hachisch et de l'aliénation mentale: Études psychologiques.* Paris: Fortin, Masson, 1845.

– *Hashish and Mental Illness.* Edited by Hélène Peters and Gabriel G. Nahas. Translated by Gordon J. Barnett. New York: Raven Press, 1973.

– *Mémoire sur le traitement des hallucinations par le datura stramonium.* Paris: J. Rouvier et E. Le Bouvier, 1841.

– *Traité pratique de la folie névropathique (vulgo hystérique).* Paris: Germer-Baillière, 1869.

Morel, B.A. *Traité des dégénérescences physiques, intellectuelles et morales de l'espèce humaine.* Paris: J.B. Baillière, 1857.

Mory, Berthe. "Dorvault et la 'Pharmacie Centrale de France.'" *Revue d'histoire de la pharmacie* 68, no. 245 (1980): 79–90.

Mufson, Claire. "France to Launch Medical Cannabis Experiment in Coming Weeks." *France 24,* 2 June 2019, https://www.france24.com/en/20190602-

france-launch-medical-cannabis-experiment-authier.

National Aid Society. *Report of the Operations of the British National Society for Aid to the Sick and Wounded in War during the Franco-German War, 1870–1871.* London: Harrison, 1871.

Neveu-Dérotrie, Victor. *De l'hystérie consécutive à l'intoxication par la morphine.* Paris: Henri Jouve, 1890.

Nicolas, Honoré. *Quelques recherches sur les effets physiologiques du chandoo (opium des fumeurs).* Montpellier: Cristin, Serre et Ricome, 1884.

"No. 2436. – Loi relative à l'exercice de la Médecine du 19 Ventôse." *Bulletin des lois de la République française* 7 (1802–03): 567–76.

"No. 2676. – Loi contenant Organisation des Écoles de pharmacie. Du 21 Germinal, an XI." *Bulletin des lois de la République française* 3, no. 8 (1803): 121–9.

"No. 7443. – Loi sur les Aliénés du 30 Juin 1838." *Bulletin des lois de la République française* (Bulletin No. 851) 1 (1838): 1005–20.

"No. 10090. – Loi concernant l'importation, le commerce, la détention et l'usage des substances vénéneuses, notamment l'opium, la morphine, et la cocaïne. Du 12 Juillet 1916." *Bulletin des lois de la République française* 8 (1916): 1154–6.

"No. 12,115. – Loi sur la vente des Substances vénéneuses, 19 Juillet 1845." *Bulletin des lois du Royaume de France* 31 (1846): 302.

"No. 27052.—Loi sur l'Assistance médicale et gratuite du 15 Juillet 1893." *Bulletin des lois de la République française* 12, no. 47 (1893): 841–9.

"No. 70-1320. —Loi du 31 décembre 1970 relative aux mesures sanitaires de lutte contre la toxicomanie et à la répression du trafic et de l'usage illicite des substances vénéneuses." *Journal officiel de la République française* (1971): 74–7.

Noirot, André. *Des troubles génitaux dans la morphinomanie.* Saint-Étienne: A. Bardiot, 1902.

Nord, Philip. *The Republican Moment: Struggles for Democracy in Nineteenth-Century France.* Cambridge, MA: Harvard University Press, 1995.

Nye, Robert A. *Crime, Madness and Politics in Modern France: The Medical Concept of National Decline.* Princeton, NJ: Princeton University Press, 1984.

– "Honor Codes and Medical Ethics in Modern France." *Bulletin of the History of Medicine* 69 (1995): 91–111.

– *Masculinity and Male Codes of Honor in Modern France.* New York: Oxford University Press, 1993.

– "Sexuality, Sex Difference and the Cult of Modern Love in the French Third Republic." *Historical Reflections/Réflexions historiques* 20, no. 1 (1994): 57–76.

O'Brien, Patricia. "The Kleptomania Diagnosis: Bourgeois Women and Theft in Late Nineteenth-Century France." *Journal of Social History* 17, no. 1 (1983): 65–77.

Odeph, Alphonse. *Abrégé pratique sur la culture de l'opium indigène, pour servir de guide aux habitants des campagnes.* Paris: Walder, 1862.

Offen, Karen. *Debating the Woman Question in the French Third Republic, 1870–1920.* Cambridge: Cambridge University Press, 2018.

– "Depopulation, Nationalism, and Feminism in Fin-de-Siècle France." *American Historical Review* 89, no. 3 (1984): 648–76.

Office Parlementaire d'Évaluation des Politiques de Santé. *Rapport sur le bon usage des médicaments psychotropes,* by Maryvonne Briot. No. 3187 (Assemblée Nationale) and No. 422 (Sénat) (Paris, 2006), 17, 357. http://www.assemblee-nationale.fr/12/rap-off/i3187.asp.

Olsen, Bjørnar. "Material Culture after Text: Re-membering Things." *Norwegian Archeaological Review* 36, no. 2 (2003): 87–104.

Onimus, Ernest. *Le Dr Charles James Campbell.* Paris: Félix Malteste, 1879.

Ozanam, Charles. *L'anesthésie: Histoire de la douleur.* Paris: Charles Douniol, 1857.

Padwa, Howard. *Social Poison: The Culture and Politics of Opiate Control in Britain and France, 1821–1926.* Baltimore: Johns Hopkins University Press, 2012.

Panchasi, Roxanne. "Reconstructions: Prosthetics and the Rehabilitation of the Male Body in World War I France." *Differences* 7 (1995): 109–40.

Parssinen, Terry M. *Secret Passions, Secret Remedies: Narcotic Drugs in British Society, 1820–1930.* Philadelphia: Institute for the Study of Human Issues, 1983.

Paul, Harry W. *Science, Vine and Wine in Modern France.* Cambridge: Cambridge University Press, 2002.

Pécarrere, Eugène. *Traité sur l'opium exotique et l'opium indigène.* Paris: n.p., 1835.

Pedersen, Jean Elisabeth. "Regulating Abortion and Birth Control: Gender, Medicine, and Republican Politics in France, 1870–1920." *French Historical Studies* 19, no. 3 (1996): 673–98.

Peniston, William A. *Pederasts and Others: Urban Culture and Sexual Identity in Nineteenth-Century Paris.* New York: Harrington Park Press, 2004.

Peter, Jean-Pierre. "Silence et cris: La médecine devant la douleur ou l'histoire d'une élision." *Le genre humain* 3, no. 18 (1988): 177–94.

Picard, Pierre. *Contribution à l'étude de l'anesthésie en chirurgie d'armée: Masque de fortune; Anesthésie simple et rapide au mélange de Schleich (et mélange modifié).* Paris: Vigot Frères, 1918.

Pichon, Georges. *Le morphinisme: Impulsions délictueuses, troubles physiques et mentaux des moprhinomanes; Leur capacité et leur situation juridique; Cause, déontologie et prophylaxie du vice morphinique.* Paris: Octave Doin, 1889.

Pick, Daniel. *Faces of Degeneration: A European Disorder, c.1848–c.1918.* Cambridge: Cambridge University Press, 1989.

Pinard, Adolphe. *De l'action comparée du chloroforme, du chloral, de l'opium et de la morphine chez les femmes en travail.* Paris: Octave Doin, 1878.

Pinel, Philippe. *Traité médico-philosophique sur l'aliénation mentale, ou la manie*. Paris: Caille et Ravier, 1801.

Piouffle, Hippolyte. *La cure des toxicomanes au Chatêau d'Orly*. Paris: Jules Céas, 1913.

– *Les psychoses cocaïniques*. Paris: Maloine et fils, 1919.

Plack, Noelle. "Drinking and Rebelling: Wine, Taxes, and Popular Agency in Revolutionary Paris, 1789–1791." *French Historical Studies* 39, no. 3 (2016): 599–622.

– "Liberty, Equality and Taxation: Wine in the French Revolution." *Social History of Alcohol and Drugs: An Interdisciplinary Journal* 26, no. 2 (2012): 5–22.

Plott, Michèle. "The Rules of the Game: Respectability, Sexuality, and the Femme Mondaine in Late-Nineteenth-Century Paris." *French Historical Studies* 25, no. 3 (2002): 532–3.

Polo, Marco. "Of the Old Man of the Mountain – of His Palace and Gardens – of His Capture and His Death." In *The Travels of Marco Polo*, 48–51. New York: Orion Press, 1958.

Poovey, Mary. "'Scenes of an Indelicate Character': The Medical 'Treatment' of Victorian Women." In *The Making of the Modern Body: Sexuality and Society in the Nineteenth Century*, edited by Catherine Gallagher and Thomas Walter Laqueur, 137–68. Berkeley: University of California Press, 1987.

Pope, Barbara Corrado. "Maternal Education in France, 1815–1848." *Proceedings of the Western Society for French History* 3 (1976): 368–77.

Popiel, Jennifer J. *Rousseau's Daughters: Domesticity, Education, and Autonomy in Modern France*. Durham: University of New Hampshire Press, 2008.

Porter, Roy. *The Greatest Benefit to Mankind: A Medical History of Humanity*. New York: W.W. Norton, 1997.

– "The Patient's View." *Theory and Society* 14, no. 2 (1985): 175–98.

Postel, Jacques, and Claude Quétel, eds. *Nouvelle histoire de la psychiatrie*. Toulouse: Editions Privat, 1983.

Pouchet, Georges. *Leçons de pharmacodynamie et de matière médicale*. Paris: Octave Doin, 1901.

Prestwich, Patricia. *Drink and the Politics of Social Reform: Antialcoholism in France since 1870*. Palo Alto, CA: Society for the Promotion of Science and Scholarship, 1988.

– "Family Strategies and Medical Power: 'Voluntary' Committal in a Parisian Asylum, 1876–1914." *Journal of Social History* 27, no. 4 (1994): 799–818.

– "Female Alcoholism in Paris, 1870–1920: The Response of Psychiatrists and of Families." *History of Psychiatry* 14, no. 3 (2003): 321–36.

Proschan, Frank. "'Syphilis, Opiomania, and Pederasty': Colonial Constructions of Vietnamese (and French) Social Diseases." *Journal of the History of Sexuality* 11, no. 4 (2002): 610–36.

Purrey, A. *Conseils aux mères de famille*. Paris: J. Roam, 1893.

Quin, Grégory, and Anaïs Bohuon. "Muscles, Nerves, and Sex: The Contradictions of the Medical Approach to Female Bodies in Movement in France, 1847–1914." *Gender and History* 24, no. 1 (2012): 172–86.

Quesnoy, Ferdinand-Désiré. *Souvenirs historiques, militaires, et médicaux de l'armée d'Orient*. Paris: Labbé, 1858.

Quétel, Claude, and Pierre Morel. *Les fous et leurs médecines: De la Renaissance au XXᵉ siècle*. Paris: Hachette littérature, 1979.

Ramsey, Matthew. "Academic Medicine and Medical Industrialism: The Regulation of Secret Remedies in Nineteenth-Century France." In *French Medical Culture in the Nineteenth Century*, edited by Ann La Berge and Mordechai Feingold, 25–78. Atlanta, GA: Rodopi, 1994.

– "Medical Power and Popular Medicine: Illegal Healers in Nineteenth-Century France." *Journal of Social History* 10, no. 4 (1977): 560–87.

– "The Politics of Medical Monopoly: The French Model and Its Rivals." In *Professions and the French State, 1700–1900*, edited by Gerald L. Geison, 225–305. Philadelphia: University of Pennsylvania Press, 1984.

– *Professional and Popular Medicine in France, 1770–1830: The Social World of Medical Practice*. Cambridge: Cambridge University Press, 1988.

– "Public Health in France." In *The History of Public Health and the Modern State*, edited by Dorothy Porter, 45–118. Amsterdam: Editions Rodopi, 1994.

Rappaport, Erika. *Shopping for Pleasure: Women in the Making of London's West End*. Princeton, NJ: Princeton University Press, 2000.

Regnier, Raoul-Louis-Auguste. *Essai critique sur l'intoxication par la morphine et sur ses diverses formes*. Paris: Delahaye et Lecrosnier, 1890.

Renneville, Marc. *Crime et folie: Deux siècles d'enquêtes médicales et judiciaires*. Paris: Fayard, 2008.

Retaillaud-Bajac, Emmanuelle. *Les paradis perdus: Drogues et usagers de drogues dans la France de l'entre-deux-guerres*. Rennes: Presses Universitaires de Rennes, 2009.

Rey-Debove, Josette, and Alain Rey. *Le Nouveau Petit Robert: Dictionnaire alphabétique et analogique de la langue française*. Paris: Le Robert, 2007.

Rey, Roselyne. *Histoire de la douleur*. Paris: La Découverte, 1993.

Richards, Thomas. *The Commodity Culture of Victorian England: Advertising and Spectacle, 1851–1914*. Stanford, CA: Stanford University Press, 1990.

Richet, Charles. *Recherches expérimentales et cliniques sur la sensibilité*. Paris: A. Parent, 1877.

Ripa, Yannick. *Women and Madness: The Incarceration of Women in Nineteenth Century France*. Translated by Catherine du Peloux Menagé. Minneapolis: University of Minnesota Press, 1990.

Riskin, Jessica. *Science in the Age of Sensibility: The Sentimental Empiricists of the French Enlightenment*. Chicago: University of Chicago Press, 2002.

– "The Defecating Duck, or, the Ambiguous Origins of Artificial Life." *Critical Inquiry* 29, no. 4 (2003): 599–633.

Roberts, Mary Louise. *Disruptive Acts: The New Woman in Fin-de-Siècle France*. Chicago: University of Chicago Press, 2002.

Robinson, Daniel N. *Wild Beasts and Idle Humours: The Insanity Defense from Antiquity to the Present*. Cambridge, MA: Harvard University Press, 1998.

Román, Gustavo C. "Cerebral Congestion: A Vanished Disease." *Archives of Neurology* 44, no. 4 (1987): 444–8.

Rosario, Vernon A. *The Erotic Imagination: French Histories of Perversity*. New York: Oxford University Press, 1997.

Roughton, Richard A. "Economic Motives and French Imperialism: The 1837 Tafna Treaty as a Case Study." *The Historian* 47, no. 3 (1985): 360–81.

Rouville, Georges Gervais de. *Consultations de gynécologie à l'usage des praticiens*. Paris: J.-B. Baillière et fils, 1902.

Sabatier, Armand. *Rapport sur la campagne de l'ambulance du midi (Marseille-Montpellier), suivi des considérations générales sur les ambulances militaires et volontaires et d'observations médico-chirurgicales recueillies pendant la campagne*. Montpellier: Boehm et fils, 1871.

Said, Edward. *Orientalism*. New York: Vintage, 1979.

Salomon-Bayet, Claire, ed. *Pasteur et la révolution pastorienne*. Paris: Payot, 1986.

Schaffer, Simon. "Self Evidence." *Critical Inquiry* 18, no. 2 (1992): 327–62.

Schleich, Carl Ludwig. *Those Were Good Days! Reminiscences*. London: George Allen & Unwin, 1935.

Schmitt, Étienne. "La pharmacie hospitalière et la vente de médicaments au public." In *Cinq siècles de pharmacie hospitalière: 1495–1995*, edited by François Chast and Pierre Julien, 230–2. Paris: Editions Hervas, 1995.

Schnapper, Bernard. "La correction paternelle et le mouvement des idées au dix-neuvième siècle (1789–1935)." *Revue historique*, no. 263 (1980): 319–49.

Schneider, William H. *Quality and Quantity: The Quest for Biological Regeneration in Twentieth-Century France*. Cambridge: Cambridge University Press, 1990.

Scott, Joan Wallach. "French Universalism in the Nineties." *Differences: A Journal of Feminist Cultural Studies* 15, no. 2 (2004): 32–53.

– *Only Paradoxes to Offer: French Feminists and the Rights of Man*. Cambridge, MA: Harvard University Press, 1997.

Scrive, Gaspard. *Relation médico-chirurgicale de la campagne d'Orient: Du 31 mars 1854, occupation de Gallipoli, au 6 juillet 1856 évacuation de la Crimée*. Paris: Victor Masson, 1857.

Sebastian, Anton. *A Dictionary of the History of Medicine*. New York: Parthenon, 1999.

Service de Santé. *Formulaire pharmaceutique des hôpitaux militaires*. Vol. 1. Paris: Imprimerie Nationale, 1917.

Shannon, Brent. *The Cut of His Coat: Men, Dress, and Consumer Culture in Britain, 1860–1914*. Athens: Ohio University Press, 2006.

Shapin, Steven, and Simon Schaffer. *Leviathan and the Air-Pump: Hobbes, Boyle, and the Experimental Life*. Princeton, NJ: Princeton University Press, 1986.

Shapiro, Ann-Louise. *Breaking the Codes: Female Criminality in Fin-de-Siècle Paris*. Stanford, CA: Stanford University Press, 1996.

Sibalis, Michael David. "The Regulation of Male Homosexuality in Revolutionary and Napoleonic France, 1789–1815." In *Homosexuality in Modern France*, ed. Jeffrey Merrick and Bryant T. Ragan Jr, 80–101. New York: Oxford University Press, 1996.

Siegel, Ronald, and Ada Hirschman. "Edmond de Courtive and the First Thesis on Hashish: A Historical Note and Translation." *Journal of Psychoactive Drugs* 23, no. 1 (1991): 85–6.

Simpson, James Young. *Account of a New Anaesthetic Agent, as a Substitute for Sulphuric Ether in Surgery and Midwifery*. Edinburgh: Sutherland and Knox, 1847.

– *Answer to the Religious Objections Advanced against the Employment of Anaesthetic Agents in Midwifery and Surgery*. Edinburgh: Sutherland and Knox, 1848.

Smith, Bonnie G. "Decentered Identities: The Case of the Romantics." *History and Theory* 50, no. 2 (2011): 210–19.

– *The Gender of History: Men, Women, and Historical Practice*. Cambridge, MA: Harvard University Press, 1998.

– *Ladies of the Leisure Class: The Bourgeoises of Northern France in the Nineteenth Century*. Princeton, NJ: Princeton University Press, 1981.

Snelders, Stephen, Charles Kaplan, and Toine Pieters. "On Cannabis, Chloral Hydrate, and Career Cycles of Psychotropic Drugs in Medicine." *Bulletin of the History of Medicine* 80, no. 1 (2006): 95–114.

Spang, Rebecca L. *The Invention of the Restaurant: Paris and Modern Gastronomic Culture*. Cambridge, MA: Harvard University Press, 2000.

Spary, Emma C. *Eating the Enlightenment: Food and the Sciences in Paris*. Chicago: University of Chicago Press, 2012.

– *Feeding France: New Sciences of Food, 1760–1815*. Cambridge: Cambridge University Press, 2014.

Steffen, Monika. "The Medical Profession and the State in France." *Journal of Public Policy* 7, no. 2 (1987): 189–208.

Sessions, Jennifer E. *By Sword and Plow: France and the Conquest of Algeria*. Ithaca: Cornell University Press, 2014.

Steinbrügge, Lieselotte. *The Moral Sex: Woman's Nature in the French Enlightenment*. Translated by Pamela E. Selwyn. New York: Oxford University Press, 1995.

Stewart, Mary Lynn. *For Health and Beauty: Physical Culture for Frenchwomen, 1880s–1930s*. Baltimore: Johns Hopkins University Press, 2001.

Strickland, Stuart. "The Ideology of Self-Knowledge and the Practice of Self-

Experimentation." *Eighteenth-Century Studies* 31, no. 4 (1998): 453–71.

Stock-Morton, Phyllis. "Control and Limitation of Midwives in Modern France: The Example of Marseille." *Journal of Women's History* 8, no. 1 (1996): 60–94.

Stoker, Donald J., Frederick C. Schneid, and Harold D. Blanton, eds. *Conscription in the Napoleonic Era: A Revolution in Military Affairs?* London: Routledge, 2009.

Studer, Nina Salouâ. "The Same Drink? Wine and Absinthe Consumption and Drinking Cultures among French and Muslim Groups in Nineteenth-Century Algeria." In *Alcohol Flows across Cultures: Drinking Cultures in Transnational and Comparative Perspective*, ed. Waltraud Ernst, 20–43. London: Routledge, 2020.

Styles, John, and Amanda Vickery, eds. *Gender, Taste, and Material Culture in Britain and North America, 1700–1830*. New Haven: Yale University Press, 2006.

Substance Abuse and Mental Health Services Administration. *2018 Key Substance Abuse and Mental Health Indicators Report.* HHS Publication No. PEP19-5068, NSDUH Series H-54. Rockville, MD: Center for Behavioral Health Statistics and Quality, 2019. https://www.samhsa.gov/data/report/2018-nsduh-annual-national-report.

Sueur, Laurent. "La fragile limite entre le normal et l'anormal: Lorsque les psychiatres français essayaient, au XIXᵉ siècle, de reconnaître la folie." *Revue historique* 3, no. 591 (1994): 31–51.

– "Les psychiatres français de la première moitié du XIXᵉ siècle face à l'isolement des malades mentaux dans des hôpitaux spécialisés." *Revue historique*, no. 590 (1994): 299–314.

– "La violence dans les asiles psychiatriques de la première moitié du XIXᵉ siècle." *L'information historique* 56, no. 2 (1994): 67–74.

Sueur, Nicolas. "La Pharmacie Centrale de France (1852–1879): Une entreprise pharmaceutique au secours de l'officine?" *Revue internationale sur le médicament* 4, no. 1 (2012): 78–100.

– "Les spécialités pharmaceutiques au XIXᵉ siècle: Statuts et fondements de l'innovation." *Le mouvement social*, no. 248 (2014): 27–46.

Surkis, Judith. "Carnival Balls and Penal Codes: Body Politics in July Monarchy France." *History of the Present* 1, no. 1 (2011): 59–83.

– *Sexing the Citizen: Morality and Masculinity in France, 1870–1920*. Ithaca: Cornell University Press, 2006.

Sussman, George D. "The Glut of Doctors in Mid-Nineteenth-Century France." *Comparative Studies in Society and History* 19, no. 3 (1977): 287–304.

Szabo, Jason. *Incurable and Intolerable: Chronic Disease and Slow Death in Nineteenth-Century France*. New Brunswick, NJ: Rutgers University Press, 2009.

Tailhade, Laurent. *La "noire idole": Etude sur la morphinomanie*. Paris: Vanier, 1907.

Taillac, Pierre. *Les paradis artificiels: L'imaginaire des drogues de l'opium à l'ecstacy.* Paris: Hugo et Cie, 2007.

Taithe, Bertrand. *Defeated Flesh: Welfare, Warfare and the Making of Modern France.* Oxford: Oxford University Press, 2010.

Terrail, Jean-Joseph. *De la morphine dans le traitement de l'hystérie chez la femme: Avantages et inconvénients.* Paris: Imprimerie des Écoles, 1889.

Thébaud, Françoise. *Quand nos grand-mères donnaient la vie: La maternité en France dans l'entre-deux-guerres.* Lyon: Presses Universitaires de Lyon, 1986.

Thompson, Victoria. "Creating Boundaries: Homosexuality and the Changing Social Order in France, 1830–1870." In *Homosexuality in Modern France,* ed. Jeffrey Merrick and Bryant T. Ragan Jr, 102–27. New York: Oxford University Press, 1996.

Tiersten, Lisa. *Marianne in the Market: Envisioning Consumer Society in Fin-de-Siècle France.* Berkeley: University of California Press, 2001.

Tighe, Janet A. "The Legal Art of Psychiatric Diagnosis: Searching for Reliability." In *Framing Disease: Studies in Cultural History,* edited by Charles E. Rosenberg and Janet Golden, 206–26. New Brunswick, NJ: Rutgers University Press, 1992.

Todd, David. "Algeria, Informal Empire Manqué." In *A Velvet Empire: French Informal Imperialism in the Nineteenth Century,* 72–122. Princeton, NJ: Princeton University Press, 2021.

Tourdes, Gabriel, and Edmond Metzquer. *Traité de médecine légale théorique et pratique.* Paris: Asselin et Houzeau, 1896.

Tresch, John. *The Romantic Machine: Utopian Science and Technology after Napoleon.* Chicago: University of Chicago Press, 2012.

"Un Français sur trois prend des psychotropes." *Le Parisien,* 20 May 2014. http://www.leparisien.fr/espace-premium/actu/un-francais-sur-trois-prend-des-psychotropes-20-05-2014-3854775.php.

Valentin, Marc. "Jean-Antoine-Brutus Ménier et la fondation de la Maison Centrale de Droguerie." *Revue d'histoire de la pharmacie* 72, no. 263 (1984): 357–89.

Van Bergen, Leo. *Before My Helpless Sight: Suffering, Dying and Military Medicine on the Western Front.* Translated by Liz Waters. Farnham: Ashgate, 2009.

Van Zee, Art. "The Promotion and Marketing of OxyContin: Commercial Triumph, Public Health Tragedy," *American Journal of Public Health* 99, no. 2 (2009): 221–7.

Velpeau, Alfred-Armand-Louis-Marie. *Leçons orales de clinique chirurgicale faites à l'hôpital de la Charité.* Vol. 1. Paris: Germer Baillière, 1840.

Vermot, I. *Petit guide de la santé: Hygiène, médecine, pharmacie.* 3rd ed. Paris: Librairie des Familles, 1878.

Vigarello, Georges. *A History of Rape: Sexual Violence in France from the 16th to the 20th Century.* Translated by Jean Birrell. Malden, MA: Polity Press, 2001.

Vila, Anne C. *Enlightenment and Pathology: Sensibility in the Literature and Medicine of Eighteenth-Century France*. Baltimore: Johns Hopkins University Press, 1998.

Vinogradoff, Luc. "'Une aberration économique et sanitaire': Début de l'expérimentation sur le cannabis médical en France, où sa production reste toujours interdite." *Le Monde*, 2 March 2021. https://www.lemonde.fr/economie/article/2021/03/01/derriere-l-experimentation-sur-le-cannabis-medical-en-france-des-ambitions-economiques-et-un-flou-politique_6071511_3234.html.

Virey, Julien-Joseph. *Des médicamens aphrodisiaques en général et en particulier sur le dudaim de la Bible*. Paris: D. Colas, 1813.

Voisin, Auguste. *Leçons cliniques sur les maladies mentales et sur les maladies nerveuses*. Paris: J.-B. Baillière et fils, 1883.

Warner, John Harley. *The Therapeutic Perspective: Medical Practice, Knowledge, and Identity in America, 1820–1885*. Cambridge, MA: Harvard University Press, 1986.

Watson, Katherine D. *Forensic Medicine in Western Society: A History*. New York: Routledge, 2010.

Wawro, Geoffrey. *The Franco-Prussian War: The German Conquest of France in 1870–1871*. Cambridge: Cambridge University Press, 2005.

Weber, Eugen. *Peasants into Frenchmen: The Modernization of Rural France, 1870–1914*. Stanford, CA: Stanford University Press, 1976.

Weiner, Dora B. *The Citizen-Patient in Revolutionary and Imperial Paris*. Baltimore: Johns Hopkins University Press, 1993.

– "Le droit de l'homme à la santé: Une belle idée devant l'Assemblée constituante, 1790–1791." *Clio medica* 5 (1970): 209–33.

Weiner, Dora B., and Michael J. Sauter. "The City of Paris and the Rise of Clinical Medicine." *Osiris*, 2nd ser., 18 (2003): 23–42.

Weisz, George. "Constructing the Medical Élite in France: The Creation of the Royal Academy of Medicine 1814–20." *Medical History* 30, no. 4 (1986): 419–43.

– *Divide and Conquer: A Comparative History of Medical Specialization*. Oxford: Oxford University Press, 2005.

– *The Medical Mandarins: The French Academy of Medicine in the Nineteenth and Early Twentieth Centuries*. Oxford: Oxford University Press, 1995.

– "The Politics of Medical Professionalization in France, 1845–1848." *Journal of Social History* 12, no. 1 (1978): 3–30.

White, Owen. *The Blood of the Colony: Wine and the Rise and Fall of French Algeria*. Cambridge, MA: Harvard University Press, 2021.

Whitlock, Tammy C. *Crime, Gender, and Consumer Culture in Nineteenth-Century England*. Burlington, VT: Ashgate, 2005.

Whitman, Elizabeth. "French Clinical Trial Disaster: 5 Critically Injured as Health Ministry Denies Test Drug Was Linked to Cannabis." *International*

Business Times, 15 January 2016. http://www.ibtimes.com/french-clinical-trial-disaster-5-critically-injured-health-ministry-denies-test-drug-2267038.

Williams, Rosalind H. *Dream Worlds: Mass Consumption in Late Nineteenth-Century France*. Berkeley: University of California Press, 1982.

Willy. *Lélie, fumeuse d'opium*. Paris: Albin Michel, 1911.

Wilson, Susannah. *Voices from the Asylum: Four French Women Writers, 1850–1920*. Oxford: Oxford University Press, 2010.

Wright, Gordon. *Between the Guillotine and Liberty: Two Centuries of the Crime Problem in France*. New York: Oxford University Press, 1983.

Yvorel, Jean-Jacques. *Les poisons de l'esprit: Drogues et drogués au XIXᵉ siècle*. Paris: Quai Voltaire, 1992.

Zimmer, Marguerite. *Histoire de l'anesthésie: Méthodes et techniques au XIXᵉ siècle*. Les Ulis: EDP Sciences, 2008.

Znaien, Nessim. "Drinking and Production Patterns of Wine in North Africa during French Colonization, c. 1830–1956." In *Alcohol Flows across Cultures: Drinking Cultures in Transnational and Comparative Perspective*, ed. Waltraud Ernst, 44–60. London: Routledge, 2020.

Zylberman, Patrick. "Making Food Safety an Issue: Internationalized Food Politics and French Public Health from the 1870s to the Present." *Medical History* 48, no. 1 (2004): 1–28.

INDEX

Milton Keynes UK
Ingram Content Group UK Ltd.
UKHW020016140824
446908UK00005B/154

9 780228 011644